Mostly Cloudy

With

Some Bright Spells

JULIETTE WILLS

ISBN-13:
978-1492337799

ISBN-10:
149233779X

ACKNOWLEDGEMENTS

This book is dedicated to Mum and Dad, or as they are more affectionately known – Dum and Mad.

Your support is commendable because I know I drive you nuts. Without fish fingers for dinner every time I come home and Dad's loose change for parrot boots and plane tickets and donkey shirts and socks with cat faces on and all the stuff that keeps me going, I wouldn't be here today. I've only ever wanted to make you proud. I love you.

To you, dear reader: thank you for buying this book. I hope it makes you laugh and cry in all the right places. In case you're wondering, the chapter headings are all songs which work with the story. You could look them up on YouTube as you read. That's right - it's a book with a soundtrack. Mentals!

FOREWORD

by Damon Hill OBE, 1996 Formula One World Champion

Juliette is a very special person. I found that out when she worked with the mechanics on my Formula One car. People really liked her, and she had real talent. Her enthusiasm was boundless, and she had us all in stitches. None of us had any idea that she was so unwell.

Formula One is exciting and glamorous, but ultimately places too much emphasis on all the wrong things. Juliette wasn't interested in the glitz and the glamour. I'd come in and find her covered in engine oil, cleaning my car or fetching nuts and bolts for the mechanics in the garage when she was supposed to be in a press conference.

Her harrowing story of her fight with chronic, crippling illness is told with brutal honesty. Only a person as brave and talented as Juliette could share such an emotionally and physically painful journey with such deft ironic subtlety. I was left stunned and saddened by her experience, but inspired by her spirit as I was when I met her. I only had a sense back then that Juliette was special; after reading her story, I now have no doubts. Her book is a reminder that we take so much for granted, and that we live by the grace of God.

PROLOGUE

November 2001

Nine hours have passed since I was brought into the operating theatre. As I jolt back to life as if waking suddenly from a nightmare I'm convinced I have been asleep for a split second. I try to open my eyes but something is pressing on them, a sensation so strange and disquieting that I begin to panic. My chest tightens. I can't draw breath. Then it comes: the pain hits me instantaneously, burning its way around my body like a raging fire.

I try to move my fingers but nothing happens. I lie rigid, my eyes forced shut, the taste of copper rising in the back of my throat. Gradually the 'beep, beep, beep' of a machine somewhere to my left becomes more rapid and it is then that the muffled sound of distant conversation stops abruptly. Someone is leaning over me; I can feel their warm fingers brushing against my cheekbones and suddenly, the weight has been lifted from my eyelids.

Somebody puts something over my face; they are telling me to breathe slowly and then I'm being turned to my left, a flurry of hands pushing into my back, the pain moving with me, worse now as it spills from my stomach and gathers under my rib cage like molten lava pouring down the side of a volcano; a burning, stabbing pain which to this day I am still unable to describe without it seeming as though it was, in some way, bearable. I'm going to die, I think, the pain so excruciating and my chest so tight I wonder if I'm about to have a heart attack.

I must have passed out because when I wake up the pain has dulled slightly. I open my eyes.

A shiny silver blanket is draped over me, the nurse tucking it around my neck and over my feet, gently placing my hands by my sides so that they too are covered. I'm shaking with cold, my teeth chattering.

'It's OK, sweetheart,' she whispers as she leans over my chest, 'the epidural wasn't in right, that's why it hurt so much.'

She pats my hand under the blanket. I glance to where the voice is coming from and see the clock high up on the wall. It's 9.03pm. My thoughts turn to where my parents are. I'm screaming for my mum; in reality it's the faintest of whispers. Nobody can hear me. The oxygen mask blocks my words and my breath simply clings to the plastic in front of my face before disappearing like a passing cloud. My eyes are heavy again and as I let them close I feel the pain subside. I take a breath, the cold oxygen hitting the back of my throat, and I let myself drift away, this time not sure if I will wake up again.

Had I known what was coming, I wouldn't have wanted to.

CHAPTER ONE
'RACE WITH THE DEVIL'
GENE VINCENT

I'm in France, somewhere south of Paris but I've no idea where as I've been asleep for two and a half hours. Uncurling from my foetal position in the bunk above the front of the truck I edge down the steps to the cab to find the sun blazing through the window, the motorway stretching out ahead as far as I can see.

'We're halfway there,' says the driver, turning to me with a grin, 'but you slept through the Eiffel Tower and if you're about to tell me that you need a wee, too bad. You'll have to hang on unless you want to go in the bushes.' I scan the horizon in a panic as my brain processes the words 'wee' followed by 'hang on'. There is nothing but concrete for miles.

'But there aren't any bushes,' I reply.

'Exactly,' he laughs.

What started off as a drunken idea - albeit a good one - was now a reality. I was on my way to Magny-Cours for the French Formula One Grand Prix, covering the race for men's magazine *loaded*. The idea was that I'd travel to France with the B&H Jordan racing team to help out in the garage for a week and generally make a nuisance of myself in front of Formula One World Champion Damon Hill. It was the best idea I'd ever had, and fortunately the editor, Tim Southwell, and racing boss Eddie Jordan had agreed.

Two bright yellow, gargantuan 40-tonne trucks, two drivers in each who doubled up as electricians, plumbers, mechanics and pit stop men, and a few million pounds worth of F1 racing cars and little old me took off from the Oxfordshire countryside bang on 10am. It was June 21, 1999, and in retrospect I can see why God deemed it the longest day of the year. As we turned off towards Dover, practically going right past Mum and Dad's house where I'd set off from four hours earlier, I rang Mum.

'I'm waving at you! We've just gone past the A224. Can you see us? As if I'm in a massive yellow truck with Damon Hill's car in the back, eating crisps and going to France and getting paid for it!'

'As if indeed,' laughed Mum, 'they could have come and picked you up on the way! Be good, be careful, don't annoy Damon Hill or get run over, and have a great time.'

After the drive to Dover, a distinctly wobbly and vomit-inducing ferry ride to Calais, driving a bit further, staying up too late and drinking far too much in a town I didn't even know the name of and a minute's sleep in some hotel, we're up again at 7am to resume the journey, and are due at the circuit in Magny-Cours mid-afternoon.

'The first job,' says Dave as we pull in to the circuit behind the guys in the other truck, 'is to clean the trucks.'

'What, after a cup of tea?' I croak hopefully, but nobody's listening. There's only one thing for it so I grab a bucket and broom thing and climb up the ladder onto the roof of the truck and get cleaning. I'm pretty sure I'm not allowed to do this under health and safety rules, but what the hell. I find myself enjoying it, despite the sweltering 30-degree heat, newly discovered vertigo and hangover. After dinner at the hotel we retire to the terrace for a drink, and are delighted to see that we have a dual carriageway out the front and miles of flat, cow-filled fields round the back. I've never been one for watching lorries thundering by so I head off to bed. As luck would have it my room faces the road. I go to bed with socks on my ears to drown out the noise. I look like a 12-year-old girl dressed for a last-minute fancy dress party as a poor imitation of Snoopy.

Wednesday, 8am, four days before the race, and we're back at the circuit unloading 40 sets of wheels, three cars, enough spares to build three whole *new* cars, and just about everything else including napkins for the motor home, industrial water bottles and a pile of other things made out of metal. By 10am it's so hot that the cup of tea I've just made myself is getting hotter, not colder, the longer I leave it. I wander out onto the circuit to see what I can do.

'What can I do?' I ask the mechanics. My answer came in the form of a ratchet thrust into my hand.

'What's this?' I ask, shielding my eyes from the sun and turning this strange metal object over in my hands. 'Is it to tighten old roller-skates? Or are we putting some pictures up?' My questions were answered over the next two hours which were spent drilling into concrete and making up the support frames on which the car's bodywork rests during engine tinkering, before helping build the pit perches which line the pit wall. Team boss Eddie Jordan and chief engineers watch the race on TV screens from here, and these things have to be put up from scratch for every race.

I break three nails and acquire two raging blood blisters, but the perches are up, and what's more, when I shove them a bit, they don't fall down. I pick up the temperature gun and point it at the track. It's a whopping 42 degrees and I'm exhausted already. I point it at my forehead, and it registers 43 degrees.

'Shouldn't I be in hospital?' I say to Dave, slightly worried that I might spontaneously combust at any given moment. I'd been feeling a bit off-colour before the trip but I just put it down to working too hard.

I'd felt under the weather ever since I had glandular fever just before and during all my GCSE exams - good timing - but looking back, I should have realised that this was different. I'd struggle to get to sleep, and when I did, I'd wake in a cold sweat, absolutely drenched, feeling as though I was glued to the bed. I knew something was wrong, but I didn't have time to think about it. I hadn't lost weight, I couldn't feel any unexplained lumps anywhere, so I carried on, putting the tiredness down to all the excitement of the job.

We leave the circuit at 6.30pm in the back of a delivery van. I ring Dad and tell him I've drilled concrete and am best friends with a ratchet. He laughs and says I've had too much sun but I bet he asks me to build a conservatory or something when I get home. After dinner at the hotel, I shower and go to bed. I can't sleep. It's 3.24am when I last look at the clock, and then the next thing I know, the alarm is going off. I've had two hours of sleep. I do not feel, nor look, very good. I walk downstairs to meet the mechanics with a face like an old paper bag. I haven't even opened my eyes properly.

'You look rough,' says Ged, one of the truck drivers. 'You should get some sleep.'

'Yeah, you'd think...' I reply, sticking two fingers up at him. He laughs, and opens the door to the minibus, ruffling my hair.

'You'll be alright,' he jokes, 'you can sleep next week.' Inside the B&H Jordan garage half an hour later I ask if I can touch one of the cars.

'You can sit in it if you want,' shrugs one of the mechanics.

I climb carefully into Damon Hill's car and stretch my legs out. The seatbelts are on and although I'm a bit small to see very well, this has got to be the most exciting five minutes of my life.

I'd dreamed about seeing a Formula One car up close but I'd never imagined I'd sit in one, let alone Damon's. Sadly I can't sit there all day and it's time to go and do something more useful, like make myself a cup of tea and find somewhere out of the way to sit down and write some notes about, uh, making tea. At 7.30am we all go over to the paddock to have a proper cooked breakfast before the mechanics get on with the rest of the morning's work. I busy myself by peering into the Ferrari garage until I'm told to move away. Later that afternoon, I spot Michael Schumacher and get all excited. The drivers arrive after the team has set up, and now it felt like something was really going on. I was as excited as I was exhausted. We arrive back at the hotel at 9.30pm. That night I went to the toilet just before bed and was pretty surprised, if not somewhat horrified, to see blood in the toilet bowl. I flushed the chain, thought I'd better check it out with a doctor when I got home and climbed into bed. This time I fell asleep as soon as my head hit the pillow.

Having been so careful in the garage yesterday, I tentatively ask if I can polish 'just a little bit' of the spare car. I'm given a can of polish and a cloth and told I can clean all three if I like. I am so excited my hands are shaking and I spray polish straight in my hair. I'm polishing Formula One cars! I want to tell everyone. I tell them. They smile politely. People stop by the garage and point. Damon Hill stops by the garage and points. I point back, thinking, 'It's Damon Hill, and he's pointing at me!'

I introduce myself, and he says, smiling, '*loaded* magazine? Really? What do you know about F1, then?'

'I know it's well exhausting, the food's great and all these people spend hours building your car and I'll spend ages polishing it only for you to drive it around the track a few times and crash it or at the very least get it all dirty again.' He looks surprised by my answer, and then shakes my hand. 'Well, you've got it about right. Nice to meet you, Juliette... I think.' He laughs, takes off his cap and runs his hand through his hair then turns back.

'Are you sure you're supposed to be in the garage?' he asks, head cocked to one side.

'Not really, but do you want your car cleaned or not?' I say, holding up the can of polish.

'OK, keep cleaning. You're doing a splendid job,' he says, somewhat bemused, leaving for his swanky hotel while the rest of us slummed it in the French version of the Travelodge.

At 11am the session starts and the track temperature is recorded at 40 degrees. The cars come in after the first lap and the tyres are already melting. I keep out of the way, writing up my notes just outside the garage, sitting on a tyre. We have lunch, I pick dropped nuts and bolts up for mechanics and hold them aloft each time someone says, 'Where did that nut go?' and write a bit more. I also wander off to see if I can spot Ferrari's Eddie Irvine, because I fancy him like nobody's business. At least that's what I was planning on doing, but at 8.30pm I'm woken up by Ged with a poke in the tummy. I'm asleep, flat on my back, on top of the tyre trolley, behind the truck. I find myself given something to do.

'If you really want to help,' says one of the mechanics, 'grab these bits on this list from the back of the truck and make a new exhaust. That should keep you quiet.'

'Uh, OK,' I say, thinking it would have been much more sensible to have asked me to make a cup of tea for everyone instead. I'm in the back of the truck, wrestling with nuts, bolts and some pipe thing. I'm just getting the hang of it when guess who pops in? Yep, Damon himself.

'Er, hello again,' he says, climbing up the steps to the truck, scratching his head and looking somewhat perplexed, 'what's going on here?'

I explain myself. 'I'm making you a new exhaust,' I answer, smiling like a lunatic and holding my hands out, showing him the bits and bobs I've been told to make it with. I don't know what else to say because this is only the second time I've met him, so I just smile a bit more, exhaust in one hand, bits and bobs in the other. He looks quite confused, possibly more concerned than the first time we met, shrugs his shoulders and walks away.

I finish the exhaust and take it to the mechanics. A little nut falls out along the way but I'm sure it's not important. Again, we arrive back at the hotel late, have dinner, and go to bed. It's 1.15am by the time I get into my pyjamas and I don't know how much more of this I can actually take. If I could just sleep all day on Saturday, I think I'd be OK.

At 6.30am on Saturday, the day when the drivers do their qualifying laps, we're already at the circuit. I'm absolutely wiped out, and I look as dreadful as I feel. I head off to find Ged to get the keys to the truck. I think it's mad that anyone would give me keys to a Formula One truck, because I lose keys all the time. But then Ged isn't my mum, so he doesn't know that. I manage to sneak a nap in the bunk and even stay snoozing through the deafening noise of the engines roaring only a few feet away. The rain is coming down and the next thing I know, all hell breaks loose and as I fall out of the truck from a great height to see what's going on, the other truckie, Dave, shouts, 'He's having trouble,' and another voice shouted in a high-pitched panic, 'Damon's coming in, he's in!'

I get out of the way just in time. Damon's car is abandoned outside the garage. Much head shaking and brow wiping is going on. The ITV television crew is clamouring for news. I ask Ged what went wrong whilst holding my eyelids open so that it appears as though I am awake.

'It looks like the exhaust split,' he says, rushing past me with a bit of burnt car. Hang on, that was what I made last night. It is at this point that I make myself scarce. I breathe a sigh of relief five minutes later when Ged tells me that it wasn't my fault as my exhaust never made it onto the car in the end because it was so rubbish it fell apart as soon as the engineer picked it up. I almost replied with the line that 'It can't have been as rubbish as this one, it just blew up!' but decided to bite my tongue for once.

The press were practically beating the door of the motor home down to talk to Damon after the incident, and I was supposed to have 15 minutes with him. He would be starting the race right at the back. Not really what you want. And not really what I wanted, either – I mean, how much of a mood would he be in and I'm supposed to interview him. Gah! I wasn't sure what to ask him, other than, 'Would you like me to make the exhausts from now on after that other one broke?'

The door to the motor home opens and Jordan's PR girl gives me the nod. 'You've got 15 minutes, Juliette,' she says, ushering me in.

'Deal,' I say, thinking, 'I'll be lucky if I can keep him talking for 15 seconds the mood he'll be in.'

I sat down. Damon had his head in his hands. There was a slice of chocolate cake on a plate in front of him. Mental note to write down thing about cake, I thought.

'Uh, eeek, that was a bit shit,' I said.

'It was exactly that,' said Damon, with a face like thunder. 'And it was the exhaust, was it not, which caused it?' He looked right at me, and I swear to God I was back in school again but this time, it was a gazillion times worse.

'Hang on. You can't get me on this. My exhaust was rubbish. Ged told me that. They used someone else's. So mine might have been alright with a bit of Sellotape round it. You can't blame me. Maybe a pigeon or something got stuck in it. Or maybe one of the other drivers put a potato up it. Did you think about that?' I said, wondering if he was going to eat the cake or not, because if he didn't want it, I'd have it. He had the grace to laugh.

'You really are quite mad,' he said, shaking his head, 'but that's good. What do you want to ask me?'

I switched on my tape recorder.

'Hang on, let's get this on the move and then I can read you my list of questions,' I said. Nothing happened. The tape didn't turn. I was horrified.

'My bloody tape recorder isn't working,' I said, 'how stupid is that?'

'Very,' said Damon, 'you'll have to make it all up.'

'Nothing new there, then,' I joked.

I didn't take notes, but told him I'd remember what he said. He teased me a bit more about the exhaust I'd made; I told him he needed to drive faster or let me have a go while he put the kettle on. We talked about dinosaurs, football and cakes. After 20 minutes, his PR knocked on the door. 'You've had 20 minutes, Juliette, that's it.'

I smiled and said, 'OK, coming' and went to put my pen down. Damon decided against it.

'She can stay a bit longer, we're talking about dinosaurs,' he said, 'and it's more fun than talking about Formula One to that lot,' he said, gesturing to the huddle of middle-aged male journalists out front.

We continued our chat, even bringing up lawn mowers.

'You could race them when you're old,' I suggested, helpfully. Sometimes we actually talked about racing. I was in there for an hour. I found him to be an extremely likeable, funny and highly intelligent man.

Later that weekend he announced that he was quitting Formula One. Blimey! I hoped it wasn't because of my interview. Or my exhaust. We leave the circuit at 12.25am. I lie awake worrying about the cars, the rain and before I know it, the alarm is going off. It's 5.30am. I'm starting to feel quite ill. I almost ring Mum to tell her how awful I feel but don't want to worry her, and besides, I've got to meet the mechanics in reception in five minutes and I'm still in my ruddy pyjamas. Flip!

CHAPTER TWO
'IT AIN'T RIGHT'
PAUL ANSELL'S NUMBER NINE

September 1999

'Ulcerative colitis,' said the consultant, leaning back in his chair and folding his hands across his chest, 'is a debilitating and chronic form of inflammatory bowel disease. The bowel becomes enlarged - inflamed, if you like - and ulcers form along the walls of the large intestine, resulting in bleeding and mucus from the back passage. The disease can affect the rectum, part of the colon and rectum, or the entire bowel from end to end, in which case the disease is referred to as Pan-Colitis. Unfortunately, your entire bowel is affected. I will put you on a course of anti-inflammatory tablets and steroid tablets. You are to take two of the anti-inflammatory tablets three times a day with food, and six of the steroids in the morning. There is no cure for colitis, I'm afraid. All we can do is try to calm the inflammation. I have to tell you that this is a disease that often gets worse, rather than better. Do you have any questions?'

I was stunned. The word 'steroids' danced in front of my eyes.

'Don't steroids make you fat? And depressed? And hairy?' I asked, wiping away a tear.

'Only in high doses,' he replied, matter-of-factly.

'I don't want to end up like Fatima Whitbread,' I muttered, 'especially since I can't even throw javelins. Is there anything I can do to help? Change my diet, try alternative medicine? Stupid Chinese herbal teas? What about an exorcism?'

At the last suggestion he doesn't even laugh a bit, just raises his eyebrows and says, 'There's nothing you can do. I wouldn't advise that you meddle in alternative medicine, Chinese or homeopathic. Just take the steroids and the anti-inflammatory tablets as directed and I will see you in three months.'

'But why have I got it? What causes it?' I bleated, wishing Mum had come in with me like she'd asked to. Ever the independent one, I had gone in on my own thinking I must have eaten a pin that had become lodged in my bottom, something daft like that.

'There's no known reason and no cure,' said the consultant, stacking my file back in a drawer by his feet. 'It can be hereditary, it could be caused by a parasite in the gut, it could be any number of things, but we don't know what causes it. What do you do for work?'

I tell him I'm a freelance journalist. He raises those eyebrows again.

'Perhaps you're stressed. It's quite a stressful job, isn't it?'

'It is, but it's good fun, too. And I can't just stop doing it,' I say, holding my hands in the air and pulling a 'don't think I'm giving up my career just because my bottom keeps bleeding' face. With that, he pushed back his chair, nodded at me as if to indicate my time was up and I walked somewhat bewildered out of the door into the waiting room where Mum was sitting reading the newspaper.

'Well? Are you alright?' she said, a half smile on her face as she folded the newspaper in half on her lap and took off her glasses.

'Not really,' I said, 'I've got ulcerative colitis. It's bowel disease. I'm not going to get better and they've put me on steroids.' I walked to the door in a daze.

'We'll have to put more money in the meter if we don't get back to the car,' I said. Mum picked up her handbag and walked over to me. She was as white as a sheet.

'Did he really say there was nothing you could do?' she asked.

'So he says. We'd better hurry up. We don't want to waste another 50p.' I've always been practical if nothing else.

That night, when Dad came home from work, we sat down and read the leaflets I'd been given. I told him about the drugs I had to take, and that I'd asked the consultant if I should change my diet or try a natural approach to controlling the inflammation.

'So he didn't even ask you what you ate?' asked Dad, somewhat surprised, 'you might be living off curry powder and worms for all he knows. Surely what you eat must make a difference?'

'That's what you'd have thought,' I replied, shaking my head, 'I mean, you are what you eat, apparently. But I haven't been eating ulcers so I don't know where they've come from.' Oh, how we laughed.

A couple of days later my younger brother, Jonathan, came into the kitchen as I was counting out my tablets for the day. He was in the midst of his A-levels and would stay up until 4am 'revising', i.e. playing PlayStation with a book open in front of him that would inadvertently be obscured by a packet of Jaffa Cakes.

'Is that a week's worth?' he asked, yawning and taking a pint of milk out of the fridge.

'I'm dealing Ecstasy pills,' I replied, 'didn't you know? Dad forced me into it to pay off his gambling debts.' This was a joke. I counted out the pills. With six Asacol (the anti-inflammatory drug) and six Prednisolone (the steroids) I took the following supplements: Glucosamine Sulphate (to counteract the damaging effects of the steroids on my bones), Vitamin C (citrus fruits and juices upset my stomach), Vitamin D & Calcium (again, to support my bones), Vitamin E (to keep my complexion healthy - if only), Vitamin B (to keep my energy levels up), Zinc (to be honest, I can't even remember what this is for), Iron (because I don't eat red meat very often and am slightly anaemic), Acidophillis (for healthy gut bacteria), Cod Liver Oil (for what, I couldn't remember).

In all, each morning I took 16 tablets, then at lunchtime and with my dinner, another two Asacol. I was sure I rattled when I walked. The vitamins cost me a fortune but I wanted to do everything I could to help my body fight this horrible disease. I cut out wheat and dairy products, convinced that gluten and lactose weren't an intestine's best friends. Back then there was no glut of internet advice but I just went on my instincts, thinking that they might be causing some of the irritation. I would have swapped my cat for a slice of hot, buttered toast and a cup of tea if asked.

I didn't realise how much of our average diet contains dairy products or wheat until I read the labels on everything before I bought it. No more Weetabix. In came porridge with soya milk. It was just about bearable with a teaspoon of honey. Out went toast, sandwiches, pasta, cheese, milk, chocolate, cakes, biscuit, ice cream and just about everything else which was nice to eat. For a couple of weeks, until I got hold of a wheat and dairy free cookbook, I was stuck. Salad is not an option in February. Jacket potatoes took over my lunchtime. How exciting, I thought, I could have beans or tuna. Or tuna or beans! Great. In came herbal and fruit teas, which I hate because they taste like bubble bath, and I excluded coffee completely because I couldn't bear to take it black. I wanted to be able to drink black coffee so I could use the 'I like my coffee strong and black, like my men' line in a restaurant. I actually preferred it weak and pale, which is more in line with the men I met. Anyway, for a few weeks I even cut out fish fingers because of the breadcrumbs.

And despite cutting out everything that's meant to be bad for you, I didn't even lose any weight, but after three weeks I began to feel better. I didn't feel bloated after dinner, I slept a bit better and more importantly, when I went to the loo, I wasn't passing as much blood.

On the rare occasion that I went out for dinner, I'd have to pick restaurants carefully, often ringing them before I left home to check that there was something on the menu I could eat. I attended a football match one night as a guest of the team's sponsor, as I was the sports writer for *loaded* which entitled me not only to a free padded seat in the stands to watch West Ham but also to a three-course meal.

At the table, I studied the menu in despair. The starter was cream of leek and potato soup. The word 'cream' was the clue that there'd be cream in that. Can't have it. With a bread roll. Nor that. Moving on to the main course, there was a choice of three - chicken korma and rice. Can't eat the korma because of the cream and yoghurt. Vegetable lasagne, the staple token veggie dish, which happens to consist of wheat, milk and cheese. The final option was steak and kidney pie. Ugh. Apart from the fact that I'd rather cut off my right hand and fry it than eat a kidney, even my own, the pie, of course, is made from flour which is derived from wheat. For dessert: ice-cream (clearly not) or cheese and biscuits (aaagh!). In short, there wasn't one single dish I could eat on the whole menu. I banged my head on the table, causing the cutlery to fall to the floor, not to mention drawing bemused looks from fellow diners. I told the PR man what was wrong.

'I'm not being difficult on purpose,' I explained, 'I just can't eat anything on the menu.'

'Nothing at all?' he asked, trying to help.

'Not a sausage. Particularly not a sausage,' I replied, sighing, 'but that's because they're made of pigs' lips and bums.' He called one of the waitresses over and I explained that I was intolerant to wheat and dairy products and could they just serve me some rice with the vegetables that came with the steak and kidney pudding?

She looked at me as if I'd asked her to hand over her purse and get down on the floor.

'Can't you have the lasagna if you don't eat meat?' she said, leaning over me and jabbing at the menu.

'It's not that I don't eat meat, although I don't eat some meat, it's that I'm allergic to wheat and dairy,' I said, thinking that perhaps if she thought I would have a fit or explode if I did eat one of their dishes, she might understand.

'Can't you have the cheese and biscuits and the soup? There ain't no meat in that.' I let my head flop back down on the table, sending bread rolls into the air.

'Forget it,' I said, 'it doesn't matter.' Dom, the PR guy, remained unfazed.

'Isn't there anything in the kitchen she can eat? 'What about egg on toast?' he said.

I interrupted him. 'Uh, without the toast.'

Eventually, the waitress said she'd see if they could knock me up some rice with vegetables or plain chicken. I apologised to everyone within earshot.

'Don't worry about it,' said the man next to me, brightly, 'I know what it's like – I can't eat hazelnuts!'

The waitress waddled off to the kitchen.

'She thinks she's in a f*cking proper restaurant, she does,' she said to the girl behind the bar, who shot me the kind of look reserved for convicted paedophiles. In the end I got fish and chips, much to the annoyance of everyone else with their soggy pies and bland lasagna. I took off the batter - duh, wheat - and allowed myself a little chuckle.

But while the symptoms of UC were slowly improving, things were going disastrously wrong elsewhere.

My face was definitely becoming rounder, one of the first noticeable side effects of the Prednisolone: my skin, usually so clear, began to itch and red patches appeared on my arms and face. I had spots, for the first time in 10 years. I'd always suffered from terrible mood swings around my period but now I felt as though I had permanent PMT. I also had ulcers in my mouth and my eyes became so dry the lids became inflamed and I couldn't tolerate wearing my contact lenses. To top it all off, I was suffering from horrendous night sweats where I'd wake up drenched in cold sweat and sometimes had to change the sheets and take a shower in the middle of the night, which was really convenient.

I was used to feeling a bit rotten, but this was more than a bit. A year earlier I'd had laser treatment for endometriosis, a condition in which the lining of the womb grows outside of the womb - nice - and attaches itself to various internal organs and muscles. For four years I was in agony for two or three days each month. The lining had attached itself to my bowel, the muscles around my spine and my ovaries, and whenever I had a cramp from my womb shedding its lining, wherever the tissue had attached itself also cramped. It was terrible, but I was finally operated on in 1998 and able to go to work and go out during my period instead of staying in bed with a hot water bottle stuck to my tummy, downing painkillers like they were going out of fashion. The summer before that, I'd had pre-cancerous cells removed from my cervix, also by laser. I was getting a bit fed up with popping in and out of hospital and having my stomach poked. Oh, and I'd had major heart surgery at four years old for a hole in my heart and you'd think that might have been enough.

I became depressed and aggressive, snapping at my friends and family and bursting into tears over daft things, although now I think about it, crying because I couldn't have my mum's apple pie and ice-cream seems perfectly rational.

One Friday night I went to a *loaded* party - never the quietest of nights out, to say the least, and drank a couple of vodka tonics. Halfway through my third, I suddenly went berserk and almost started a fight like someone on the Jerry Springer show. I wasn't aware of what was going on at all. I thought somebody had spiked my drink. I felt a surge of adrenalin rush through my body; I thought I could take on the world. My head hurt. I felt sick, and my friend Charlie took me back to her flat. Within minutes I was fast asleep. When I woke up the next morning, I had no recollection of the latter part of the evening. I was mortified when she told me what had happened. I realised it must have been a reaction to the steroids.

'I went bananas,' I told Mum the next day, 'like Hulk after he had too much Gamma. Although my clothes didn't burst and I don't remember pushing cars over or rescuing bewildered lady scientists from laboratory fires, but I might have done. Better get this morning's papers and have a look!'

I was living at home with my parents in Orpington, Kent, which for some people might sound a bit weird. After all, I was 27-years-old and as far as I was aware, not suffering from any mental illness (although Mum would say that was debatable) which prevented me from living on my own. I had a good reason - I was saving up to buy my own place, and I *had* left home before. 'Several times,' as Dad would say, raising his eyebrows.

My early experiences of 'leaving home' consisted of a huge tantrum, then a walk down the garden path, half way down the road (or up it, just to mix things up a bit) and sitting on the pavement, sulking. I had a happy home, but I wasn't a very happy child. Mum and Dad were great parents and I have only good memories of being little – such as Mum and her mum taking me to the village shops to choose some sweets before feeding the ducks and playing on the swings, or Mum brushing my blonde hair in front of the fire after a nice bath.

Dad, despite suffering with a slipped disc and arthritis, would give me 'Juliette-Eating Camel' rides around the living room, which meant him crawling on all fours chasing me, then me riding on his back, squealing, 'Faster, camel, faster!' I had great birthday parties where he'd wear his Incredible Hulk T-shirt and chase all my friends around the garden, scaring them half to death. Obviously he'd be in prison if he did that these days, but that was the '80s and that's why it was brilliant, because dads could pretend to be Hulk and pick one of my friends up and pretend to throw her over the garden fence in a rage while they were screaming and laughing their heads off and not have to worry about someone calling the police on them.

Up until I went to secondary school, I used to ride my bike or go on my skateboard to meet him halfway home from work. I only had to cross one (very safe) road and I'd wait at the bottom of the hill for him to come around the corner from his train. When my brother was born, I used to take him with me. Even our cat, Whizzy, used to come with us sometimes. We were always incredibly close and although we didn't have much money back then, I really didn't want for anything. I had all the love and attention I could have wished for.

Outside of home, things were a bit different. I didn't like nursery, didn't like mixing with other children and really didn't like being told what to do. By the time secondary school came around, I was absolutely insistent that I wouldn't go to the all-girls' school in a neighbouring village, because 'it will be full of girls, and girls don't like football and are mean to each other.' A pretty good insight for a 10-year-old, no?

Mum insisted that we went to the open day. Despite the head teacher saying, 'Even though it's out of your catchment area, we'd be happy to take Juliette if she passes the test', I insisted that I wouldn't go.

My parents looked at each other and said, 'You've got to go to school somewhere!' and I said, 'Can I go to the all-boys' school instead?'

In the end, Dad wrote a letter to whoever decides where you get to go to school and said I was too clever for the rough school and wanted to join Coopers, a mixed school in the same posh village as the girls' school, but with boys in it. I don't think that's what Dad wrote, exactly, but he did a good job at persuading them to take me.

My brain worked reasonably well with certain subjects - English, French, German, but not with maths and science. Halfway through revising for my GCSE exams I came down with glandular fever. Subsequently, I did next to no revision as I was so ill and dosed up on Solpadeine and Lucozade for the exams. Mum waited outside in the car to take me back home to bed as soon as I'd finished each exam. My results were disappointing but no worse than expected - no A's but a good spattering of B's and C's and a hysterically funny F for maths. I think it stood for 'f*ckwit'.

My parents wanted me to stay on another year at school to re-take my maths GCSE; I said I'd rather burn myself with cigarettes. The argument was that I wouldn't get a job without a pass in maths, and my typically petulant answer was that I didn't want a job where I *needed* a pass in maths. I developed a phobia about anything to do with numbers and even now can't write phone numbers down properly when they're read out to me. The thing is, I'm really good at basic maths as an adult – the important stuff, like paying mortgages and bills and working out restaurant bills and percentages and never going overdrawn. I just can't do fractions or use a protractor, or tell you how long it'll take a man and a half to fill a bath and a half, but I don't think I'll ever need to.

I went to the local college to study for a Private Secretary's Certificate, a two-year-course squashed into nine months. It was full time, 9am-5pm which came as a shock as I thought I'd get to sit around in the canteen all day eating doughnuts and learning to smoke. I learnt shorthand (well, how to write it but not once how to read it back correctly), how to type quickly and how to decide where to put pot plants in a prospective boss's office. It was 1989, not 1949, so I was quite surprised at the old fashioned teachings of it all and promptly didn't listen very much. I still passed 'with distinction', which is hilarious because I went on to be the worst secretary ever.

I didn't have a clue what I wanted to do with my life other than stroke tigers or stalk footballers. Mum had talked me into it as 'it's always useful to be able to type' and as always, she was right, despite the sentence sounding like it had come out of a World War II booklet for young ladies.

My first job was as a secretary at The Mirror Group on *The Daily Mirror* newspaper when Robert Maxwell was in charge. It was an extremely high pressured environment, my first time in London, and I hated it within five minutes of starting. I had very little to do all day and then at 5pm someone else's boss - the advertising director - would dismiss his secretary and pile a load of work on my desk. I never really understood that but it stank. I wasn't getting home until 8pm, so it was a long, unproductive and very dull day. I wasn't learning anything other than how slow clock hands move when you do nothing but stare at them all day. I was just being shouted at which was tantamount to abuse.

One day, when Robert Maxwell called to speak to my boss who was out of the office, he called me a 'useless little cow' because I couldn't get my boss on the phone - 'because, Mr Maxwell, he's not bloody here!' and slammed the phone down on me. I was a bit of a Goth back then, all long black skirts with horrible fringe bits hanging off and 12-hole black Doc Marten boots, and believed in witchcraft, so I put a little curse on him after lunch. Just after I left The Mirror Group two months later, he 'fell' off his yacht and drowned. His death made front page news - on his own newspaper. Ah, the irony.

By the age of 18 I'd been through another two secretarial jobs (the second of which ended up with two slaps and me going out to buy my boss a sandwich and never coming back) and finally I settled on a great job in an international advertising agency.

I absolutely loved the job, and even the commute was easy. A long, nasty walk through industrial estates and alley ways to get to the station, but a mere 25 minutes on the train to Victoria, and a little stroll around the corner to the office, which was in one of those fancy big squares made up of beautiful Regency properties. I made a lot of friends - all a good few years older than me - and settled in quickly. I still felt, however, that I needed more out of life. After six months there I left home to move into a flat share with a good friend from work, a mad German girl called Susanne who only ever ate peas for dinner.

Susanne lived in Manor House, a horrible, run-down area of North London. There were more tower blocks than you could shake a stick at and it was the sort of place where you wouldn't want to walk anywhere on your own after dark. Or before dark, for that matter.

It did, however, have one draw. It was only a couple of miles from Tottenham Hotspur Football Club, the team I had supported since birth. Although the whole area was nasty, I felt a strange kind of security and familiarity as I'd been travelling to my team's ground, White Hart Lane since, I was 14.

Dad had always worked six days a week, Monday to Saturday, so we went to midweek games as often as we could. Dad and I were either completely enraptured by each other's company, or we couldn't bear to be in the same room. It was mad. At football, however, we just bonded like crazy and Dad would take me whenever he could. I think I was the son he never had, at least until he actually had one.

After a summer of living in the house, shared also by the landlord (a real creep of a man who ate cold new potatoes straight from the tin and regularly got caught spying on Susanne or me through the keyhole in the bathroom) I'd had enough. I also missed our cat so much I couldn't bear it any longer. I wanted to save some money instead of throwing it away on rent to live somewhere so rough that the streets had been cordoned off to stop kerb-crawling.

In the autumn of 1990, after England's sensational World Cup performance, the ad agency landed the ad campaign for Brut aftershave. No big deal, you might think, except that the most famous footballer in the country, Paul 'Gazza' Gascoigne was signed up to advertise it. It meant that Gazza would have to do a photo shoot for the bus stop ads and billboards, and that two account managers who worked opposite me would be going along. I spent two days making tea and coffee and running errands, begging to be allowed to come along and meet him. I think they said OK just to shut me up, and maybe because I'd already said I knew where it was being shot and I'd resign and go anyway and stand outside. I bribed their secretary to take over my workload for a few hours by telling her I'd do all her work for a week. Everyone could see how excited I was and nobody had the heart to say no.

Gazza was lovely - extremely professional, jokey and daft like we all know he is - but above all, very down to earth. He couldn't believe how famous he'd become in a matter of weeks. I sat on his knee for a photo and ever the practical joker, he feigned injury and cried out that he'd pulled a hamstring. I leapt off in horror - after all, he's a Tottenham player! - and he let me believe it for a few seconds, then gave me a hug and posed for a photo with me. It was one of the best days of my life and I floated back to work - eventually - on cloud nine.

Although I loved my job, I'd been there a year and had started to get itchy feet, and not the kind of itchy feet you can buy a powder for. I wanted to do something else, something creative and before that, I wanted to travel. I'd been typing up the copywriters' ads for a few months whilst covering for their secretary, and had a terrible habit of changing their scripts a bit here and there, and nobody seemed to notice. I couldn't be bothered to do a copywriting course because it was at a college miles away in Watford (Watford! I'd sooner have commuted to Nepal) so I moved back home and saved just over a grand in a couple of months. My granddad gave me a top-up for 'having the guts to go, good for you!' and I was ready. I didn't want to go to America on my own but nobody else had the money, much less the desire, to come with me.

I put an ad for a travelling companion in a style magazine called *Sky*. I'd asked for 'someone adventurous and mental in a good way to travel around America with me. Must have some pocket money and an interest in football, not cannibalism'. I had three replies, and thought they were all waste of time, including a letter from one girl in Liverpool who said she didn't have any money, but would have loved to join me because I sounded hilarious and she was sure we'd have a good time. Eh?

Eventually, in June 1992, I set off for Florida to meet Alan, a 21-year-old Tottenham fan from Surrey who'd placed an ad in the same magazine a couple of months later, which I'd answered. He apparently had lots of letters but most of them were from weirdos (his words, not mine) and he thought my letter was 'funny and mental', so he binned all the rest and rang me two days later. We met up in a pub in Victoria station and although I didn't actually like him very much, he looked a bit like the actor Matt Dillon if I squinted through one eye and put my hand over the other, so I decided I'd go with him.

Three weeks later we'd met up just once more, half-heartedly planned a route around the East Coast of America, which basically consisted of me holding a Biro and drawing circles around places I liked the name of or had read about with haphazard lines linking them together. Alan had then flown to Florida with his friends for a fortnight. Meanwhile, I packed, re-packed, packed again until I only had hand luggage and one sports bag (which appeared to be entirely full of contact lens solution) then flew out to meet them all on the last day of their holiday.

We took the Greyhound bus up the East Coast via Virginia to New York, where we blew most of our money on a helicopter ride over Manhattan whilst staying in the YMCA, then Chicago, Niagara Falls and back down to Florida where we spent the last three weeks of what turned out to be a three-month, not six-month trip, on Treasure Island on the west coast. We were the only guests in a small motel on the beach run by an affable old chap and his wife, and had the pool to ourselves, apart from when a huge stork came to say hello. It was very chilled out, we were running very low on cash because we'd spent more on hotels and food than we had anticipated (mainly because the places recommended in The Rough Guide were true to its title - rough - and during the last week we lived off McDonald's and Budweiser beer, which wasn't exactly healthy but hey, it was cheap and like I said, 'Hell, all Americans live like this!'

I 'celebrated' my 20th birthday by learning to smoke Marlboro Reds whilst dangling my feet in the lake behind the motel, my toes being nipped at by flying fish as they flipped in and out of the water. It was midnight, nobody was around and the only sound I could hear was the lapping of the cool, clear water against the wooden slats beneath the pier. The stars were shining like I'd never seen before and I soaked up the peace and quiet, grateful for the fact that there wasn't another person in sight. I had a cold beer beside me and I was alone - Matt Dillon had gone for a stroll along the beach. It was then that I decided I couldn't go back to secretarial work.

It came down to two things - animals and magazines. I loved reading, bought piles of magazines every month from football ones to fashion magazines, and I also loved animals to the point that I risked disease by cuddling a fox which had been run over outside our house and nursing a dead bird in my jumper for a weekend when I was about seven. I knew working in a zoo was a limited option - the money was dreadful and I was already used to a good wage, didn't want to live at home forever to be able to work at London Zoo. There was also the problem that I'd failed biology and maths at school and I think you need those so you can work out what animal it is and how many of them have gone missing after you forgot to lock the gates. Saying 'They were furry, and had legs, but I don't know what they were because I can't do biology and I don't know how many there were in the first place because I can't count', wouldn't cut it. That left magazines. I couldn't bear to go back to college to do A-Levels and then a degree or journalism course, so I decided I'd give myself six months to wing it and if it hadn't worked, find something else.

My parents met us from the airport two days later, we dropped Matt Dillon off and all of a sudden I knew I'd miss him, despite the fact that we argued every day. What made up for it was that we shared the same warped sense of humour and a liking for police shows (*COPS* was the best) and beer. We had become an item, as Mum would say, during the trip, because we did fancy each other and we did both support the same football team, so it seemed like a good idea. It also saved on hotel beds and gave us something to do when we were too poor to do anything else.

We'd spent almost 24 hours together, seven days a week for three months, and then no sooner did we land than that was it, nothing. It was really odd. We spoke on the phone a couple of times but I never saw him again. I often wonder what he's up to and whether he thinks about me and how much I nagged him about stealing my cotton buds.

CHAPTER THREE
'WILD SIDE OF LIFE'
CHARLIE FEATHERS

I did have to do some temping when I got back to London but I combined it with working part-time on The Spur, a Tottenham fanzine. I worked for two days a week for nothing for the editor in a cramped 'office' in Notting Hill that was as hot as a greenhouse. I'm sure had I been in the same kind of environment in Malaysia I'd have been knocking out 100 pairs of Nike trainers by the hour.

I wrote match reports and book reviews and helped sell the magazine outside the ground on match days. I knew it was what I wanted to do full time but I needed to get paid for it, so I picked on my favourite football magazine, *90 Minutes*, and wrote them a letter. I said I'd do the cleaning and even brush people's hair after making them tea, anything to get a foot, and maybe my hands, in the door. I got an interview exactly six months after that night on the lake. As luck would have it, they were looking for an editorial assistant and wanted someone who could type fast (thanks, Mum!) and who knew how to answer a phone. It was more important to the editor that I had already been working in a media environment which meant long hours and high stress levels (and no lunch hours) for the past couple of years, and that I'd got a bit of my travelling bug out of the way. I was up against another girl once we were down to the final two. Apparently she had bigger boobs than I had and blonde hair, but she was an Arsenal fan and not as funny as me ('of course she isn't,' said Mum) so that settled it.

Our office was located next door to *loaded* magazine, a new launch which knocked the socks off the publishing world in 1995 with its tales of debauchery, praise of cigarettes and alcohol and celebration of all things men like to do and see.

Things in the office were, to put it mildly, a little off the wall. IPC Magazines operated a total no-smoking policy yet every morning I'd get to my desk and find cigarette butts in my *90 Minutes* coffee cup, the milk gone from the fridge and sometimes a trail of blood or unidentifiable fluid (beer, sometimes... often worse) from the *loaded* office to the toilets which were just around the corner from my desk. There was always something untoward going on next door, and our afternoons were often interrupted by one of the staff asking us to help test biscuits or knives for a feature.

One morning the police arrived at *loaded*'s door. There was much rushing to the loo and flushing of illegal substances down toilets, but despite every surface being covered in Rizla packets and porn, all the law enforcement officers wanted was a copy of the magazine. Life, as you can expect, was never dull, even if it did smell a bit stale sometimes. I remained sensible to the point of ridiculousness at this time in my life, turning down tickets to Oasis' first gig and after show party with the *loaded* lot to go home and water the garden because Mum and Dad were away. On the same night, whilst watering the hydrangeas and runner beans I had a call from the then Liverpool footballer Jamie Redknapp, inviting me to meet him at his hotel the next evening 'for a lemonade'. I'd interviewed him over the phone at work the day before and he'd asked for my number. I couldn't understand why he asked for it but I didn't question it; back in 1994 he happened to be one of the Premiership's best players, along with being so handsome it was untrue. Now, I won't elaborate too much, but although Dad had banned me from taking the car out (because every single time I backed it into the garage to put it away I scraped the wing mirrors) I sped off into the night and duly drank my lemonade whilst being unable to speak to Jamie because he was super famous and super good-looking. I could have done with something a bit stronger than lemonade - I left about three hours later with a very surprised expression on my face and it didn't go back to normal for about three days. And yes, I scraped the wing mirrors. Sorry dad!

At least I went that night. Another time I said no to a celebrity party because I had some broccoli in the fridge that would have gone off if I hadn't have eaten it that night. Hello? Honestly, it's true.

That summer I booked a holiday with my friend Rachel and two other girls. It was a fortnight in Gran Canaria - not my choice at all - I'd wanted a nice, quiet-ish Greek island but unfortunately I'd been at the football when they'd booked it. Off we went, and within three days I'd met an 18-year-old who was 'working' out there as a DJ, and sort of fallen in love. Oh dear.

I was 23 at the time. Ross told me he was 20 because he thought admitting that he was 18 would have 'put me off'. He was hilarious, and I enjoyed his haphazard company, when he felt like joining me on an evening out. He was from Leicester. I lived in Kent. It had 'holiday romance' written all over it, and nothing more.

I went back to work after the holiday, and just as promised, a month later when he returned to England, Ross called me. I was both astonished and expecting it; it's hard to explain. I went to see him at his parents' house and fell in love not just with him, but also with his mum. Everyone thought it was a bit weird that I was dating a teenager (he came clean about two months in, I just found him even more attractive because he'd stay younger for longer) but he was the funniest person I'd ever met, so why not?

Rachel and I moved into a hideous flat in Stamford Hill, back on the doorstep of my beloved Tottenham Hotspur Football Club. The inhabitants of Stamford Hill fell into three main categories - orthodox Jews, crack heads and us. The first I didn't have a problem with, they would pretty much do everything to avoid us, the second I did, as they did pretty much everything to hassle us. I must have needed my head examined, moving back to North London considering I already knew I hated it, but as I spent all my money going to watch football I thought I might as well be only 10 minutes away from the ground and save on train fare and journey time.

On the first day that we moved in, Rachel and her boyfriend were unpacking while I cheekily went to White Hart Lane to watch Tottenham play Manchester City. My friend, Kit Symons, whom I'd interviewed countless times for *90 Minutes*, was playing for Man City at the time and got me a pass for the Players' Bar after the match. I looked dreadful, unlike all the other bleached-blonde women standing around in their designer suits - it's really not that far removed from the TV show *Footballer's Wives* - and it was a windy day so my hair was all over the shop and I'd got rubbish clothes on because I couldn't find anything to change into when we got to the flat because it was all in bin bags.

I arrived in the bar straight after the match so I knew I'd have to wait around before Kit had got showered and changed. Nobody else seemed to be on their own and I felt a bit awkward, so I took ages to go to the loo and put a bit of lipstick on and tried to make my hair look less windswept with tap water and the hand dryer, which only made it look even worse.

I went red about a hundred times during the next half an hour as Tottenham players walked into the bar - every time I made eye contact with one of them I'd get all silly and hot and start shaking. I'm not exactly the vampy, go-get-'em kinda gal, more the 'Eek! He just looked at me and smiled!' sort, which is a shame because one player who I'd been besotted with for eight years did, in fact, look over and smile in a fairly 'come hither' way and I simply turned away and ignored him. What an idiot (me, not him).

Anyway, I said my hello to Kit and a goodbye a few minutes later, after all that, as the team had to board the coach back to Manchester. As I was leaving I bumped into Tottenham player Sol Campbell and introduced myself. I'd interviewed him over the phone a couple of times and thought I'd say hello. I thought I was shy but he was even worse. He asked where I lived and I said, 'Down the road in a nasty flat as from this morning', and he said, 'Oh, I could have given you a lift but I'm going the other way to my mum's for dinner.' I thought it was a bit crap that he didn't just say he'd give me a lift anyway, but I said goodbye and walked out to the car park and down the road to the bus stop. I must have been there about 15 minutes when a car pulled up in front of me. Someone wound down the window and I thought they were going to either kidnap me or drive-by shoot me, but as I peered into the car from a safe distance, I saw that it was, in fact, Sol Campbell and he was offering me a lift. He said he'd felt mean and came to find me. I thought, 'How cool is this, getting a lift home from our centre-half?'

Sol agreed to come in for a cup of tea and it was only then that I thought, 'I haven't warned Rachel and she'll think it's mad.' I was right. We walked into the flat. I explained the mess and put the kettle on, getting out my Tottenham mug especially for him (in retrospect I think that might have scared him a bit). I walked into my bedroom where Rachel was putting my bed together, bless her, and Sol poked his head around the door behind me. Upon seeing a 6ft 2in black man in the doorway she promptly dropped the screwdriver and squealed, just as I was announcing, 'Look! It's Sol Campbell, he's come in for a cup of tea, how mad is that?'

She went white, then red, then mumbled 'hello' and shot me a look that said, 'What?!' and I went to the kitchen and made his tea. We sat in the lounge, which was vile, and made polite small talk about the game and how nasty our new flat was and all the way through he drank his tea with the teabag still in it. I've never forgotten that, I could only think, 'Ugh, he's going to swallow the teabag, choke, and die in my nasty lounge, and then we wouldn't have a centre-half!' He left quite quickly, probably because I kept saying, 'Look! It's Sol Campbell! He's drinking tea in our flat!' and laughing hysterically like a hyena on crack. He took my phone number and rang a few times and even invited me to his 21st birthday party, which was insane, but we never met up again until I went to a press conference at Tottenham a couple of years later when he had hit the big time, was playing for England and he barely said hello!

That spring, IPC Magazines held their annual Editorial Awards. It was a big posh affair, dinner, wine and everyone dressed up to the nines. Except I'd stubbed my toe running up the stairs at home that week, which meant I could only wear trainers. My best friend, Declan, the magazine's designer, was chatting to me, wine and cigarette in hand after dinner, when the awards bit started. We were still chatting, drinking and smoking when my name was read out by a big, booming voice that sounded like The Wizard of Oz behind his curtain.

'And now, nominations for the Best Newcomer Award...' and there it was: my name, along with five other nominees. How funny! I went red, and half watched the short bit of film about the nominees that showed some of their work. I felt a bit sick.

The Wizard of Oz boomed: 'And the winner is... Juliette Wills!' I spluttered my wine over my knees, looked at my editor, Paul, and made a 'Huh?' face. I had no idea what I was meant to do as it was the first award of the night, and I was plastered. Already. Because the wine was free, and I put in so many hours that went unpaid that I was drinking about six months' worth of overtime in alcohol.

The lads on the *loaded* table stood and cheered, and our table followed suit. I was still stuck to my chair. A spotlight picked me out, and Paul said, 'Go and get your award, you daft cow!' and so, wine in hand, I limped around the tables and chairs, wishing the spotlight would go and find a spider or a burglar or something, and leave me to it. I was still holding my glass and looked on in befuddlement as I was handed a framed award certificate thing, and an envelope. And then a microphone. I turned to look at the audience and then, instead of a 'Thank you everyone for your kind cheering, thank you to my editor for nominating me, thank you to starving children in Africa,' I instead did a bow, almost fell on my face, stood up, squeaked 'Yay!' and raised my glass, stumbling back down the steps again.

In May, right at the end of the football season, another big night was on the cards. IPC held their Football Magazines Awards party. I was so excited in the run-up to it that I could barely breathe. I put a dress and high heels on (the toe had healed) and even brushed my hair. I thought I'd died and gone to heaven – Premiership footballers were everywhere, and there were no bouncers, police or gates stopping me from getting to them. I thought I was going to have a stroke I was in such a state of delirium. And it was free booze again! Ian Astbury from The Cult was there. That was mad. I was a bit drunk (what a surprise) and kept telling him, 'I love She Sells Seashells, best song ever, drove into Vegas listening to it!' while he kept saying, 'It's 'she sells sanctuary'. Not seashells. Sanctuary.' I wasn't having any of it.

Everywhere I looked there were pop stars or footballers. I thought I was going to implode. Damon Albarn from Blur asked to borrow my lighter, and only later on did Declan tell me that 'he was chatting you up, you idiot' but as usual I had failed to realise that and thrown him my lighter across the table and then asked somebody else to retrieve it when it showed no sign of coming back. I've never been one for reading signals.

TV presenting comic duo Ant and Dec were there, and I thought that was hysterical. I had a little chat with them and told them Rachel and I kept a poster of them on our kitchen wall and that every time we dropped some food, like a mushroom slice, or a pea, on the floor we stuck it to their face on the poster. So far Ant had a bit of mushroom and a pea for eyes and Dec had a bit of lettuce for a nose. They backed away. However, a few hours later when I everyone I knew had gone home without offering me a space in their cab, I asked Ant if I could jump in their chauffeur-driven affair.

'But we live in Fulham, pet,' he said in his Geordie accent, holding my shoulders to try and halt my swaying, 'and you live in North London.'

'Oh, bothered!' I remember mumbling, 'I'll just stay at yours then.'

I grabbed hold of Ant's jacket and threw myself into the car. They didn't exactly have a choice, and I ended up sitting on the sofa in a crumpled heap next to Ant watching GMTV and talking about football. Dec made us a cup of tea and looked bewildered and went to bed. I was stone cold sober as the sun came up and wondered how the hell I'd ended up at Ant and Dec's when I clearly remember telling Rachel I'd get a cab home with her at 1am.

I then got a taxi back to my flat at 8.30am when all the kids were on their way to school. Ant came down to the flat's entrance to see me into the cab, no doubt to make sure I really had left, and all these kids were walking past. One of them spotted him and shouted, 'Oi! Ant and Dec!' which I thought was weird because it was only Ant, but I'm guessing they're such a famous pair that you don't say one without the other, a bit like shouting 'Morecombe!' without 'Wise!' or 'It's a Ronnie!' for one of The Two Ronnies. I got in the cab, fell asleep and ended up paying £35 to get home as it was rush hour and took forever to cross London. I had a shower when I got in, went to bed for an hour then got up and went to work. I wasn't sick but I felt terrible. My editor said 'What time do you call this? Where have you been? We're really busy!' and I replied, 'about two o'clock, and I've been at Ant and Dec's so you've got to forgive me because that's the funniest thing ever,' and to a roar of laughter, I was duly forgiven.

There was never a dull moment in my job. One afternoon I looked up from my desk to see Darth Vader. Well, Dave Prowse, the bloke who played him. Sadly he wasn't in costume as a) he wasn't there because of Star Wars and b) I'm not sure he actually has the costume anyway. He had popped in for a photo shoot as part of a promotion with Snickers giant bars or something, and he stopped for a cup of tea. Sweet.

'Did you have a good day?' asked Mum over the phone that night.

'Yes,' I said, 'I met Darth Vader.'

In December 1996, a new girl band called The Spice Girls exploded into the charts. I liked them. At my age, it wasn't really cool to admit that, but I'd never really been one for caring what anyone thought about me. We decided they'd make a great cover for the Christmas issue of *90 Minutes*, dressed up in football kit. Naturally, as I was the one who was a bit obsessed with them, I got to do the interview. I had a chat with Mel B (Scary Spice), Mel C (Sporty Spice), Emma (Baby Spice) and my favourite Spice Girl, Geri (Ginger Spice). I was a bit excited, and commented that I couldn't believe she could stand up straight because her boobs were so enormous yet her feet were so tiny.

'Your feet are mental small,' I gasped, pointing at her toes, 'that you could wear hedgehog shoes! Or baby shoes.' Geri looked a bit scared, and waved Victoria (Posh Spice) over while she went off to have her lunch. If anyone's interested, Mel B and Geri had sausage and mash. Mel C had sushi and Emma had hummus, salad and pitta. All apart from Mel C smoked. Cigarettes, I mean, nothing sinister. But you could tell that their PR didn't want anyone to write about that. I mean, these girls were role models for a new generation. You couldn't say, 'Baby Spice chugs all day on Silk Cut!' could you?

I liked Victoria instantly. She had a slight awkwardness about her, and was the shyest of the group. She kept pulling at the hem of her dress, saying that she didn't know why she always had to wear such short skirts.

'Because you have a tip-top pair of legs?' I suggested.

'The other girls have got good legs,' she shrugged, 'but we've all got our 'thing' now, and mine seems to be the tight dresses and heels.'

'It could be worse,' I said, 'you could be 'Homeless Spice', just imagine what they'd dress you in then.' She laughed, smoothed her hair and nibbled on a couple of dried dates. That's all I saw her eat all day, and I felt a bit sad for her. She was clearly incredibly self-conscious despite her killer figure which she obviously felt needed trimming down. It didn't. I felt like a big lump next to her, and I was only a size 10.

I'd brought along some photos of footballers to see if the girls showed an interest in any of them. I'd forgotten to ask the others, so I pulled out the envelope in front of Victoria, and explained that I wanted a thumbs up or a thumbs down depending on their attractiveness. We got a thumbs down for the first four - and quite rightly, as I'd picked the ugliest players I could think of - and she looked as if she was beginning to tire of my exciting charade. I pulled out the last one.

'What about him?' I asked, 'he's going to be one of the best players in the world, and he's got a nice floppy fringe.' I was holding a photo of David Beckham. She grabbed the photo.

'Thumbs up, then?' I asked, seeing her eyes light up.

'God, yeah,' she replied, 'he's lovely! Who is he?' She was smoothing her hair down again.

'No point doing your hair,' I said, 'it's only a photo, he can't see you! His name is David Beckham. He plays for Manchester United. He's good already, and he's only young. Handsome, no?' Victoria snatched the photo from my hands.

'I'm going to keep that,' she whispered.

'If you want to meet him,' I said, 'why don't you ask Mel C to take you to Old Trafford? She knows her football. You're pop stars, so you'll get tickets, no problem.'

'What's Old Trafford?' she said.

'It's the name of Manchester United's ground. Go up for a match with Mel C, then go and talk to him afterwards in the Players' Bar. I'll put it in the magazine that you fancy him so he already knows and that'll be it, job done. You can thank me later.'

'I will,' she smiled, 'I'm going to ask him out for dinner, that's it.'

The article came out two weeks later. Victoria met David in the players' lounge at Old Trafford a few weeks later. The rest, as they say is history. And, no, I never did get a thank you!

After being burgled twice in Stamford Hill, Rachel and I both went back to our parents' homes. Again. I was saving for a deposit on a flat even though I wasn't even sure where I wanted to live (but I knew where I didn't want to live - Tottenham). I'd been at *90 Minutes* for four years as Staff Writer, and decided to go freelance, which meant I was working from home now with my computer haphazardly set up in the lounge and I slept in the box room with Whizzy the cat, while Jonathan, who was 16 at the time, had my old bedroom. For six months my belongings were in storage, at a friend's house, in the loft, all over the place. I did sub-editing on magazines like *FHM* and *Maxim*, went to *loaded* a couple of weeks a month to sub-edit there and wrote football and music features for *Melody Maker*, *Mixmag*, *loaded* and *Goal*, a new football magazine set up by IPC just before *90 Minutes* closed.

I interviewed England and Chelsea superstar Frank Lampard when he was at West Ham United. I had recently got back together with Ross after a few months' break, and our relationship was a test in itself, just because he didn't know from one week to the next if he was visiting me in West London, North London, Orpington or somewhere else he was yet to hear about. He'd also just moved from Leicester to Hull to go to University. Trust me, nobody wants to spend time in Hull unless they really, really have to. I made the trip a few times, but I struggled with staying in a crowded student house full of uh, students. Ugh. Anyway, back to Frank Lampard. He asked me on a date, and I turned him down because I loved Ross. Despite saying 'no' (and it wasn't easy, believe me) he called me a few times and even rang from Milan when he was playing with the England Under-21 team. He soon lost interest, which is a shame, particularly as Ross dumped me quite spectacularly about a week later. D'oh! When people say they lived their life with no regrets, they have clearly never turned down a date with Frank Lampard.

I knew I didn't want to rent in London again, and unless I won some money or married a Sheik I wouldn't be able to buy anywhere in London either. We thought long and hard and then my parents decided that Dad's redundancy money from his last job as a service engineer with Sainsbury's would no longer sit in the bank but would go into a new house. They traded in their three-bed semi for a four bedroom house in a nicer area, opposite a nature reserve and, as Dad would tell everyone, 'with a garage and room for *three* cars on the drive!' Mum told me I'd better stay there for at least a year to make the move worthwhile, and that the small bedroom could be used as my office. I was over the moon.

A typical day saw me up at 8.30am, eating breakfast on the patio, our cat, Pebble, keeping me company (Whizzy, sadly, was no more after her first summer in her new garden. We'd had to have her put down at the respectable age of 17, two days after Princess Diana died. It was quite a week for mourning). Pebble was chosen from a cage in a local animal rescue centre, and was pretty lovely. I'd take next door's Labrador, Holly, for a long walk through the woods, and on the way I'd feed the horses and the sheep. I had a favourite sheep who got more carrot and apple than any of the others because he always said hello as I came up the hill and shouted to him, although he didn't strictly say 'hello', he kind of burped. If he'd said 'hello', obviously I would have rung a circus or something and sold him for a fortune as 'The Hello Sheep - He Honestly Says Hello!'

I'd come home, do a couple of hours of research or writing, have dinner, see friends, go to bed. I was 26-years-old, enjoying a great career, and had saved almost everything I earned from writing to get enough for a deposit on a flat.

One day I was upstairs in my room, sitting on the floor with the telephone and a tape recorder. I was in the middle of an interview with the late walrus-shaped singing sensation, Barry White. I'd just asked him if he had any pets when Mum shouted up the stairs.

'Juliette, how many fish fingers do you want? Four or five? You can have five, there's an odd one left if you don't!' and I had to put my hand over the mouthpiece and shout back, 'Mum! I'm on the phone to Barry White!'

I resumed the conversation only for him to ask what in God's name a fish finger was and how come I could eat four of them? To say I had a strange 'average' day was putting it mildly. Oh, and he had two Alsatians, in case you're wondering. And loved to barbecue fish but couldn't 'cook nothin' else for shit'. Bet you didn't know that, eh?

On my birthday, an almost unbearably hot day in July, I took the train to Brighton for the day with a friend. I'd always loved the seaside, but had never been to Brighton as a child. I thought it was brilliant. It had pretty much everything that London had – great shops, great restaurants - but at the end of it, there was sea. How mad is that? I'd been a few times over the years and always wished I didn't have to get on a train when the sun began to set. On a whim, and without the benefit of hindsight, I decided that's where I would live.

It had been two months since I was diagnosed with ulcerative colitis, and the effects of the steroids had yet to take hold. It was a cold, dreary day, not ideal when looking at a place as a prospective habitat. Leo, whom I'd met while freelancing on a women's magazine at IPC had accompanied me on the trip as her parents lived in Brighton so we could stay the night. We spent the day peering in estate agents' windows, asking for details on flats and eventually getting around to why I was thinking about moving there when I didn't know a soul.

'I don't know,' I said, sipping on a Black Russian (cocktail, that is, not man), a few hours later. 'I just think I fancy a bit of seaside, a few seagulls waking me up in the morning, decent shops right on the doorstep and you can get those hot doughnuts on the Palace Pier.'

'But won't you be lonely?' said Leo, looking as though I was bonkers. 'What will you do with yourself?'

'Make bags even though I can't sew, read magazines, count chocolate biscuits, sleep, watch the football, throw myself off the pier, make a secret camp in the helter skelter with some hedgehogs. I basically want to live in the helter skelter. I could collect stray animals, pretend the phone's ringing when it's not. Go on the rollercoaster just because I can. Get my fortune read. Every day. I don't know. But considering the barman's just given us a free round, it's looking more and more likely by the minute that things will work out.'

Said barman, in fact, had taken the £20 note from my half-heartedly manicured hand, turned to the till, opened it up, and lifted out two £10 notes, which he handed back to me. Now, like I said, maths has never been my strong point - I can't even remember how old I am sometimes - but I knew he'd made a mistake. He had nice eyes so I told him what he'd done.

'You've given me two tenners,' I said. 'Have you been helping yourself to the gin all day or are you just really bad at counting?' He laughed and winked at me, not a cheesy foreign waiter wink, a nice, shy, 'I'm a little bit naughty' kind of wink.

Four Black Russians later the bar was closing. The barman kept looking over as we were putting our duvets (otherwise known as puffa coats) on. He had a really, really handsome, cheeky face. I remembered I had a few business cards in my bag so I flung one at Leo and said, 'Give that to barman who can't count and let's go,' pulling her out of the door as she thrust the card in his hand. He looked bewildered.

'It's not mine!' she shrieked, 'it's hers!' And with that, we stumbled out of the door.

Men usually wait until the Wednesday after a Saturday night to call you for the first time. Tuesday is a bit too early (you look a bit keen), Thursday is a bit late (you look like you don't care). Mark called on Monday. We talked for an hour. He made me laugh. A lot. I told him I was riddled with a hideous disease and had to take tablets which made me a bit mental, and even that it was something embarrassing and that I might get all ill on him. He wasn't in the least bit fazed. I think I was in love with him by the time I put the phone down.

The day after he called me he fell down some slippery steps at work and dislocated his shoulder. I guess he was bored and invited me down to see him, so 10 days after the night we met I got on the train to Brighton and I went to meet him, hoping he was as handsome as I had remembered and not, in fact, an obese dwarf, because due to the cocktails he kept letting me have for free, I couldn't be sure.

I was early. My eyes were darting all about the station until I realised the person walking confidently towards me, his pace quickening with every step, must be him. I think my jaw dropped. He was the most handsome man I'd ever seen. Well, the most handsome man I'd ever seen who wasn't in a film. I tentatively kissed him on the cheek. He wasn't prepared for it, almost sidestepped me and I fell into a bus shelter and hit my head. Good start. We went for a drink in a pub halfway between the station and the sea. The fire was lit, he ordered a Guinness and took a sip at the bar, coming back to the table with a Guinness moustache which he wiped off with the back of his hand after I'd pointed it out. I wanted to do it. I could feel myself getting hot and blamed the fire. He smoked roll-ups. I held his hands across the table. I took off my cardigan. I was so hot and excited that I had to sit in the pub bare-shouldered for an hour despite the fact that it was snowing. Outside I mean, not inside.

We left the pub after an hour and went for a pizza too late to be called lunch and too early to be dinner. I cut up his food because his arm was in a sling. I helped him with his coat, the empty sleeve flapping about in the cold wind as we stepped outside. It was dark already, yet it was only just gone 5pm. I started to think about getting home at the same time as I thought about wanting to stay.

We walked to the seafront. I asked him if he thought we'd kiss today. We were on the beach in front of The Grand Hotel. I was shivering. He shrugged off his coat and with his left hand, put it around me, and pulled me to him. I couldn't look him in the eye. My heart was beating so fast and so loud I was convinced he could hear it. Cars were passing above us, a few people must have walked past but I remember it as though time stood still. When I close my eyes I can almost feel the cold wind on my face and in my hair all over again. We stood together, my arms around him inside his jumper, pressing against his T-shirt and feeling the warmth from his back work its way down my hands. Maybe 20 seconds passed and then we both started laughing.

'You'd better get on with it,' I said, 'I'm bloody freezing.'

He did. He just brushed my lips with his at first, then stopped, looked at me for a moment, smiled, and kissed me again. It was - and I have had my fair share of kisses - the most wonderful kiss I have ever had. He had this walk, a kind nonchalant gait about him. I can't explain it, but I thought it was really sexy. I walked behind him whenever I got the chance so that I could watch him.

We got a taxi back to his house. I'd imagined it to be some student tip, but it was nothing of the sort. He went to the back yard to chop some wood for the fire. With one arm. Really. He made some tea *in a pot*. It was all very old fashioned and proper. I sat nervously on the sofa, my arms outstretched in front of me as I warmed my hands before the fire. As the flames wrapped themselves around the logs I wondered how I would bring myself to leave. He walked into the room carrying two mugs, kicking the door shut behind him. He set down the tea, pushed up his sleeves and took my hands in his, first rubbing them then kissing my fingers. He asked me to stay. I said no. He didn't push it.

It was starting to get late. He rose from the sofa to get our coats, taking my gloves out of my bag and putting them on my hands. He took the bus to the station with me, and I got the train back up to Victoria, then another one down to Orpington. When I arrived home, I came through the front door and declared to Mum, 'I'm in love. I'm totally, utterly, head over heels in love.' She sighed and rolled her eyes. I went upstairs to call him to let him know I was home. We talked for an hour. I went to bed but I didn't sleep.

The next three months flew by in a blur. I'd drive down to Brighton on a Saturday morning and if I didn't have any work lined up the following week, I'd not go home again for four or five days. Although the colitis didn't go away, I didn't have any of the symptoms that I had been told to expect. The stomach pain and diarrhoea, the rushing to the toilet up to 20 times a day, it never happened. I thought it was really weird. I'd read up a lot about the disease and they were always the symptoms described. In fact, I had the opposite problem - I was always constipated. Oh well, I reasoned, typical that I had to be difficult.

I was so happy at that time that my illness took a back seat. Being in love was a fabulous distraction and I believe that Mark was doing me the world of good, even reminding me to take my tablets and thinking up wheat and dairy free dinners for me. I had him all to myself then, and I couldn't have been happier. I would often lie there wide awake as he slept soundly behind me, my hands around his hands around me. I would lie perfectly still, frightened that if I moved it would all have been a dream.

One day I interviewed a footballer I was absolutely mad about who was playing for London Premiership side Fulham.

'That's the man for me,' I thought, a big handsome bloke with nice blue eyes who scores goals. Well, he would have been if I wasn't in love with someone else.

During lunch he asked me if I had a boyfriend and I even went as far as to say that I was engaged. I was so nervous I couldn't eat my food for thinking what it would be like to kiss him. He smelled wonderful, was dressed impeccably, he made me laugh and well, was stinking rich and played football. And he had a thick Yorkshire accent - my favourite.

I finished my wine and asked for a lift back to the station. He suggested going for a drink. I said I had to get back. He kissed me on the cheek and told me to take care. I watched him drive off and stamped my feet like a three-year-old then rang my friend Helen to tell her what had - or hadn't - happened. I told her I was so in love I wasn't interested, or at least I wasn't interested enough to ruin what I had. She said, 'Willsy, I think you've lost the plot. Either that or you're proper in love!'

Mark and I stayed in on New Year's Eve, 2000. The Millennium. Blimey. It was all a bit too much, trying to decide what to do, so we decided to do as little as possible, that way we wouldn't be too disappointed. He spent all afternoon making a four-course dinner from scratch, munching on my mum's Christmas Specials - her fabulous sausage rolls and mince pies. I didn't have to do a thing, other than watch him roll out the pasta, make the soup, whisk this and blend that. It was all a blur to me but he seemed to have everything under control. I spent all afternoon getting ready and worrying whether I could drink champagne with all my tablets bouncing around inside me. I put on a proper slinky dress and high heels.

I sat on his lap to eat my pudding (a perfect, homemade crème caramel). At midnight we climbed the stairs to the attic to watch the fireworks from the window. He held me tightly - more to keep me upright than anything else, looked me in the eyes, sighed and, after a pause of around three hours, got to one knee and said: 'I could murder one of your mum's sausage rolls.'

I put an offer on a one-bedroom flat in February. It was 10 minutes' walk up a very steep hill from the seafront on the opposite side of town to Mark's place. When my offer was accepted my parents came down to look at the flat as I had no idea about checking damp bits and plumbing and all that kind of dad stuff. It soon transpired that Dad didn't either, but I wanted them to reassure me I was making the right decision. Mum and I were in the bedroom measuring up for the curtains and trying to work out where all my shoes would go (Me: 'On the ceiling, from string?' Mum: 'It's time to stop buying shoes!'), Mark was in the kitchen with Dad talking about where to put the fridge and the washing machine.

From that day, things started to change, but I wouldn't notice the signs that he no longer loved me, or perhaps never had, until weeks later.

Whilst waiting for an exchange date on the flat, I was at home when I came down with gastroenteritis. I cried in despair at the pain, but more at the fact that I was supposed to be interviewing Hollywood movie star Denzel Washington for *loaded* that same day. He was in a hotel in Mayfair, waiting for my questions. I was at home chucking up my internal organs while my questions were being faxed to the office so that someone else could step in at the last minute. To say I felt hard done by is an understatement.

With the colitis already running riot through my system, the gastroenteritis knocked me for six. I couldn't keep anything down, even a sip of water, so I couldn't take my steroids aside from anything else. I was bleeding from one end, puking from the other, diarrhoea in between and sometimes all three at the same time. Eventually, I managed to take the steroids with just enough water for them to go down and stay there, and that's how I spent the first three days. After a week of total agony I returned to Brighton half a stone lighter - I'm sure I threw up a lung somewhere along the line - thinking I'd be clear of germs, but two nights later when Mark sat bolt upright in bed, pale, shaking and feverish, I knew he'd got it. I have a lifelong fear of vomit - myself, bad enough, makes me cry and flap hysterically - someone else, well, I can't be in the same room let alone hold their hair back or mop their fevered brow. A bloke was sick on the train near me once on the way home from work. I was so horrified I got up, walked across the seats (with people on them), got off at the next stop and ran down the platform so that I could get on in a different carriage, far, far away, then decided that wasn't far away enough and just waited for another train. No, I'm not good with vomit.

This time I sat on the bathroom floor with him in his pyjama bottoms, held him in my arms, disinfected the toilet so he'd at least be holding on to a clean toilet seat and lay in bed with him as he sweated, shook and cried out in pain. I kept him warm, I brought him water and held it to his lips at 4am when he wanted a sip, I changed the sheets, I had ice-cold flannels at the ready whenever his temperature rose and I did this for two days. On the third, his dad came to pick him up and take him back to his house in Surrey. I had to drive back Kent to pack for my next trip – and what a trip! This time I was off to the Australian Grand Prix, again for *loaded*. As much as I was mad about not being able to interview Denzel Washington, I was glad I'd been ill that week and not this one. I did not want to cancel a trip to Australia. As Mark got in the car I turned to go back inside the house to gather my things before driving home. He wound down the window.

'I love you,' he shouted as the car turned the corner. That was the last time I'd hear him say those words.

The Grand Prix season kicked off in Melbourne in March 2000, and the night before I flew out I couldn't sleep with the excitement.

Now, most people I meet think my job is glamorous. I would like to put them straight. Interviews with footballers are usually conducted on a freezing cold February morning, in the middle of a muddy field, where I'll have been standing for an hour waiting for their training session to finish. Often their PR representative or agent sits in on the interview, waving a hand and shaking a head should you so much as ask them anything about their personal life, such as 'how are you today?' or 'do you live in a house?'

If I'm lucky, I get to sit in the canteen and take my gloves off long enough to press 'record' on my tape recorder (which, as I've already mentioned, usually doesn't work). Most interviews also tend to take place up north, and so involve four-hour train journeys (that's from London which, of course, I have to get to in the first place), cabs from stations to the outskirts of the world and all over again on the way back. I have to pay for the tickets and taxis upfront, and get the money back around two months after the article is published. Oh, and on a wheat and dairy free diet, getting anything to eat is a nightmare, as it's all coffee and sandwiches and burgers and chocolate and cakes. It takes forever to get home and I always seem to just miss a train and end up stranded, usually at Crewe.

I can tell you that 24 hours in economy class being served pork fried rice that I won't eat for breakfast is not in the least bit glamorous either, but hey, I'm on the way to Australia so who cares? At least that's what I think for the first hour, after that I just get fed up with sitting down. After 10 hours I'm almost in tears. I have nobody to talk to and I'm feeling really claustrophobic.

I've read three books and managed to miss four films by not having the ability to tune into the correct channel quickly enough. After 13 hours and a three-hour stopover in Singapore at 5am with only my bag to chat I tried to sleep, upright on a plastic chair with my hand luggage tied around my ankles for security. Needless to say, I just ended up sitting upright in a plastic chair with my hand luggage tied around my ankles for security. By the time I got to my hotel, a five-star marble block in the centre of Melbourne, I was losing the will to live and desperate to make conversation with someone other than an air hostess. No offence, but I wanted to talk about something other than whether or not I had fastened my seatbelt.

The blonde, drenched-in-make-up receptionist tapped her false nails on the keyboard in front of her, pulled a face and brightly informed me that my room was booked for the next night, not this one.

'Er, but it can't be,' I said, 'it should be booked from tonight until next Tuesday. I check out on Wednesday.' I put my bag down and rested my arms on the marble desk.

'No, Miss Wills, it's most definitely from tomorrow night. And I can't fit you in because we're totally booked up. You could try our sister hotel. I'll call you a cab,' she said, making it sound like it was a question rather than a statement, as Australians are wont to do.

I got to the other hotel and checked in. It was 1.45am Australian time, but I couldn't work out how long I'd been travelling or even what day it was here, let alone at home in England. I'd told Mark I'd call him to let him know I'd arrived safely but worked out that it was the same time at home, so he'd be asleep, so I took a shower and went to bed. And my, what a bed! I slept until 10am the next morning, checked out and got a taxi back to the hotel I was supposed to be staying at in the first place.

As I opened the door to my room I realised that I didn't have a room, I had a suite. It had a proper stainless steel kitchen in it, with a dishwasher and a washing machine. And things in the fridge. And a bowl of fruit. Real fruit! And a bar of chocolate. And peanuts. And crisps. And huge, soft, white towels. And a bathroom the size of a small island. The bed was so wide it took me half an hour to crawl across it. Well, almost. I had two balconies. I had to sit down. It was amazing. On the bed lay a package from the race sponsors, Fosters, containing T-shirts, baseball caps and sun cream. There was a map of the track, how to get there and a watch, fleecey jacket and wallet, which I immediately put in my suitcase for my dad. I've lost count of the amount of promotional freebies I've brought home for him. He'd wear a Barbie T-shirt if it was free.

The next few days were spent at the racetrack. I'd be up at 7.30am. I'd shower, go for breakfast on the hotel's terrace with the photographer, the pair of us melting in the 100 degree heat. We'd watch the sessions, photograph fans in daft outfits, have some lunch and not too much wine, try to avoid burning under the midday sun (I didn't do very well at that), then head back to the hotel, shower, and go out for dinner. We ate lobster, drank champagne and cocktails (the exchange rate was phenomenal and we had £40 expenses per day!) and I didn't want to go home. We had a barbecue on a roof top terrace at a friend of the photographer's, and spent a lovely afternoon lazing on the beach. I would have happily stayed for six months if it had been possible.

The photographer left two days earlier than me, so I went to Melbourne zoo and took two rolls of film of koalas and kangaroos. The weather was glorious and I felt fantastic. I even visited Ramsay Street, where *Neighbours* is filmed, in the hope that I might stumble upon one of the actors that I fancied. Sadly, they were filming the coffee shop scenes that day, so I didn't get to stalk anyone, but I did sit in the middle of the road and let a tourist take a photo of me for my mum, who openly admits to watching it every day despite her not having had a lobotomy that I am aware of.

I flew home, but not without some bother, as I'd missed my flight by an entire 24 hours. How? The flight was at 1am, so I checked in at 11pm the night before... on the date of the flight. Luckily I got booked on a spare seat and just had to endure three hours in Singapore, I think on the same plastic seat as last time. This time I actually managed to sleep for a few hours, and when I came through the front door, Mum said, 'Mark's called three times already and I said you'd be in just about now. He said he'll call back.'

I was shattered. 'You look as white as ever! I thought you'd have a tan!' said Mum, putting the kettle on and hugging me with one arm whilst taking my bag off my shoulder with the other. I unloaded gifts, dirty washing and camera films full of koala pictures, then the phone rang.

I knew Mark was at a friend's wedding that day. We had arranged to meet at Victoria station the next day, despite my stupid jet lag. He'd be working his last day at a temporary job in London and I'd be staying at his friend's flat with him in the centre of town for a few days. Meanwhile, I started two weeks' work on a women's magazine on the Monday, so I'd have the luxury of being able to walk to work and come home to someone who'd have already made the dinner. I thought we'd have a great time pretending we lived in this huge mansion flat in the middle of town and spend every night catching up on all the things we'd missed thanks to stomach bugs and being on opposite sides of the world.

He rang me from the wedding reception a couple of hours later. He was drunk. He told me it was like a Mafia wedding - the bride was Sicilian - and that he'd never been to anything like it in his life.

'Does it make you want to get married?' I asked, not sure if it was a joke or not.

'No,' he answered softly, 'no, it doesn't. But I'll tell you what,' he continued, 'the girls, the bridesmaids, are absolutely beautiful. See you tomorrow.' I heard giggling in the background then the line went dead. I felt sick to my stomach and just stood clutching the phone for a few minutes. I should have gone with my instinct and stayed at home the next evening, but ever the martyr, I didn't.

When two of my trains were cancelled and the next was delayed I *really* should have known things weren't going my way and gone home. By the time I got to Victoria station I was 40 minutes late. I ran to where we were meant to meet, laden with bags, but he wasn't there. I called the flat. No answer. I called home, he hadn't rung to see where I was, nor had he called my mobile. He didn't have one, so I couldn't call him.

I stood there for 10 minutes wondering what to do when I felt a tap on the shoulder. I turned around. A stranger stood beside me with his hands in his pockets. He said hello. It took me a moment to recognise him. I'd never seen him without a smile on his face. He looked thin. His face had changed shape. He'd had his hair cut and it didn't suit him, it was too short. He had new jeans on and I remember wondering why he hadn't paid me back the money I'd loaned him instead of buying clothes.

'You look different,' I said, still holding the bags, him still a foot away with his hands firmly rooted to his pockets.

I waited for a kiss. Or an answer. Or anything. His left hand reached out. I put down one of the bags and went to take his hand. He pulled it away, picking up the bag, and started to walk towards the taxi queue. I caught up with him.

'You look different,' I said again. I felt sick.

'I feel different,' was all he said before turning away. As he stared out of the window I knew he wasn't looking at anything in particular, he just couldn't look at me. The first tear hit my cheek without me even realising I was crying. I brushed it away with the sleeve of my coat. He may as well have been a hundred miles away.

Back at the flat, I found him in the bathroom, cleaning his teeth with a towel around his waist. I stopped myself from wrapping my arms around him, kissing his broad shoulders, feeling his soft skin on my cheek. I didn't know what to say, so I didn't say anything. He spat the toothpaste into the sink and turned off the water.

'Are you sleeping in with me?' he asked. 'I don't know,' I said, genuinely confused. 'I don't know what you want me to do. I don't even know why I'm here.' He hadn't said a word to me since we met at the station. I felt the tears rolling down my face. I was leaning against the bathroom door and I could feel a breeze against the back of my heels. I had taken my Converse and socks off and left them in the lounge. My feet were freezing. That was all I could think about.

'My feet are cold,' I said.

'Come to bed then.'

And so I did. And I lay there, on my back, arms by my side, tears rolling like they do when you're laid flat, from the corners of my eyes, across my cheeks, gathering in a tiny pool on my neck. I couldn't be bothered to lift my hands to wipe them away and they kept coming. I wasn't making a sound. He lay on his side, away from me. I knew he was awake. I sat up.

I was out of bed now, pacing the room in my knickers and one of his T-shirts as I hadn't brought anything to wear in bed because I never did.

My arms were folded tightly across my chest and I shivered and shook because I was cold and I was scared and I was so incredibly sad. I suddenly felt as though all I had in my life now was this horrible disease, that it was destroying everything, that I could blame it for this. He'd made me so happy I had almost forgotten I had it, and now, both physically and mentally, it was *all* I had.

I was in the corner of the bedroom, sitting on the floor, knees to my chest, head to one side, all the tears going in the same direction, exhausted and ripped apart and sick and hurting and scared and alone. He wasn't really here with me. I felt like I was choking. I went to the bathroom, splashed my face like they always do in films and banged my head against the door a couple of times like they generally don't. I did it again and then I punched the door. I fell to the floor sat upon the cold, hard tiles and cried as hard as I could until there was nothing left, and climbed back into bed.

It was 5am when he turned over and put his arm around me. I was wide awake and I reached for his hand and held it gently, afraid that if I squeezed too hard I'd wake him and he'd realise he wasn't meant to touch me because he didn't love me. I must have been shaking so much he woke up anyway.

'You're shaking,' he whispered.

'I know. Why are you cuddling me?'

'I want to,' he answered, his face pressed against my neck just like it be used to when everything was OK. I undid my fingers from his and put my hand high on the pillow.

'You're just trying to make me feel better,' I said, but it only made me feel worse.

'I don't know what I want, Juliette,' he mumbled, and turned away.

I watched the sun come through the curtains until my eyes began to sting and then I got out of bed and made some camomile tea like he always made when he couldn't sleep. It was then that I remembered that he'd made camomile tea in the middle of the night, then sat downstairs for hours at a time and not come back to bed until it was almost dawn for the past few times I'd stayed with him. He'd not been able to sleep in the same bed as me for a long time because he'd known this was going to happen. It was 8.30am. I went into the lounge and rang Mum and cried some more, then got ready for work.

It was a beautiful morning, but as I walked down an almost empty Oxford Street, it felt like a dark cloud was about to burst. Not above me, but inside me. Minutes earlier Mark had stood just outside the front door of the flat and pulled me towards him.

'It'll be alright,' he said, 'just give me a couple of days.' He kissed me on the mouth. He tasted of toast and coffee. I watched him shut the front door, and I knew it was over.

I got asked to leave the office at lunchtime. It was fair enough, I was in pieces and couldn't concentrate, plus I had the production editor from *loaded* calling to ask about the Grand Prix piece I was writing up.

I couldn't *not* take their calls as they were on a deadline and needed to know what I was planning to write, but I was also meant to be working for someone else. I was due to have a meeting that evening with Tim, my former editor at *loaded* who had gone off a couple of weeks previously to work on a secret project. I liked and respected him a lot and I'd known him for years so I rang him from outside a pub in Soho, just around the corner from where I should have been working, and this is what happened:

'Hey, Tim, it's Juliette. Are you at the restaurant now? Good. Can I come over in a bit? OK. See you in an hour.'

I found him at the bar of a fancy member's club, the kind of place where a waiter puts an olive or cashew nut in your mouth for you instead of you having to bother doing it yourself. I ordered a vodka and tonic (double) and sat down. I hadn't had any lunch so I ate all the bar snacks with the manners of a hungry runaway, listened for a while to what was being said about my new role in this new company and when he stopped talking and waited for an answer to something I hadn't really heard I found myself with a great new job starting in two weeks' time. I bought some totally impractical red ankle strap stilettos just for the hell of it. I don't know whether I was celebrating a start or commiserating an end.

At home I sat up on the kitchen table like a little kid and told Mum about it all, trying to keep things in order but getting completely mixed up. One minute I was laughing and the next I was in her arms sobbing while she stroked my hair and gently rocked me back and forth like she used to when I'd fallen off my bike and hurt myself.

Mark called that weekend and told me he didn't love me anymore. That he probably never had. He said sorry. I said nothing, and hung up. I tried to pick up the pieces and get on with my life but I found it so hard. I was sure he'd met someone else at the wedding but didn't have the balls to tell me. I was tired. I cried all the time. I felt really stupid, being so upset, I mean, he hadn't died or anything, but some days I wished he had, because then at least nobody else could have him. I couldn't bear the overwhelming despair that seemed to just engulf me.

I went to see my doctor. He put me on Diazepam. It worked in so far as I stopped feeling anything, but I couldn't write or even concentrate enough to drive without almost having an accident. I was only on the pills for three days and I think I almost got run over about sixteen times. My colitis became ferocious, and I was losing a lot of blood again. I'd dropped the steroid dose to four from six, but knew I had to up it again to try and calm the inflammation. I wasn't in any pain. I thought it was odd that my only symptom was the bleeding, but I just thought, 'be glad,' and that was that.

One night, I decided to see if the footballer I was so interested in was still in the slightest bit interested in me. I really needed cheering up, and I'd decided that he was the man to do it. It took me a large glass of Merlot and an hour to get the confidence to pick up the phone. I dialled the number, swaying ever so slightly as I did so.

He answered thus: 'Ey up, Jools, what's with the change of mind?' in his Yorkshire accent.

'My boyfriend dumped me, so I need cheering up.'

'He's an idiot,' he said. 'Wednesday alright? I'll ring you and tell you where in the afternoon.'

Wednesday came, and I took the train up to London. I was so nervous I was shaking. I met him in a bar in Covent Garden. He drank two brandy and cokes in the time it took me to make up my mind whether to have lemon in my vodka tonic. We made small talk - 'you look well handsome' (uh, me to him) and 'how's the hamstring' (also me to him) and then he suddenly leaned over and kissed me full on the lips.

I was so excited I almost passed out. I was wearing my new leopard print coat, high-heeled red ankle boots (the rest of my outfit decidedly un-sexy - jeans, black shirt) and I've never been one for tall shoes at the best of times, but he had to grab me around the waist as I swayed off balance for a moment or two. During dinner I kept giggling like a lunatic and apologising for it (I was excited) and rang Helen from the loo, saying, 'I'm eating lobster and chips and mayonnaise and really fancy bread with Geoff Horsfield, what a dream!' and cackling down the phone. We took a taxi back to his place in Wimbledon as I'd accidentally on purpose missed my last train and not accidentally happened to bring my toothbrush, spare knickers and some make-up remover with me.

His hamstring seemed to be holding up just fine, although I don't think his manager would have been too happy at the 50kg weight it was supporting in the hallway. Suffice to say, I had a very enjoyable night, and then morning came; bright golden sunlight streaming through the curtains and across the bed, engulfing him in some kind of weird but well deserved full body halo. We walked to the car. He pointed his key thing at a black BMW, naturally, with cream leather interior and fancy wing mirrors that folded in electronically. It was brand new and reeked of leather. He dropped me off at the station at 9am and went off to training in his football kit, training top on inside out and hair which said 'Gaffer, I was clearly on the sauce and entertaining a lady and did not get an early night in preparation for today's training.'

I made my way back to Waterloo on the tube, then took the train from there to Petts Wood, picked up my car and drove home. I got in at 11am, dishevelled but with a big smile on my face. I took off my heels, made some breakfast and told Mum (almost) all about it. I got a text message from 'The Horse', as he's known, saying: 'Had a good night. Hope you enjoyed it. I know I did. See you soon x' which made me blush profusely. Sadly, just after that he was sold to Birmingham City and I never saw him again. Just my rotten luck!

A couple of weeks later I moved into my flat in Brighton despite coming to the conclusion that I actually didn't want to. I'd gone through with it in some kind of blur, not really thinking about what I was doing. In retrospect I was cutting off my nose to spite my face - too proud to go back on my decision to live there and I wanted Mark, somehow, to know that I had done it anyway. I think he had got cold feet because I was moving to Brighton rather than just visiting him. I wouldn't have expected him to live with me – at least not for a long while, as I liked my space and there wasn't much of it in my little flat – but I'm sure he thought that would be my next move, and got scared by it.

Mum, Dad and Jonathan helped me move in, carting boxes by the hundred up and down three flights of stairs. What should have been an eventful and joyous occasion ('she's finally moved out, and this time it's permanent!') was, instead, a huge anti-climax. I didn't really want to be there, and I think they knew I didn't really want to be there. I put on a brave face, and they waved me goodbye at 7pm. I couldn't help but start to cry as they disappeared round the corner to the van, and then I found myself sobbing uncontrollably. I wanted to ring my brother and get them to come back for me, take me home, just sell the flat and stay with them. I was in a state of total despair and it was only at that moment that it hit me like a freight train right in the pit of my stomach - I didn't know anyone. I had no life here. What had I done?

A week after moving in, unpacking, crying, exploring the beautiful park which was only two minutes walk from the flat, taking photos of the helter skelter and genuinely wondering if I could actually live inside it, finding that Topshop was within walking distance and enjoying my view of the sea from the lounge window - albeit with my head right out of the window and twisted like an owl's - spending hours on the phone to my friends and parents pretending everything was OK, I started my new job, working with Tim at this internet company in London. It was meant to be a full time position, but I found the journey from Brighton exhausting after only a couple of days.

I'd be up at 6.30am, leaving my house at 7.30am to walk the mile and a half to the station - and in my part of town, that means stumbling down the steepest hill seen since, well, *Hill Street Blues*, and at the other end, practically climbing up the pavement like Spiderman. Flat roads are scarce in Brighton, to say the least. I'd scramble for a seat on the invariably delayed train to Victoria, try and keep my face out of fat men's armpits on the tube to Warren Street, then have a five-minute walk to the office. Eventually I'd get to my desk and promptly fall asleep. I was not a star employee.

There was a trip to Belgium and another to Eindhoven during which I wrote and presented a Euro 2000 preview for football fans, which was four days and nights of solid filming from 8am until 1am or 2am, sleeping in the back of the people carrier between destinations and throwing up on the ferry. A few weeks later a team of us went away to Budapest for a week to a hideous rock festival, where I wrote and presented music and travel pieces for the website. It was non-stop hard work, but good hard work. The beer was amazing and only 20p a pint and although I wasn't meant to drink it (of course, it's derived from wheat - gah!) I allowed myself the occasional pint at the end of a hard day, my vitamins making up for it. I was knocking back more pills than Ozzy Ozbourne.

The Hungarians did a lovely job with corn on the cob and spit-roasted chicken, watermelon and banana shakes (non-dairy) and knocked up a lovely peanut brittle, so that was essentially my diet for seven days. I think I covered all my food groups, one way or another. I got a decent tan, saw Oasis play live on the last night, fell down some steps in a posh hotel in front of Liam Gallagher and got blind drunk with my colleagues in a strip club at 4am. So drunk, that at one point I was in the cage with one of the dancers, threatening to take my T-shirt off. I had been loudly bemoaning that actual lack of stripping - for a strip club - as none of the girls took anything off, other than their coats. I woke up so drunk the next morning that when I stumbled into the bathroom in the hotel and could see everything, as opposed to my usual blindness without my glasses, I thought I had drunk myself sighted. I rang Fiona, one of the production team.

'I've drunk myself sighted!' I croaked, 'I can see! I can see!' Five minutes later she walked in and pointed to my empty contact lens case, then at my bloodshot eyes.

'Do your eyes sting?' she asked me, holding up the lens case.

'Loads,' I replied, blinking to try and ease the pain.

'That'll be because you left your lenses in, you idiot.'

I'd racked up trips to Barcelona, Melbourne and France for Grand Prix races, and now it was the big one - Silverstone. I found myself in a fancy evening dress at the Silverstone Ball, held the night before Saturday's qualifying. It was a black tie affair (for the men, not the women) and I relished the opportunity to actually look nice at something to do with F1, for a change. All the drivers would be there, plus a few crap so-called celebs. I wondered if I'd be able to get a little interview with one of the drivers. I knew Damon and Heinz-Harold Frentzen, and I'd briefly met Michael Schumacher and Eddie Irvine, a man with so much spare testosterone I'm sure that's what powered his racing car. I drove up to Silverstone, checked into the hotel and hung up my dress while I took a shower. I'd spent the whole time in rubbish clothes when I was 'working' in the Jordan garage, covered in oil, with my glasses on and no-make up, nor sleep. Tonight I wore a vintage late '70s electric blue, floor-length dress and ridiculously high vintage silver sparkly sandals. I'd spent about 10 minutes on my hair and make-up and was quite happy with how I'd scrubbed up. I'd also had a fringe cut in at the hairdressers that week. It was enough of a transformation that nobody I knew from F1 actually recognised me.

At one point, towards the end of the night, I was clutching a champagne glass in one hand and a cigarette in the other when I heard my name being called from somewhere near the floor. It was coming from under the table. 'I can't be so drunk that I'm hearing voices,' I thought to myself, 'let's investigate.' I lifted up the tablecloth and was rather surprised to see somebody very famous crouching under the table, beckoning me to join him.

'Quick,' he said, 'before someone sees you.' It turns out he'd been under there for 10 minutes, whisper-shouting my name every time he caught a glimpse of my sparkly sandals.

'What are you doing?' I asked, scrabbling under the table and bringing my knees up to my face.

'I'm waiting for you,' he said, 'for a kiss!'

I was dumbfounded, to say the least.

'Eh? What do you want to kiss me for?' I asked, 'you're a gazillionaire racing driver and there are models everywhere you're supposed to be fighting off. Are you mental?'

He cleared his throat and said, 'Juliette. At the end of the day, I may be very rich, but I'm still a man. That's all it boils down to. You look beautiful tonight. Can I please kiss you?'

I duly obliged. Just a little one. I mean, I'm not the kind of girl to mess about under tables, ordinarily. Unfortunately, while this exchange was going on my cigarette was burning a hole in tablecloth. I could smell it. I opened one eye, and saw it.

'I've set the table alight!' I squealed, pushing him off me, 'and I'm wearing vintage, a poly-mix, too, it'll go up like a bastard!'

I doused the smoke with my champagne (what a waste!) and scrambled backwards from under the table, hitting my head along the way. I popped up right in front of a middle-aged couple clutching an autograph book. I presumed it wasn't for my benefit.

'Uh, hello, I dropped my cigarette, hence the burning,' I said, unconvincingly, pointing at the floor where a little puff of smoke still lingered.

'We're waiting for one of the drivers, to get their autograph,' said the lady. 'There's only one we haven't seen.' She told me who they were after. I blushed profusely.

'Have you seen him?' she asked, tilting her head to one side and eyeing me suspiciously.

'Absolutely definitely not. I mean, you can see that he's not here. He could be under the table, hiding, but he's not. I think he went to the bar, he likes a drink, so he does,' and pointed as far in the opposite direction as my arm would allow.

'That bar,' I said, seeing nothing but a wall. They traipsed off, straining their necks to spot him. I poked my head under the table.

'You can come out now, but you should go to the gents and wipe my lipstick off your face,' I told him. I left him to crawl out. I presumed he'd made it out from under the table when I spotted him heading for breakfast in the paddock at qualifying the next morning looking a little sheepish.

That summer I'd also begged for, and been obliged, a trip to the Monaco Grand Prix. It wasn't bad. There I was at 8.30pm in the evening sitting with the photographer in a restaurant whose owner had mistaken us for a couple. He'd moved the table and chairs down to the seafront so that we could enjoy a romantic dinner for two. I wasn't going to argue. I'd taken off my sandals and left them up the beach a bit, so that the waves could lap at my feet. It was bliss. I had just ordered my steak dinner, and I was on my second glass of Cabernet Sauvignon and in a pretty good mood, as far as moods go. Especially considering if I'd left my shoes behind me on Brighton beach, they'd have been stolen and put on eBay before I'd be on my main course. As much as I was feeling nostalgic and somewhat saddened that this would be my last trip, I was also hugely excited. I'd always wanted to go to the Monaco Grand Prix, and here I was. It was my job. It was ridiculous that I was getting paid to be here.

It had started so well, but the rest of the weekend descended into chaos. Our tickets and pit lane passes had gone AWOL, and a broken down boat thrown into the equation meant the photographer and I missed the qualifying session and found ourselves running through the town to get to the track in 100 degree heat, although obviously the roads were all closed off due to the impending race. It took us three hours to make our way to the track. My feet were killing me, and my stomach wasn't feeling too clever either. Instead of watching the race from the sponsor's yacht as planned, we were now right on the starting line behind a wire fence, paying £250 for the privilege (you've got to love company credit cards). It was a restaurant full of Ferrari club members. We could see this because every single person was male, about 45-55 years old and dressed head to toe in Ferrari merchandise. I think I had some salad, but I can't remember much. I do know that at one stage I had one foot on a table, the other on a chair, and was hanging precariously by my fingers from the wire fence. Nice. Not quite what I'd had in mind. There were three false starts, so at least we saw some action, but I'm not sure the fumes contributed too well to the food.

After the race we gate-crashed a champagne supper on somebody's yacht, as you do, then I went gambling in Monaco's finest casinos with a hideous, red-faced man who looked like a huge baby and dressed like Prince Charles, like all very rich men seem to do. He seemed intent on taking me back to his yacht at the end of the evening, so I let him think he could, simply by not saying that he couldn't. That was all the encouragement he needed to ply me with booze at £35 a glass and give me money to spend on the roulette table. I was beginning to think that I could forge a new career out of this, but alas I just got really drunk and made a show of myself.

Knocking Cristal all over the roulette table and cackling every time he lost his chips, I was having a ball. I even won 500 francs and in a pleasantly drunken stupor, then managed to shake off the huge baby man somewhere between Giorgio Armani and Louis Vuitton and stumble my way along the edge of the harbour to the sponsor's yacht, sleeping and dribbling up top under the stars. I wasn't in a bed or even in a room, I was simply in a heap on top of the boat, clutching my handbag and supporting my head with my cardigan placed strategically atop a box with some old rope in it.

I don't even know how I got there, but I seem to recall wandering about in the harbour, looking for a Foster's flag and once spotting it, thinking, 'well, that's me home', despite the fact that I was actually booked into a B&B in Nice.

The next morning I awoke to a complete stranger standing above me, shouting at me in French. I mumbled a 'pardon moi' and clutching my pounding head, stumbled off the boat. I had, in fact, been on a private yacht. The Foster's yacht was parked up next door. I had an hour to get back to Nice before we left for the airport. I was a bit confused as to how I would do anything other than stand there and cry. It was then that I spotted British driver Jenson Button in the distance, so I headed over to him and asked for a snapshot as he loaded racing driver type stuff into the boot of his car. Considering he'd had a terrible race, then add to that the fact that I must have reeked of booze, had slept outside and was still in last night's clothes, he was extremely obliging. Hoorah for Jenson Button! I then pushed my luck by asking if he could give me a lift to Nice, and I as he politely said, 'No, sorry,' I knew he wanted to scream at me to do one.

I spotted a man I'd met before at a press thing and asked if I could tag along to the station. He seemed unafraid and said yes, and even bought my train ticket I was clearly inept. I jumped in a cab at the other end, and once in the hotel I managed to throw my things into my case and get downstairs just as the PR lady was, I think, about to call the police. 'I'm here!' I said, tripping over the step and falling to my knees, 'don't panic!' Clearly, and with good reason, she had been. I was now officially a *loaded* writer. They were *all* a nightmare for the PRs!

I spent the summer 'working', i.e. sunbathing in the park opposite my flat, occasionally writing ideas down and sometimes even talking on the phone. I stood a bit more in front of the helter skelter, and also rode on the Ghost Train, just because I could. I was basically living the life of a teenage runaway, but with money. I fed Hula Hoops to mutant seagulls the size of pigs, talked to the ducks, wondered why I wasn't getting a tan (because I was still using the sun block factor 420 which I had been given in Australia) and finally realising my mistake at the end of September. One seagull, which I named Steven, would knock on my bedroom window with his beak every evening at tea time, and I'd give him some bread and try to cuddle him. One evening the window was open and there he was, squawking on my windowsill!

I was as lonely as hell, though. I had been kidding myself when I thought I could live happily in a town where I knew nobody. I talked to people in shops, but anything more than 'hello', 'please' or 'thank you' and they looked at me as though I was a bit mental. I'm not surprised. So I got myself a hamster to lift my spirits. She was lovely – the colour of honey. I called her Babylegs. I took her out of her cage every night and let her run riot in the bath or in her plastic ball. She wasn't really one for cuddles, so I was lucky if I got a little stroke before putting her back in her cage. Whenever I drove up to my parents' place for a couple of days, I'd take her with me. Strapped in the backseat of the car, I'd have to yell 'hang on!' when we turned corners. I made her bedding out of dried up, ripped up scented baby wipes rather than straw. She was the new love of my life and I talked to her constantly (the poor thing!).

One afternoon, I'd gone to the park. It was something I did as often as work permitted, and there was nothing more enjoyable than reading a book or working on some ideas for work stuff in the sun, surrounded by seagulls and ducks. On this occasion, though, as I attempted to sit up from sunbathing, I got a sharp, shooting pain in my left hip. The next day, the same thing happened. On other occasions, I'd just feel a bit stiff, and it'd be a real effort to sit up. I couldn't just 'get up' anymore.

I didn't really dwell on it at the time, and later, when it would get worse, I suppose I had already become used to not feeling right, so by the time I told my doctor about it, it was pretty bad. Once, I tried to sit up and it took me a good 10 minutes. It then hurt to go from sitting to standing. I was desperate for the loo one day in the park, and it usually only took me three minutes to get home but this time I was in a panic that I wouldn't make it. I didn't know why I was getting the pains, but I guessed it was something to do with my colitis. Then I thought, 'well, I know I failed my biology GSCE but I'm pretty sure my colon isn't in my hips, so it can't be that.' I put it to the back of my mind, as usual, and got on with things. My doctor didn't have any answers, so I just took painkillers.

I went up to London now and again for work, but mainly developed ideas and features at home because I found the journey so tiring. It was hard to explain my illness to my boss as I looked absolutely fine. At one point he even said, 'There's nothing wrong with you, what are you on about?' to which I had to say, 'sorry I haven't got a rash or anything to show you but it's my insides that are ulcerated, not my outsides.'

To say you're exhausted doesn't really cut the mustard. Nobody seemed to notice that I wasn't there and anyway, so I kept quiet and hoped they wouldn't start calling out my name and wondering where I was.

I wrote a column for *loaded* which paid the mortgage each month and saved up half my earnings from the internet place, not for a rainy day, but for what would turn out to be a rainy rest-of-my-life. I read books and magazines, half-heartedly came up with ideas for novels which never got past the first paragraph, let alone chapter, and decorated my flat.

I saw a new consultant at the hospital in Brighton who agreed that I should stay off the steroids as I appeared to be in remission, and I joined an Ashtanga yoga class which did wonders for my energy levels. Top that lot off with a visit to a nutritionist who made me stand with my arms outstretched while she put test tubes with labels saying things like 'coffee' and 'oranges' upon them, declaring me 'allergic!' or 'OK' to each one, and I was doing just about all I could do. She told me to give up oats as well as wheat, anything acidic (most fruit, some vegetables), sugar and salt.

'What am I going to have for tea?' I asked, in disbelief, 'feathers?' She wasn't sure what to make of that so instead she sent me home with some leaflets which all seemed to be telling me what I couldn't eat. Again. I decided that her methods were questionable, at best, and that you can't really tell if a person has a food allergy by pushing their arm up and down.

A month later Leo and her boyfriend moved down to Brighton from London, buying a beautiful regency flat in the centre of town. At last I had some company. Not that hamsters aren't great company, but the conversation tends to be a little one-sided.

Around this time my nutritionist suggested that we go a step further with the enquiries into my health problems.

'OK,' I said, a little unsure as to what she would suggest, 'what's next?' I had every right to be apprehensive. She told me that in order to analyse the goings on inside my gut, I'd have to pooh into a cardboard tray, push it into a test tube and leave it upon her doorstep in a box.

'It's then going to go to a lab in the Rocky Mountains for analysis,' she explained, as if that made sense. That night, I duly did as instructed, although poohing into a cardboard tray in the bath wasn't as easy as it sounds. It was quite revolting, even by pooh standards. It was put on a plane bound for the Rockies. Apparently the levels of a certain bacteria in my gut called klebsiella showed signs of a disease called ankylosing spondylitis. I read it all, understood some of it and put it away. I lay awake that night wondering who the hell picks through pooh for a living?

CHAPTER FIVE
'ROCK 'N' ROLL BLUES'
EDDIE COCHRAN

November 2000

I lived on the top floor of a three-storey Victorian conversion. The ground floor flat was rented, the second floor was owned by a woman who kept herself to herself, and who was a little bit odd. She'd never say hello to me if we passed in the street or bumped into each other picking up our post, and would scuttle away like a beetle if I so much as chirped, 'morning!'

This I could live with, but what started to happen next I could not. It began with her walking out of her flat at 5am, stomping down the stairs, slamming the front door so hard that my bed shook and repeating the sequence on the way back in five minutes later. She'd then do it all again for around an hour. I once heard that front door slam 17 times between 5.30am and 6am. After that, she'd start moving the furniture around in the flat, dragging chairs and tables across the floor underneath where I slept.

She'd fling rubbish out without bags - I once stepped outside to find a chicken carcass in the middle of the path - and do her best to drive me insane with noise, either from the Hoover which she'd leave in one position in the room while she went out for an entire 24 hours or the television, which again, she would switch on, turn up to full volume and then go out for hours on end, slamming the doors as she went. At one point I removed the fuse from the fuse box in the hall but she just banged on the floors or the ceiling instead.

After a week or so, the furniture moving and door slamming would start at 2am or 3am and go on past 6am. I would go to bed at midnight, read for a while, turn out my light and wait for sleep to come. It wouldn't. I would lie awake until three or four in the morning, waiting for the noise to start, fall asleep for an hour or so and then be woken up by the door slamming just as it was time for me to get up and go to work. I was at least trying to put an appearance in at the office two or three days a week.

I tried talking to her, but she wouldn't open the door. I left notes outside, but she ignored them. One evening I came home to find her in the hallway outside my door, shaking and talking gibberish about being locked out. A few hours later she started banging on the downstairs neighbour's door, screaming to be let in and shouting across the street that we wouldn't let her indoors.

The police arrived. I was in the middle of getting ready to go out, standing halfway up the stairs in a towel with wet hair and an omelette frazzling away. So desperate was I for company that I'd got myself a blind date through *The Guardian* newspaper's 'Soul Mates' section. Honestly, I had no other option at that point. At least it got me out of the house. The police said that she had run off when they turned up, that there was nothing they could do about the noise, the door slamming, unless she actually threatened me. The fact that she was wearing her bra over the top of her jumper and had no shoes on didn't seem to alert them to the fact that she was as mad as a bag of frogs.

'Unless you're in danger or she's in danger, there's nothing we can do,' they said. The downstairs neighbour moved out a week later, worried about the effect all the noise was having on her pregnancy. Things didn't get any better and I wasn't sleeping at all. I wrote another note, this time not pulling any punches, and when she opened her front door at 5.40am, I lay in bed waiting for the abuse to start. A minute later she was banging and kicking my front door, screaming obscenities. I got out of bed and called the police. I told them she was threatening me.

'I live here on my own,' I said, 'and I can't go out without going past her door. What if she pulls a knife on me? She's a big lady, you know, like that mentalist nurse in *Misery*. I don't stand a chance.'

'Well until she does actually pull a knife there's nothing we can do. Ring us if she actually threatens you.'

'Well, that's just brilliant', I said, 'I'll call you from A&E when they're trying to stitch up a few stab wounds.'

What constituted a threat if it wasn't someone completely unhinged and three times your size, clearly off whatever meds they're meant to be taking, banging on your door, screaming abuse? I called the office and told them I wasn't well.

Strange things were happening around me, too. I was in the bath that night when a picture flew off the wall and hit me on the side of my head, just above my eye, before dropping into the water. But it didn't fall off the wall, it flew - with quite a force. The picture hook was intact, and if it had just come loose, it would have fallen straight down into the bath, not travelled the length of the bath at the same height as my head. It was pretty freaky, and it hurt a bit too. The bleeding stopped after half an hour or so, but I was pretty shaken up. I'd had my eyes closed and my head halfway under the water when it hit me. The thought that it might have knocked me out, so I'd have probably drowned, wasn't particularly comforting.

I felt dreadful. I hauled myself into work a couple of days later and fell asleep at my desk, red-eyed and unable to concentrate. In the end, it didn't matter as just before Christmas the company announced losses of millions and made us all redundant - without pay. I packed several large bags and went to Mum and Dad's, desperate for some rest and some peace and quiet. Luckily I'd saved quite a bit during the time I'd worked there but even so, I was facing Christmas with no job, a home I didn't want to go back to and an illness which left me feeling completely shattered. I went for a pre-Christmas drink in London three days before Jesus' birthday with Leo and our friend Kirsty. Halfway through the evening I suddenly had to put down my gin and tonic. I was doubled up with chest pains. They literally took my breath away. I went to the toilet, held on to the sink and, gasping for air, was unable to breathe without the pain searing through my ribs, my stomach and my chest. I tried not to panic, but I probably did a little bit. It gradually subsided, and I made my way back up the stairs to the bar.

'I have to go home,' I said to my friends, grabbing my coat, 'I feel really weird.' I didn't bother trying to get a cab - after years of going out in London I knew it would be quicker to walk.

At Charing Cross station the pain started up again. I was really struggling for breath. I had to sit down on the station concourse. For some reason there are no chairs or benches, so late at night the station is full of people leaning against shop windows, propping themselves up on their elbows on the floor or crouching down whilst they try and put away their Burger King fries before getting on the train. At this time of year, a lot of passengers are so drunk they fall over on the platform and stay there. Girls are always crying about men being bastards while the men throw up in the corner by the ticket machine. Suffice to say, I didn't attract any attention crying and clutching my chest. I must have just looked like I'd had too much to drink or was suffering from acute melodrama. I waited 10 minutes for the train, got a seat by the window, leaned my head against the glass and quietly cried all the way home. It was a very, very long 25 minutes.

By the time the train pulled into Petts Wood station the pain was even worse. I stumbled to my car and got in. I was crying hysterically by this point, my whole chest tightening with each breath. It was horrendous. I felt like I was being gripped in a vice, or hugged really hard by a bear who didn't know his own strength. I drove the three miles home like the clappers, parked the car with a screech of brakes, grabbed my bag and rang frantically on the bell. It was 10.30pm. Mum opened the door.

'Mum, my stomach's killing me, I think I need to go to hospital,' I cried, sort of collapsing on the hall floor. I couldn't even collapse properly. 'I'm rubbish,' I said, holding out my hand so that she could help me up, 'I only half collapsed.'

'Charlie!' she shouted to Dad, leaning down to hold my hand, 'get your coat on, get the car keys, your daughter's not very well.' Dad came out of the lounge looking terrified. He asked what was wrong, and I told him. I could hardly get the words out and I was struggling for breath. They got me in the car, and Mum asked what happened and why I hadn't rung from Charing Cross. 'Your dad would have driven to London to pick you up if he'd had to,' she said, stroking my forehead.

'Mum, he'd have had a nightmare getting there and I got a train almost straight away. He couldn't have got there as quickly as that if he had his own helicopter.' Mum shook her head.

'You should have rung,' she said, 'I can't believe you drove home.' She said it so quietly that it was barely audible.

I wasn't seen by the triage nurse for an hour and a half. I sat on a plastic chair in the waiting room, doubled up in pain and sometimes lying on the floor because it was more comfortable. I was in tears the whole time, and I can tell you now that it takes a lot to make me cry. Well, pain-wise it does. I cry my eyes out at adverts for sad mobile phones and at films with animals being heroic in them. And you should see the state of me when I watch *E.T.* And if I drive past a dead fox or badger. You get the idea. When I was eventually seen by the nurse, because I could just about answer her questions without passing out, I'm entered as non-urgent. My head is spinning as I answer her questions. With each answer, I gasp with pain. I tell her I have colitis, that it could be a bowel perforation. She looked blankly at me.

'The doctor will call you in when he's ready,' she said, 'but we've had an emergency so it could be four or five hours. You might want to try a pain killer in the meantime.'

'I've had some Nurofen,' I said, 'it's not working.'

'Try this, it's a pessary. Stick it up your bottom; it should start working within 20 minutes or so.'

Mum sent Dad home to ring my brother who was at the local pub with his girlfriend and expecting a lift home. I went to the toilet with Mum waiting outside the cubicle, asking if I was alright every three seconds. I fiddled about and eventually completed the task. How unpleasant.

'It's like a tampon,' I called out, 'only you're less committed because there's no strings attached.' I could practically hear Mum roll her eyes and shake her head on the other side of the cubicle. I walked out of the toilet, exhausted, and said I wanted to sit and wait, and if the pain went away, I wanted to go home. I was not prepared to sit on a plastic chair and cry my eyes out in front of strangers any longer than I had to. After 15 minutes the pain slowly began to subside. After 20 minutes I felt only a slight ache from where my muscles had been cramping. I stood up and told the receptionist I was going home.

'I don't blame you,' she said, consulting her computer screen, 'it looks like we're backed up for at least six hours.'

I rang Dad from my mobile.

'Can you come back, Dad?' I said, my breath visible in the cold night air. 'I've had enough of sitting here, I want my bed.' Dad picked us up and I went straight to bed. I have never felt so exhausted in all my life. At 3am the pain started again, and this time there was no messing about. After around an hour of lying there trying to call out for Mum who was asleep in the next room, I just lobbed a book against the wall instead. That did the trick. She flew into the room and took one look at me and gasped. She called the doctor. I could hear her side of the conversation.

'Yes, it's an emergency, and I'm sorry to call but no, it can't wait until tomorrow. We've already been to A&E tonight. No, she's not a patient at your clinic now but she used to be.'

At 4am someone I didn't know turned up, had a look at me, felt my stomach, shrugged his shoulders, said absolutely nothing, and prescribed me some tablets. He gave me some sort of pill to take there and then.

'Is this an E?' I half laughed. 'Am I going to start dancing round the room and telling everyone I love them?' Mum shook her head in despair at my inappropriate response, something I was becoming quite adept at.

'Er, no, it's a painkiller,' he said, and with that, he disappeared into the night leaving a prescription for something stronger which would have to be collected tomorrow, from the hospital pharmacy. The pain didn't really go away, it just moved around. If you can imagine wringing out a sopping wet towel, twisting it and squeezing it as hard as you can to get the water out, that's what it felt like inside. I couldn't get out of bed that morning. It felt as though I was glued to the mattress, like some invisible weight was pushing me down. I felt so heavy. I ached from my head to my toes. Mum brought me up some breakfast so that I could take the tablets which Dad had gone to get first thing. An hour later the pain was worse.

'I'm so tough,' I whispered, 'that I should be on *Europe's Strongest Man*, pulling tractors and setting fire to myself.'

Mum rang the doctors and got an emergency appointment that afternoon after surgery. The doctor, a miniscule Chinese man wearing head to toe beige and tiny spectacles which kept slipping down his nose, was surprised to see me.

'But you were at the hospital last night and you had a visit from the locum who gave you a prescription,' he said, looking at my notes as if I'd come along for fun.

'Yes, and she's worse,' said Mum. Just in case they weren't getting the idea, I continued, in a pathetic whisper of a voice.

'It's Christmas Eve tomorrow. I don't want to be sitting in A&E all night with idiots from office parties who've fallen off the photocopier with their trousers around their ankles or swallowed a bauble when we should be at home stuffing the turkey.'

'I can get you an appointment with A&E so that you are examined and X-rayed,' he said.

'You should have had an X-ray last night in case it is a perforated bowel,' he continued, tapping his pencil on the desk.

'I told them that,' I sighed.

The doctor wrote a quick letter to the hospital explaining my situation and telling them to whisk me through as it was urgent and I needed to be seen immediately.

'So we won't have to sit there all night?' asked Mum.

'No, no! A doctor will see you as soon as he is free. No waiting, this is very urgent. As I said, it could be a perforation,' he smiled.

We went home to have something to eat. Well, Mum did. I reasoned that if I needed something doing to me, it'd be best if I hadn't eaten.

I was seen by the first doctor who merely took my note away an hour after turning up. It was 7.18pm; I have the print out saying so. Mum and I waited, and waited. I slept, my legs curled up on the chair, my head in Mum's lap. I told Mum to go home and have a cup of tea, watch some TV, and that I'd call when they'd seen me. She told me not to be so daft, that she wasn't going anywhere. We read 100 year-old magazines about farming and fishing and railways - why don't they ever have normal magazines about shoes and celebrities and lipstick in hospitals? - and sighed a lot. So much for being whizzed through.

At 11.15pm, four hours after we arrived, I was seen by the second doctor. I had an X-ray and blood tests. There was dried blood on the wall next to where I lay on the bed. A doctor came along and offered Mum a sandwich. Another nurse came past and made her a cup of tea. I didn't want anything, except to get my blood test results and go home with some tablets to make me better.

At five to midnight the doctor came back with the results. My liver function tests were high (I told him I'd been drinking rather a lot of red wine each night for the past few weeks to try and dull the sound of my mad neighbour) and I had some mild scoliosis of the lumbar spine but other than that, everything was 'normal'. Nobody was explaining the pain.

'You might just be constipated,' said the doctor, 'the X-ray doesn't show much. I'll prescribe you something for the cramps, it should help.'

Half an hour later a nurse appeared with a packet of paracetamol and some painkillers used to treat period pains. I almost laughed. 'I'm sorry to sound so demanding but have you got anything stronger, like a bottle of brandy, or maybe some bleach?'

'Just try them,' she sighed, looked exasperated, 'you never know. We need the bed.'

We got home at 12.30am. Dad put the kettle on. I went up to see Jonathan. I could see that he'd been crying. He was sitting amongst a pile of work - he was now in his first year of a media degree at University - but I knew he wasn't doing anything.

'Are you OK?' he said as I pushed the door open and sat on the edge of the bed. 'I mean, I know you're not OK. What is it?'

'I don't know,' I said, sitting down on my old Tottenham Hotspur duvet cover. 'Nobody seems to know what to do or what to give me. It's like they think I'm having a panic attack, not actual pain. But don't worry,' I said, holding his hand, 'I'm your big stupid sister. I'll be OK.'

He put his hands over his face and peered out from behind his fingers, shaking his head.

'It's not fair,' he shouted, not at me, not at anybody. 'Why can't anyone help you?'

'I don't know,' I said, holding his hand, because I didn't.

Spring 2001

The pain stayed with me, though now it came in the early hours of the morning as opposed to the night. These weren't symptoms of colitis. At around 5am I'd wake up on my side, unable to breathe properly. I couldn't turn over. Any slight movement sent white-hot pain through my right side, from below my shoulder to my hip, a shark bite shaped area of pain. Whenever I tried to move anything other than my head, it felt as though somebody was tightening barbed wire around my ribs. After a donkey had kicked me in the back. Sometimes, it was a different pain, deeper, more central, in my spine. That I described to Mum as 'like someone has whacked each vertebra with a toffee hammer, all the way down my back.'

For two or three hours I'd lie there, unable to move, scared out of my wits. Sometimes, through sheer exhaustion I'd go back to sleep for a while. I'd wake up at 9am or 10am, and the pain would still be there, but fading. It would take 15 or 20 minutes for me to get out of bed by slowly sitting up on my side, and gradually pulling my body to the edge of the bed with my hands whilst gasping in agony. I didn't have the energy for a scream. I would then tentatively stand up, and more often than not be on the receiving end of a horrendous stabbing pain throughout my left side as I put my foot to the floor. I would hobble to the bathroom in tears, leaning against the walls as I went, then go to the kitchen, swallow some pills - by now my doctor had prescribed me Tramadol, a powerful painkiller - and wait for it to work.

An hour or so later I could walk around my flat, still in pain, but not in agony. By then I could have a hot bath, which seemed to help, get myself dressed – slowly, and not with a bra because I couldn't stand to wear one as it was so uncomfortable around my ribs, and then two hours after that I would be able to leave the house and walk into town or drive to Sainsbury's without having trouble breathing or standing straight, clutching my side as though I'd been stabbed. I felt spaced out, not right, unable to focus on anything. My days just disappeared in a muddle of trying to feel well enough to do normal things. Sometimes, though, it didn't get better and I'd be unable to get dressed because I couldn't bend down to pull my jeans up or put my socks on. I gave up on those mornings, and stayed in my pyjamas for hours, having a bath to try and ease the pain (not with my pyjamas on, obviously) then finally managing to get dressed as it was time to go to bed and put my pyjamas back on.

Clothes lay scattered on the floor, and if I dropped something, that also stayed there. It got so bad that I bought a 'grabber' from the Sealife Centre; one with a shark's head for the grabbing bit. It was meant to be for kids, obviously, but I used it to pick up things I couldn't reach. Well, I say I used it, but it was rubbish. I attempted to use it, refusing to let Mum buy me a proper one, because 'old people use them, and I don't want to'. How daft is that? But then when I think about it, it's not that daft. Not being able to bend down and pick things up off the floor was the reality. I just didn't want to admit it.

Needless to say, I wore my pyjamas a lot, but before you have visions of me looking all sweaty and ill in dirty pyjamas, I had several pairs so that I was always clean, if not dressed. Every night I would go to bed, exhausted, and wake up with the same pain the next morning. I couldn't have felt lonelier. It was overwhelming, but still I didn't ask anyone for help, or admit how much pain, both physically and mentally, I was in. It was that masochistic streak again, just propelling me to do the opposite of whatever I really wanted to do. I think I saw myself as a failure if I admitted defeat, so it wasn't an option. If Mum and Dad had known how bad I really was, they'd have come and picked me up, put me under the care of better doctors and consultants, and looked after me. Instead, I struggled on, alone, incapable and exhausted. I still don't know why I dealt with it like that. Nobody would have thought any less of me for asking for help, but I couldn't bear to. It's the biggest regret I'll ever have (aside from moving to Brighton in the first place and not going out with Frank Lampard when I had the chance, or Geoff Horsfield the first time he asked me).

I went back to the doctor, a different one this time. He was more sympathetic than my usual doctor, wanting to work out why I was getting this pain rather than just handing out tablets to dull it. He examined my back. I told him I was also getting joint pain, which had started up as I got out of bed, in my lower spine and hips, and that sometimes I couldn't walk. He thought it might be rheumatoid arthritis, and prescribed some different tablets, though not painkillers.

'These are fairly mild anti-inflammatories,' he said, scribbling something down on his prescription pad, 'and so should attack the inflammation directly and reduce it, so that you don't need painkillers. Try them for a week or so and let me know how you get on.'

I really needed these to work. I'd planned a trip to Memphis in April for Dad's 60th birthday present. We are all Elvis fans and I knew Dad would love to go to Graceland, he's just too tight to spend the money himself. I owed them a couple of thousand from an extra bit of deposit they'd loaned me for my flat, so I talked it over with Mum back in February and decided that it was a great idea. At the time, my pain was manageable. As the trip grew closer, it was not.

I decided to go through with it as I'd lose a lot of money if I cancelled, plus I thought, 'I can't not see Elvis's house.'

'You know your father,' Mum had said on the phone, 'He'll love it. He'd talk about it but never do anything about going and he'd never spend the money. Do it.'

We managed to keep it a secret for almost a month, although Mum had almost slipped up a few times. I wrote Dad a poem in his birthday card explaining what his present was. Each line in the poem was from an Elvis song, so it took him a while to work out what was going on. When he did, he was, as we thought he would be, completely stunned.

I was all packed and drove back to their house the day before we were due to fly. I'd given up on the Tramadol tablets because they made me, well, aggressive and depressed, if you must know, and was now on new ones - Voltarol - which seemed to be working. I still had some pain but it was easing off and I some mornings I almost felt OK.

Along with some clothes I packed the tablets, the anti-inflammatories which I'd been on since I was diagnosed, some cereal, two packets of soya milk and my vitamins, hoping customs weren't looking for a family of three Elvis fans to investigate. The flight was uneventful, we changed in St. Louis... and our internal flight to Memphis was cancelled. And so was the next one. It was 10.30pm by the time we arrived at The Heartbreak Hotel on - you've guessed it - Lonely Street. We were shattered. I'd booked us a weird kind of room where my parents would have the bedroom with en-suite and I'd sleep on the pull-out bed in the lounge as if I was five. That way we were only paying for one room and Mum wouldn't worry so much about me being ill if I was only in the next room. Well, it wasn't even a room, it was more like a half-baked slatted door through which I could hear Dad watching Elvis movies on the 24-hour Elvis movie channel. I was doing the same.

'It's non-stop Elvis,' said Dad through the slats, 'how cool is that?'

'Very,' I replied, 'although unless it's just my TV, we've seen *Clambake* four times already tonight.' I turned out the light and went to sleep.

On day one I felt OK. By day two I could feel the pain coming back. By day three, I couldn't get out of bed again. I didn't want to worry Mum and Dad so I just pretended I wanted a lie-in. Breakfast in The Heartbreak Hotel was dreadful anyway. It was OK for Dad, who polished off a couple of doughnuts and a cup of coffee each morning ('but I'm on holiday!' he'd wail when Mum pointed out that he may not make his 61st birthday at this rate) and Mum managed to find some cereal. Well, as near to cereal as you can get in America - unidentifiable flakes of stuff covered in sugar with extra sugar round the edges, topped with some more sugar and some full-fat milk. Nice.

Obese Americans stared at me on the first morning as I filled a polystyrene bowl with my own non-sugar coated cornflakes and added my soya milk. You'd have thought I'd come down to breakfast wearing a T-shirt saying 'I *heart* Hitler' from the looks they were shooting in my direction.

'It's milk, but not as they know it,' whispered Dad, so high on donuts that he was now confusing the Heartbreak Hotel with the Starship Enterprise. I picked up a banana only to discover it was plastic. Eventually we located a real bowl containing real fruit by which time I was almost delirious with hunger so took every banana I could find. Which amounted to a grand total of two. Oh well. Dad then stuck them on his head like antlers - no more sugar, please! - then we proceeded to reception to get instructions on how to get to Graceland.

'Are y'all drivin'?' asked the enormous, dour-faced clerk, passing a wet wipe over her telephone receiver, almost breaking into a smile, but more likely just suffering from wind if she'd partaken in the hotel breakfast.

'No, we're walking,' I replied. The look of bewilderment on her face led me to believe that nobody had ever said that before. I was bewildered too, but at the size of her. I'd never seen anyone so fat. I stepped away from the counter in case she tried to take a bite out of my arm.

'Walkin!' she bellowed, 'you guys are crazy!' She shook her head and pulling out a pen and paper.

'I'll draw you guys a map, it's a long way, that's for sure.' Three seconds later and she's drawn two lines, one with a star on, the other with the word 'Graceland' on, and pushed it over the counter to me.

'So you're here,' she said, tapping her pen at the star, 'and Graceland, well, you take a right outta here and ya'll get over the road and y'all find it on your left,' she said, looking exhausted from getting a whole sentence out without pausing.

'OK, great. How long will it take to walk there?' I enquired, wondering how long my hips would hold out.

'Uh, I don't know,' she said, shaking her head, 'folk don't walk round here,' waving her hands in the air and concluding with the advice that: 'Y'all would be better gettin' yourselves a hire car, people,' before answering the ringing telephone with a nice big 'Yo!' Americans invented a lot of things, but walking wasn't one of them.

Around six minutes and less than half a mile later we walked into the Graceland ticket office, which resembled a multi-plex cinema foyer only without the ice-cream and popcorn, though everybody in there looked like that's all they'd eaten since the day they were born. It was only 10am yet there were hundreds of people milling around in their XXL T-shirts, picking up tickets for the Graceland Platinum Tour at a bargain $35 and contemplating nipping back to the hotel for another doughnut to see them through the queue. As it was April, and not August, it was neither too hot nor particularly crowded, but I don't think it would have made a difference what month it was as to how fat everybody was. Still, they could always live off their reserves while they waited in line.

Preconceptions of Graceland were thus: it would be vast and imposing, it would be hidden down a dirt track far from the eyes of passers-by, it would, in the hallway, have the stairway blocked off by a red rope and at the very top, an electric blue velvet curtain tied with gold braid keeping visitors from getting to Elvis's bedroom. Actually, the first two were preconceptions and I couldn't have been more wrong - the house, although hardly small, wasn't the sprawling mansion I imagined it to be. The strangest thing about Graceland is that it is visible from the road, a handsome mansion set back from the highway and surrounded by greenery. That we would be able to see Graceland from the roadside was something I hadn't taken into consideration simply due to the fact that you do not expect such a famous house to be so, well, obvious.

The third preconception was actually a mad dream that came to me two weeks before we left England. I'd seen photos of the outside of Graceland many times - the classic photo of Elvis outside his new home leaning against his new Cadillac - but never the inside. In the dream, which left me in a right old pickle, I had taken a job as a cleaner at Graceland - as you do. Whilst on my rounds, complete with wheelbarrow (I have a vivid, if not slightly disturbed imagination), French maid's outfit (Elvis would have liked that, I thought to myself) and a pile of cheese (not sure where that fits in, to be honest, probably to do with me being on a dairy-free diet) I happen upon a door which is slightly ajar. I turn the handle, and parking the wheelbarrow and its load of cheese, take a step through to a long corridor. At the end of the corridor - which was, incidentally, a replica of the hotel in *The Shining* - there are some stairs, blocked at the bottom by a thick, blood red rope. By now I really have forgotten all about cleaning and cheese, and approach the stairs. As I look up all I can see is this electric blue velvet curtain, from floor to ceiling, along the top of which runs a thick, gold braid. Unclipping the metal catch on the rope, I climb the stairs, my heart beating faster with every step. Downstairs I can hear the other maids (did they all have cheese or were they delivering other foodstuffs? I never did find out) chatting, so quicken my pace. At the top of the stairs I push aside the curtain to reveal Elvis' bedroom. I'm in the doorway, he's listening to a tape of birds singing, sitting on his huge white four poster bed in a cream and red silk Western shirt and dark blue jeans, with his back to me, head down, looking at something in his lap.

I walk into the room until I come to be at his right hand side, and see that he's holding a postcard from Australia, a picture of a kangaroo on the front. He hears me approach and looks up, and I see that he's circa 1968, and he's looking pretty good.

'Hi,' he says, softly, smiling that wonderfully genuine smile. He pats the bed next to him, motioning for me to sit down. I perch next to him, my hands in my lap, and say hello. I ask him how he is.

'I'm OK, darlin', he answers, 'did you bring my cheese?' I tell him I left it downstairs in the wheelbarrow. This, of course, doesn't faze him because it is a dream. He takes my left hand and looks into my eyes.

'You wanna watch a movie or sumthin'?' he asks, tracing the outline of the heart line on my left hand with his index finger.

'Uh, OK,' I say, 'but what about the cheese?'

'Forget about the cheese, baby' says Elvis, 'let's cuddle up and watch a movie.' He presses the top of his head and a TV appears from nowhere, the screen showing we're halfway through *Jaws*. Brilliant.

He turns and puts one arm around my waist, the other arm he lifts above my head and strokes my hair. Then he kisses me gently on the lips, his eyes closed. He pulls back and smiles, says, 'I'm gonna have a rest now, honey, you be sure to come on back tomorrow and watch a movie with me. Maybe we'll kiss a while if that's OK?'

'That'd be grand,' I say, stood up now and waving goodbye. Elvis disappears and I find myself at the foot of the stairs, the image of the blue velvet curtain the last thing I remember before I wake up.

I don't think about the dream again until we reach the front steps of the house. The air is calm. It's a fairly cloudy day, one which I had hoped would be gloriously sunny as would befit a visit to The King's Palace.

It is eerily quiet, despite the presence of the 15 or 20 visitors who mill about the driveway taking pictures. They're talking but I don't hear them. An immensely handsome Palomino horse thing grazes in the paddock as a gentle breeze blows his mane this way and that, and as we approach the front door, I almost begin to cry. Part of me doesn't want to go in, doesn't want to invade Elvis' privacy. You know, as if he's still in there, trying to eat his breakfast in peace. It seems wrong to trample through his home.

Dad is close to tears. Momentarily we hold hands for the first time since I was a little girl and walk together through the front door. Each visitor is provided with headphones though which they listen to a pre-recorded tape of the 'Graceland tour', an audio guide to go with the visuals, which gives you basic information on Elvis' home, and, later, his career, the narrative relating to specific areas of the house and/or times in his life.

I can't put into words how it feels to walk around Elvis Presley's beloved Graceland. If you can walk around that house without a lump in your throat then you are surely not an Elvis fan, but a voyeur, a simple tourist whose visit is borne out of nothing more than curiosity, a way to pass the time on a long car journey through Tennessee.

And then I see it - the red rope, the stairs, and can hardly bear to look up. Mum sees it first and when she gasps, I guess either the curtain at the top is blue or Elvis himself is standing there.

Dad says, 'blimey,' and I look up to see an electric blue velvet curtain, floor to ceiling, with gold braiding along the top. This is too weird, but I didn't see my wheelbarrow full of cheese and I didn't get a job as a cleaner, despite asking for one.

We were in Elvis' kitchen. It was all a bit overwhelming.

'We're in Elvis' kitchen!' I bleat at Mum, clutching my chest, 'as if!'

Although you are actively encouraged to pass through the rooms as quickly as possible, there's no poking you with a cattle prod or being shot at from the security guards should you wish to linger for a couple of minutes beside his enormous round fake fur bed with built-in stereo, nor are you asked to move on when you find yourself rooted to the spot as you stare dribbling at *the* '68 Comeback show leather suit.

It was an unbelievable place to be - surrounded by Elvis's most famous outfits, not replicas, the actual originals. There were hundreds of Elvis's stage outfits to marvel at, suits which looked so stunning without Elvis inside them that it's hard to believe folk didn't have heart attacks just simply glancing at him on stage. In short, the tour was magnificent. The last port of call, appropriately, is the meditation garden where Elvis, his mother Gladys, his grandmother Minnie May and his father, Vernon, are all buried. Though this wasn't his anniversary month, floral tributes laid down by fans from all over the world created a wonderful carpet of colour in the garden, and I'm glad to say that every single person who walked around that special place, even the kids, were quiet, respectful and genuinely moved by the enormity of what they were seeing. A few tears were shed, and although there was a sense of overwhelming sadness, you somehow felt in your heart that Elvis Aaron Presley was watching it all from heaven, somewhat amazed that people were still turning up to look around his house and have a nose at his clothes 25 years after his death.

I had pulled a tiny speck of carpet off the wall in his hallway (yep, the wall) and put it in my jeans so that I would forever have a bit of Elvis's house with me, except that I couldn't locate it when we came outside. Dad raised his eyebrows as I rummaged frantically through my pockets looking for a speck of green fluff.

'It was so tiny it probably blew away. You're daft,' he said, and he wasn't wrong.

Determined to come away with something other than photos of his leather suits, gold jacket, gold discs and round fluffy bed, I picked up a leaf from the path near the stables instead and kept that between the pages of my book.

We visit Sun Studios, where Elvis cut his first record, and I sat on the spot marked with tape where he stood and sang. It made me cry with joy, so Dad took a photo. He cried with joy when he stood on it so I took a photo of him. It went on like this for some time. We then had a root beer, which we drank even though it was disgusting, in the cafe next door where Elvis and Sam Phillips, his producer, would drink root beer.

'Well, root beer is horrible,' announced Mum. We all agreed on that.

I was meant to be driving us to Mississippi the next day. I had driven in America before – back when I was 21 I'd gone on holiday to LA, Vegas and San Francisco with my friend Rachel and if you can drive there, you can drive anywhere. Actually, I couldn't drive there very well at all, now I think about it. I mounted a pavement in Beverley Hills and busted a wheel in San Francisco. Plus we screamed a lot on the highway because it was so scary. And we got lost, like, all the time. Plus we thought Vegas to San Francisco was a three-hour journey. It wasn't. Oh, and when we did drive through Death Valley, we had no water except for two small bottles of Evian, hadn't checked the radiator to make sure there was plenty of water in it, and only had some chewing gum, Guns 'n' Roses CDs and cigarettes. We were extremely ill-prepared for anything. Also, I drove with one foot on the dashboard, reading a book because the roads were so straight and there was no on-coming traffic.

Still, I seemed to have forgotten all that, at least until careered through red lights on a railroad crossing with a police car right behind me. I whizzed through as the barriers came down, the police car trapped behind it. I hadn't seen either - the crossing or the police. Dad looked like he was about to have a coronary.

'Um,' he said, tapping me on the shoulder from his seat in the back, 'you do know that was a railroad crossing and that there was a police car right behind you, don't you?' to which I replied, 'Really! That's mad, I didn't see anything!' and zipped through another red light. I soon remembered that traffic lights in America are above, rather than in front of you. I made a mental note to keep one eye in the sky, and one on the road. God, I hated driving in America!

The roads in Tennessee aren't as bad as those in LA, where I had to negotiate about 12 lanes of traffic whilst screaming my head off in a blind panic, but they're still difficult. For me. We set off for Tupelo, Elvis' birthplace, bright and early that morning.

Tupelo was beautiful, and what's more, it was a warm, sunny day. We took photos on the porch of his wooden house - a very much repainted, restructured and made-to-look-better-than-it-was wooden house, which I don't think was even in the spot where his house even was, but never mind - and admired the amazing scenery, the reds and yellows of the trees set against the clearest blue sky I've ever seen. It was so tranquil. Unfortunately that was where the fun stopped, as that night we stayed in some weird motel where gangs of bandana-clad black guys played deafening hip-hop and openly dealt drugs - and women, referring to them as their 'bitches' and 'hoes' - outside of our rooms. I was in one room, Mum and Dad in the other, both of us on the phone saying, 'Uh, should we go outside and tell them to keep the noise down or just not?'

In the morning we headed out of Tupelo for Shiloh. Dad is obsessed with history, particularly American history and the Civil War, and it has been his dream for as long as he can remember (probably as long as he wouldn't think of going) to visit the Shiloh Battleground, home of the famous uh, battle. At Shiloh. Shows what I know. I can't say as Mum and I were that thrilled at the prospect (me: 'it's just going to be a field, isn't it?' Mum: 'yes'), but the weather was glorious and as it turned out, Shiloh was, indeed, incredible. A nine-kilometre drive around the park where the battle took place was interspersed with signs every few yards. I was driving at around six miles an hour, rather like those old men who end up on the news after finding themselves driving the wrong way down the M1 in their motorised wheelchairs having just popped out for some milk.

Each time we approached a sign, I stopped the car, and Dad got out and stood, hands on hips, in front of the sign, and read what had happened upon that spot however many years ago it had happened. He'd get to the end, pull a face which said 'Yeah, I knew that,' which he always did, look up into the sky and all around, and get back in the car. It went on like this for about four of the nine kilometres, until I screamed, 'Dad, will you just read it out of the window, this is driving me bloody mad!'

After three days (well, it felt like it) we left Shiloh. Dad was over the moon. I'd taken photos of him in front of statues, of him lying in the grass pretending to be wounded, pictures of a lake called 'Bloody Lake' where hundreds of men met their deaths, and which, on this hot day, reflected the crimson leaves of the trees surrounding it as though their blood still ran through the water. It was eerie, yet beautiful. As we'd got the park fairly late in the day, nobody else was around. Dad, he would later recount to friends and family, and on some occasions complete strangers at the till in the supermarket, had had the place to himself.

'I've seen Elvis's house and I've lay on the ground at Shiloh. That's all I need. I'm the happiest man and the luckiest dad in the world. I've got the best daughter anyone could have.'

He had a point. I am pretty great.

CHAPTER SIX
'I'VE GOT NOTHING WORKING NOW'
ANN COLE

I must have been in remission because the joint pain had subsided considerably, enough for me to join the local gym at the end of May. I laughed out loud as I filled out the form because I've always been totally against the idea of running along a bit of rubber, sweating next to strangers when you could run around the park or along the seafront instead and sweat on your own. Trouble was, I knew that unless I saw a personal trainer and actually got them to tell me to come in, I'd never do anything. I was slim, but I wanted to tone up and I thought it was about time, now that I had time, to do it.

OK, I confess. I went to have a look around and two things persuaded me to join up - a very, very handsome instructor and a swimming pool which was warm and shallow enough to stand in without flapping about. I have a real fear of deep water and as a teenager would lower myself into the deep end of the swimming pool, swim a length to the shallow end, then get out and run (and invariably slip over) to the deep end and start again. I couldn't bear the thought of running out of energy at the deep end as I'd almost drowned when I was 10 years-old on an ill-supervised school trip to France, so I would get into a right old panic if water went above my chest. The sight of what looked to me like the baby pool was most welcome. Mr Instructor was switched on to full power flirt mode that also helped my signature find its way on to the membership form.

'I'll see you at seven tomorrow,' he said, 'don't be late.'

I went back at seven the next night and was gently put through my paces by the instructor who I'd decided was too handsome to be allowed out to work and should be locked up by the council. I feared a heart attack before I even got on the treadmill.

'Now,' he said, writing something on his clipboard (probably 'note to self: this girl is an idiot'), 'I don't want your heart rate going above 70. I don't want your blood pressure to go too high.'

'Well in that case may I suggest you leave the room, mister,' I cackled, Barbara Windsor style. He laughed and rolled his eyes.

'I make the jokes around here, Juliette,' he said, with the authoritative tone of a headmaster scolding a pupil, and went downstairs.

As soon as he'd left the room I stopped breathing in and let my tummy go. Such relief!

I went to the gym every other day. I was also going to Ashtanga yoga classes in town twice a week, which I thoroughly enjoyed. In short, I was as fit as a fiddle, apart from having ulcerative colitis. My tummy was toned and I had no rushing to the loo, nothing like that, so you'd never have known I was ill. I could walk up the steep hill to my flat without struggling for breath.

'You need to be motivated to come here three times a week,' Instructor God told me.

'Uh, don't worry, I am,' I insisted. I swam in the warm baby pool, sat about in the Jacuzzi avoiding brushes with other people's limbs - usually by getting out as soon as somebody even looked like they were remotely heading in my direction - and cleared out mild hangovers in the steam room. I had no problem keeping up my fitness levels - the only stressful moments came when I saw someone else's hair in the shower plug. Ugh! Once, the shower curtain stuck to my shoulder as I was under the water and in my attempt to shake it off my skin I fell out of the shower. Class. Other than that, I quite enjoyed it.

Twice a week or more I'd do a 40 minute work out before swimming 50 lengths. When I didn't fancy the gym, i.e. every day, I'd swim 100 or 150 lengths. Before you think I must be some kind of closet Olympic athlete I hasten to add that the pool was only about three feet long. Still, I was getting really fit and more importantly, Instructor God - all six feet four and 15 stone of him - would come and say 'hello' whenever I had the pool to myself. One day he even came into the steam room for as long as he could stand it to have a chat.

Two days before my birthday I was floating about in the pool, pretending to be dead to see if Instructor God would come and rescue me with the kiss of life or just scoop me out of the water with the giant fishing net thing, when he came in and shut the door. He asked me what I was doing at the weekend.

'It's my birthday,' I told him. 'I've booked a little boat and some old bloke who might well be Captain Birdseye and some friends are coming down from London and we're going to sit on the boat and eat from a giant platter of fish-fingers - maybe - and drink gin and tonics and we'll try not to fall overboard and then we'll come back and sit on the beach and watch *Gladiator* on the big screen on the beach because they're showing it. On the beach. On the big screen.' There was a pause while he took it all in.

'Uh, OK,' he said, kneeling down at the side of the pool while I kept everything but my shoulders well under water.

'Is that a belly button ring?' he asked, looking under the water.

'Either that or a fish hook,' I said, realising that after all my exercising I didn't need to hold my tummy in any more.

'Why don't you come along on the boat on Saturday?' I asked him, without even thinking.

'I'm working 'til eight,' he said, 'but I would have loved to.' I think he meant it.

'Shame,' I said, 'I won't even get a birthday kiss, then.'

'You can have it now, if you like,' he said, turning back to the pool and smiling. 'I'm here now and my knee is all wet. It seems a shame to have a wet knee for nothing.' Somehow, despite the fact that my legs had turned to jelly, I did that weird underwater stride to the side of the pool and bobbed up and down a bit whilst fiddling with my ponytail.

'Come here, then,' he said, leaning towards me, 'I'm not coming in.'

I swam to the edge of the pool and stood looking down at the water. I had my eyes scrunched up and was about to break into a giggle when he leant down and kissed me on the lips. A proper kiss on the lips. I thought I was going to faint, which would be inconvenient as I would have drowned. I went bright red. He wished me a happy birthday for Saturday and reminded me to come in and see him before I went on the boat. Happy birthday to me indeed!

I'd started jiving lessons in the summer. I went on my own, was paired off with a man who'd been dancing for about thirty years and that was how I spent every Sunday night for eight weeks. Off my head on painkillers some weeks to get through it, naturally, but it was worth it. Between lessons I'd go to rockabilly gigs with my friend Aaron and what with going to the gym and swimming, I was pretty fit. The pain had come back, though. It came in stabbing form half way through dancing one night, and continued throughout the next day. I took painkillers before, during and after classes, still pushing myself beyond what any sane person would do.

I'd finally found myself a friend in Brighton. His name was Jon, and he was also a freelance writer who worked for *loaded*. He was concerned that a fellow writer with a penchant for Elvis might be lonely, and could he help. Jon got exciting jobs such as flying to LA to interview Robert Downey Jnr or Kate Beckinsale or other Hollywood big guns. We got on like a house on fire, mainly because he was a bit weird, like me, and we'd talk for hours about nonsense. I persuaded him into coming along to a rock 'n' roll club in Shoreham, about 10 minutes from Brighton. It wasn't really my scene but I had hoped I might me someone under the age of 95 there. I stood on the sidelines and accompanied Jon out to the foyer every time he wanted a cigarette, which was pretty much all of the time. And that's when I saw him.

Battered motorcycle boots, turned up jeans, key chain in his pocket, fag packet in his rolled-up shirt sleeve, all jet black greased up quiff and sideburns and olive skin and chiseled cheekbones. He looked like he belonged in a fifties B movie, the guy who'd beat up on Elvis and stub his cigarette out on his blue suede shoes. I was instantly besotted. I kept looking at him, I thought he looked like he was married with 10 kids and lived in a caravan or something. Jon told me he looked like he was with a woman with long dark hair who stood next to him and glared at me whenever I dared look over and so that was that.

I tried not to stare at Mr B Movie but I couldn't help it. He was ace. I watched him jive, and it took my breath away. As Jon and I were leaving, I wondered if I'd see him again. Turns out that I would, in an obscure little pub near Eastbourne two weeks later.

There I was, sitting at the table nursing a Coke and a packet of bacon Frazzles waiting for Aaron to turn up. The door opened, and as I looked up to see if it was Aaron, I gasped a bit. It was him! He came straight over, and after introducing himself - 'me name's Rolie!' he said brightly, he told me to get a pen and write down my number so that he might 'take me to some rock 'n' roll clubs'. As I shot up from the table - I needed no encouraging - he blurted, 'I'm not tryin' to chat you up...' to which I replied, 'that's a shame,' and headed for the bar, my cheeks turning crimson as I felt his eyes burning into the back of my head.

We had our first date two weeks later and despite his pompadour leaving grease marks on my suede cushions I thought he was pretty cool. A couple of sandwiches or even a flask, a packet of crisps, a sausage roll, a blanket and perhaps a location short of a picnic - but he seemed like decent bloke and smoked like James Dean. As long as he didn't drive like James Dean I figured we'd be OK.

All we had in common, however, was a love of decent music and the fact that we were both available and also liked bats. You can imagine the struggle to find common ground if that's all you come up with, but so what. I'd seen him jiving that first night and I never thought I'd say anything as flouncy as this in my life, but he was fantastic. Me, fancying a bloke because he can dance. He'd drop to his knees in front of a lady and as he spun her round, he'd be up on his nimble feet again before she knows what's going on and she'd spend the next minute and a half being flung around the dance floor like a rag doll. I wanted to be one of those women but I'd only had three lessons.

'There's plenty of time to get good,' he'd say, and there should have been.

We were also not sleeping together. I was eating more biscuits because of the strain but I reckoned it would be worth it.

'November 10th,' I told Rolie, 'I can give in then. We'll book into that fancy hotel in Brighton with the Bettie Page room and do it all night then eat Walker's Tomato Sauce flavour crisps and I'll have a Tia Maria and some Matchmakers.'

A month before our special date I went off on a rock 'n' roll weekender at Hemsby, in Norfolk, with my trusty sidekick, Charlie (whom I'd met while working at *loaded*. Charlie was a fashion intern with a love of vintage clothing and rockabilly music and we'd instantly clicked), and a group of rockabillies who arrived at Mum and Dad's place in convoy. They parked their cars - a beautiful blue Plymouth, a black Cadillac, a black Consul and a Ford Roadster in a line stretching from next door's driveway to four houses down. I was rushing about indoors making sure I had packed everything, though there wasn't much I could do about it if I hadn't as I'd packed in Brighton and had come up the night before. Charlie had got the train down from London and I'd picked her up, come back home with just enough time for a quick cup of tea before everyone arrived. While Aaron loaded our bags into his car, squashing them between his drum kit and bemoaning the fact that we'd got so much stuff 'for one poxy weekend' as he called it, the others, most of whom I'd never met before, took it in turns to traipse in and out of the house in their biker boots to use the toilet. I don't know what the neighbours made of it all but 15 rockabillies (most of whom were covered in engine oil and tattoos) roaming around their driveways must have made for fervent curtain twitching. Once we were all set, each huge American car turning on somebody's driveway to the occupants' horror, we set off for Hemsby.

Seven hours and six breakdowns later, we arrived. To keep costs down, Charlie and I were sharing a chalet with Aaron, Andy, Frog and Rob. Charlie and I had one room, Frog and Rob the other, Aaron and Andy would fight over the sofa bed in the living room. The next three days and nights flew by, a whirlwind of vodka tonics, bacon sandwiches, hangovers, dancing, loud rockabilly music and a haze of cigarette smoke. And that was just in the chalet. I had given up smoking (though 10 cigarettes a fortnight barely qualified me as a smoker in the first place) when I had gone through the pre-cancerous cells on my cervix stage, and I can honestly say that there's nothing smokier than 3,500 rockabillies under one roof. Bleuch!

I'd been on painkillers all weekend. In fact, I'd been back on them for the last two months. I'd tried diazepam, co-codamol, Tylex, Nurofen, Remediene, Voltarol, amitriptyline and just about everything else imaginable in between. Nothing seemed to work. My doctor was sympathetic, but there was no real sense of getting any proper help. She just read from a list of painkillers and tried me on a new one each time I went back complaining about the current one. I found, however, that by the time the night came around and my painkillers had had all day to take effect, half a little bottle of vodka loosened me up enough to be able to jive. Well, of sorts. I'd been in so much pain every day for the last 10 months that I'd forgotten what it was like to be able to do the simplest things - get out of bed, shower, walk to the shop and pick up a paper. Here I was at a weekender, trying to keep up with everyone else and wondering why I was having such a hard time of it. I think that's the first time I realised that I'd have to slow down - but at the same time as realising it, I was denying it. In fact, I was doing more than that - I was ignoring it at my peril.

On the Saturday morning I'd given up trying to sleep. Frog snored like a walrus with flu and I could hear him through the paper-thin walls, Charlie talked in her sleep and Aaron and Andy came crashing through the door at 7am, slightly the worse for wear, and decided it'd be a good time to play the drums. With saucepans. I felt well enough to head out to the site shop for a copy of *The Guardian*, and shook the paper until The Guide, the going out/staying in supplement, fell onto the table. My first feature for them was the cover feature on R&B/rock/pop goddess Kelis. I was positively beaming. I read that, had a coffee and some breakfast but as I stood up to take my cup to the sink, my left hip completely seized up. I cried out in pain, Aaron flew out of bed to come to my aid and sat me down again. I swallowed a couple of pills and waited. Aaron brought me another cup of tea and a slice of toast, and sat with me until I felt a bit better. Twenty minutes later I stood again, nauseous from the codeine, and this time it still hurt, but I could move. I didn't mention how utterly sick I felt and hoped it would pass. It didn't. We decided to go into town for a few bits and pieces and he said he'd carry me again if he had to.

He had to.

On the Sunday, I started the day with painkillers and breakfast, then painkillers and lunch, then more painkillers until I couldn't actually feel anything at all, good or bad, and bought a wonderful vintage cocktail dress which was so tight that midway through a jive that night it ripped at the shoulder, the black fabric hanging limply down my right arm like a wounded bird. I hurried - as best you can in high heels - back to the chalet to put on my jeans, and just as I put the key in the door I felt the first stabbing pain in my stomach. I just about managed to open the door before I doubled up in agony.

I didn't make it back to the hall that night. Instead, I crawled on all fours across the dirty carpet to the bathroom. Ten minutes later I'd managed to stand half way up, wash my hands and face and clean my teeth. I took off my earrings. I undid the straps on my shoes. What fabulous shoes they were. I'd bought them in Memphis. They were original 1950s ankle-strap stilettos, black, with an orange mesh bit holding my toes in, a black and orange pom-pom type affair on the front, and black leather ribbons that I tied up around my ankle. I put them beside the bed, pulled on my pyjamas - this was October and I was freezing, despite having brought my leopard print throw with me - and lay down under the duvet. The pain seemed to be subsiding. After taking a call from Charlie on my mobile - 'have you got lost again?' - I went to sleep. It was 1am.

We drove home on Monday morning, bleary eyed and pale of face.

All of us had sore throats and were losing our voices, despite the fact that only two of us smoked. I felt terrible. Packing my things, which has never been my strong point as Mum would tell you, took forever. I seemed to be winding down; it was as though my batteries were wearing out. An uneventful drive home down the motorway through the rain saw us arrive back in Orpington at teatime, just as Dad was coming home from work. Charlie had to go back to East London, so Dad gave her a lift to the station.

The next day I was supposed to drive back to Brighton but I couldn't get out of bed. Mum brought me some painkillers and a cup of tea. I eventually got out of bed with her help an hour later. I sat in the garden and cried. Mum brought me the paper, fetched me drinks, and kept my painkiller intake topped up.

'There's no point in taking them,' I told her, 'they only work with vodka, just below overdose level. On their own they just make me feel drowsy and sick. I can't drive on these.'

'You can't drive anyway,' she said, rubbing my shoulders and stroking my hair, 'your dad will have to take you home tomorrow. I'm going to do fish fingers tonight. Your favourite.' Good old Mum, putting the world and my pain to rights in one easy grill-to-plate step.

The next day it took me half an hour again to get out of bed and down stairs. Once I'd had some breakfast, walked about a bit, all hunched and clutching my back, my bones began to loosen up.

'I'll go in a while,' I told Mum, 'tell Dad I'll be OK.'

Dad was at work. He called at 10am.

'How's my poor girl?' he asked Mum.

'She's doing a bit better,' she told him, waving at me to come over. I took the phone.

'Hi, Dad,' I said, 'you OK?'

'Nothing wrong with me,' he said, 'I'm just worried about my little girl. Are you OK to get home?'

'I'll be fine,' I lied.

'Love you, baby,' he said. I kissed my mum, dragged the cat indoors to save her being run over, shouted goodbye to my brother who was still in bed, and drove home, grimacing and gasping all the way, glad that the majority of the journey was on the motorway which meant I didn't have to press my left foot down to change gear, as that sent shooting pains up my leg into my hip. The pain was playing havoc with my frown lines, too.

'November 10th. Bloody hell, that's ages away,' I said to Rolie that night. He'd come over after work, covered in sawdust from his carpentry work. He looked about fifty until he'd had a shower and done his hair. I've never seen anyone scrub up so well.

'I'm going to book the room tomorrow,' I told him.

'Well book it right up, sweetheart!' he laughed, coming out of the bathroom and into the kitchen and putting his arms around my waist. He kissed me on the back of my neck. I loved that. I was washing up. 'Let me do that,' he said, and took over.

'You have a sit down. Had your tablets?' he asked. I told him I had and sat down to some stupid television. While there wasn't much going on in his head, I did at least feel like he was able to take care of me. He never let me carry anything heavy, or even light, and he always opened doors for me and brushed his tobacco off the passenger seat of the car before I got in. I couldn't really ask for more. Plus, he was incredibly strong so he could carry me to the sofa, carry me to bed and probably, given half a chance, carry me everywhere with him all day, every day.

Rolie left for work at 7.30am. He sat on the edge of the bed and kissed me on the cheek.

'I'm off to work, baby,' he said, stroking my hair, 'you look beautiful. I love you. Phone me later.'

I smiled, but didn't open my eyes. As he shut the bedroom door, I let the tears flow at last. I had been in unbearable pain since 5am, the whole of my right side going into spasm. I couldn't move. Eventually, I managed to turn over, gasping in agony as I did so. It took forever, a fierce, burning pain shooting through my body as though I was being sliced open with a hot knife. I made it to the living room on my hands and knees and rang my doctor.

I swallowed a couple of pills, and still on my knees, dragged myself to the bathroom, leaned up to the taps and ran a hot bath. I lifted myself into the bath, stiff as a board, and slowly lay down in the water. Gradually the pain subsided, and I managed, just about, to get out of the bath, get dressed and kind of stumble, limp and grab walls and fence posts, lampposts and almost passersby all the way to the surgery, a trip which usually takes 10 minutes tops, but today took 40 minutes.

My GP asked me what was wrong. I told him that I still had the joint pain, still had the muscle pain, that I was exhausted, in agony, in despair. That I'd been to see my consultant at the hospital a month previously, and been in so much pain I had to get a porter to take me to his office in a wheelchair (that was true). That even then he still wouldn't get me any crutches, because, and I quote, 'you haven't actually injured yourself as such, and it's not my department.' All he had suggested was that I go back on the steroids. I refused. Certainly when you are told a scan shows you are suffering from onset osteoporosis you don't want to be put back on the tablets which caused it in the first place. I couldn't understand why nobody would help me.

'I'm going to try you on these tablets,' said the doctor, producing his prescription pad from a drawer. He was an affable man, all rosy cheeked and smartly dressed unlike a lot of doctors who look as though they've just woken up from a three week sleep in a hedge. He handed me the prescription and wished me luck. I thanked him for listening. It was the first time anyone in the medical profession had done so.

I started on the tablets immediately. Usually I'd read through the side effects and do's and don'ts, but this time I didn't. I just took one.

'Hopefully,' said my doctor, 'these will work overnight to reduce the inflammation and you'll wake up pain free.'

I didn't believe him, but it worked. The next morning I woke next to Rolie and as I opened my eyes, I turned to him and pinched his nose to wake him up, because I can be mean like that: 'I'm not in pain,' I whispered. That was the first time in months that I'd been able to turn over, let alone say I wasn't in pain. It felt like a miracle. I was absolutely amazed, and got out of bed at the same time as him and made him a coffee, waving him goodbye as he headed to work.

The next week passed by quickly. I had a big project to do for work - another 16-page supplement for *loaded* which I had to write from scratch at home then edit on screen in the office once I'd had the copy approved by the client.

On the Wednesday that I travelled up to London I felt a bit strange. I had to go to the loo twice at the station in what can only be described as archaic toilets that looked like they were part of an exhibition at The London Dungeon. My tummy didn't feel right. I wasn't in pain, but just uncomfortable. I put it down to stress. There was a lot of money riding on this project and it had to be finished in the next two days. I'd been working around the clock to get it done, on one day working from 8am to 6pm then starting again at 8pm and working until 4am. I was, unsurprisingly, exhausted.

When I arrived at the office to find that hardly any layouts from the freelance designer were ready for me to look at, I wasn't too pleased. What a waste of time and energy that I didn't have. I struggled just to get through some soup at lunchtime, and went home. As luck wouldn't have it, the trains were delayed and it took three hours to get back to Brighton from Waterloo. I'd left my house at 8.45am. It was 7.45pm. What a waste of a day. I was so tired I went straight to bed after calling Mum and telling her what a disaster this project was turning out to be.

'You sound stressed out,' she said, 'have you been up late, writing?' I told her I had. She tutted.

'You know it makes you worse,' she said, 'you should take it easy.'

'Mum, I said, 'If I take it easy I don't get paid.' She knows that as well as I do, so she wished me luck with it, sent my dad's and the cat's love (really) and hung up.

The next day, I awoke not with the same pain as usual but with stomach ache. Rolie had had a bit of a tummy bug the week before and I thought it must be that.

'I can't believe it's coming on now,' I said to Helen over the phone, 'I've got to finish this bloody job tomorrow but I feel awful.'

We chatted some more about the usual things - men, shoes, football, and I got on with the last few bits I was writing at home. The client, despite not knowing much about the *loaded*'s core readership or the editorial style and content of which I was pretty much an expert having written for them for four years, kept making petty changes to the copy. I'd sit at my computer, get a phone call from the marketing woman at the magazine to say she was emailing some of their points they had raised and then set about ploughing through 16 pages of copy adjusting headings and swapping sentences about. It was tedious and unnecessary and I was getting really, really pissed off.

I cooked some dinner but couldn't eat it. I still didn't feel right. My glands were up and I had a headache. I took my medication, rang Rolie, told him I'd see him on Saturday and went to bed.

It was Friday. The plan was that I'd go into work for 10am, work right through, and then meet my friend Stav (a tailor who was the spitting image of Elvis circa 1968) for dinner in Islington before I headed back to Brighton.

I felt dreadful. I had no appetite, which was unusual for me. In fact, unusual doesn't come into it. I've always had an appetite. It had been a hard day, and to top it all I'd been running back and forth to the toilet half the time. I made it to Islington to but felt worse than I had before I'd got on the tube. We had dinner at a Thai place. I couldn't eat much, nor concentrate on anything he was saying. I was nauseous, feverish and had stomach cramps. I felt so bad I just wanted to be at home. I told him how sorry I was but that I felt really unwell, and he got the tube back to the station with me and saw me on to the train. How I didn't think this was the colitis going nuts is beyond me. I should have gone straight to hospital, not out for dinner.

'I'm sorry to cut the night so short,' I said.

'Marry me, Juliette!' he said, grabbing my hand and pulling me towards him, 'come to Cyprus with me when I move back there and marry me. We can eat olives and get you a tan.'

'Uh, I'll let you know,' I replied, somewhat taken aback. The train doors shut. Honestly, I thought, my life is ridiculous.

CHAPTER SEVEN
'LIVE FAST, LOVE HARD, DIE YOUNG'
FARON YOUNG

I didn't think I could feel much worse, but when I woke up on Saturday, I did. I still drove to Rolie's in the afternoon but had to stop twice on the way to go to the toilet in revolting petrol station toilets. My stomach felt like it was going to explode and I was feverish and felt really faint. I have no idea why I drove there. I popped some painkillers when I got to his house and we actually went out dancing. Honest to God. Well, I sat around and drank apple juice, he jived with other women, I got a bit jealous, I danced for a bit and sat down again, feeling queasy. He was worried about me. I was worried about me. I felt absolutely dreadful. We slow danced and I cried on his shoulder. Even Gene Vincent's *Unchained Melody* couldn't cheer me up. That was when I knew I was ill.

On Sunday I was in a worse state. I'd been up during the night, passing more and more blood. I no longer had the joint and muscle pain, but was suffering from such strong stomach cramps that I felt worse than I had when I had suffered from endometriosis a few years earlier, and I thought that was as bad as it could get.

We went to a boot fair on the Sunday morning - Rolie's favourite pastime aside from smoking and drinking. I don't know why I agreed to go - I suppose because I don't like admitting defeat - and I'll never know why he wanted to take me. I could barely walk I was so weak. We came home within 15 minutes as I needed the toilet. He got annoyed with me; I got annoyed with him because he thought I was being melodramatic. I lay on the settee and he brought me some soup that I'd made at home in the week. I fell asleep. I stayed that night, and left on Monday after he'd gone to work, the 40-minute drive home done in a mad panic, with stabbing pains in my stomach and such bad nausea that I thought I might pass out whilst driving. I was relieved to be home in one piece, but I knew I needed to get to hospital.

I rang Mum then called the doctor. They asked if I could come in. I said I couldn't leave the house as I was in agony and had to be by the toilet. They said they'd send someone round tomorrow. I checked my emails. There were changes to be made to the copy I'd already finalised on Friday. I sat at my desk and worked for the next hour or so, sipping water and wishing I felt hungry because I certainly felt faint. I emailed the changes through and lay down on the sofa and sort of whimpered, like an injured animal. I didn't know what to do. I was in such pain I couldn't even cry properly because it hurt so much. When I think about this now, I can't believe I felt so bad for so long, and didn't get Rolie to take me to hospital. I don't know why I didn't ask for help. I'm sure most people, if they were bleeding from their back passage and had agonising stomach cramps, a head which felt as though it was about to explode and a raging fever, would probably do something about it.

I watched daytime TV for the first time since I had glandular fever and missed school at 15. Daytime television is crap. I laughed inwardly at the adverts offering me loans, washing powder and help if I wanted to sue someone for something that was my fault. I wasn't that ill that I could watch talk shows, so I switched it off and went back to my computer. As I sat down, I screamed out in pain and abruptly stood again, then spent the first of many hours in the bathroom not knowing whether I was going to throw up or pass blood. Either way, it was blood. A lot of blood. I called Rolie at work where he was converting a barn, as you do. I left a message and asked him to come to my place that night, as he was supposed to go back to his place in Eastbourne after work. When he turned up I was in tears, wrapped up on the sofa, shaking with cold and fright and in agony despite having swallowed some incredibly strong painkillers an hour earlier.

'I'm worried, baby,' he said, kneeling down beside me, 'what's up?'

'Blood. It's just blood. Loads and loads of blood,' I cried.

'What do you mean? Where are you bleeding?' he said, panicking, cradling me in his arms. He smelt of wood shavings, tobacco and sweat.

'Look in the toilet,' I said, 'I'm sorry it's so grim but that's what's coming out of me. How horrible is that? It's been like it all day. My stomach's killing me.'

He went into the bathroom, muttered something to himself and flushed the toilet. He walked back into the lounge, rubbing his forehead, as white as a sheet. He made me a cup of tea and himself some dinner. I'd already spoken to Mum and told her I was feeling terrible, that I didn't know what to do. I'd reminded her of the time I'd called a doctor out a few months before and he'd told me I had indigestion and that I was 'being silly'. He said he didn't know much about colitis but that 'muscle pains weren't a symptom.'

'I can hardly draw breath,' I'd whispered, clutching my right side. He wrote me a prescription after I begged him for some painkillers and threw it on the table.

'I can't get the tablets,' I cried as he walked down the stairs to the front door. 'I can hardly move, how can I go to the chemist?' He carried on down the stairs and as he disappeared out of the door, shouted, 'You're having a panic attack, you silly girl.'

I rang the surgery after he'd left, spoke to my doctor, explained what had happened and as if by magic, the chemist brought the prescription round that evening. After that, I never bothered ringing the doctor when I was in pain, I rang Mum for an over the phone cuddle and took whatever painkillers I had to hand in the kitchen. I guess this is why I just tried to manage on my own. Because when I did ask for help, I didn't get it. And the doctor? He retired about a week later. Shame he didn't do it a week sooner.

I went to bed at eight and took another couple of pills. Rolie came to bed at midnight, cuddling me gently but it hurt to have his arm across my body. I went to the toilet and passed thick, red blood four times between 10pm and 2am. I woke up at 5am and couldn't get back to sleep. At 7am Rolie got up for work, trying not to wake me. I tried to speak to him, to tell him I was awake, but nothing came out. I started to try and sit up. On his way out of the door, he popped into the bedroom to kiss me goodbye. I couldn't even muster the energy to tell him to stay. My eyes were shut and my head was spinning.

At 7.45am I made it to the living room via the bathroom. I had a raging temperature, would be baking hot one minute and freezing cold the next. I had a really sore throat, and a mouth full of ulcers. At 8.10am I rang the surgery and made sure they were sending me a doctor round in the afternoon. I'd managed to get myself in to the bath, but had trouble getting out. I sat in the bath for over an hour, until it went cold, shaking and feeling as though I would faint at any minute. The doctor arrived with a medical student, the three of us a crowd in my living room. He asked if I'd come to the surgery for some blood tests. I said I could hardly get to the bathroom, so no, I wasn't up to it. He fiddled around in his doctor's case and took out some plastic vials, and said he'd take the blood samples now, having finally realised that I wasn't in a fit state to leave the flat.

The doctor sat down beside me as I pulled my dressing gown tighter and suggested I think about having an operation for my illness 'in a year or so. We can talk about it. It's the only cure. You won't have any more pain, and you'll get your life back.'

'But... I'll have... a colostomy bag,' I said, struggling to get the words out.

'No, no,' he assured me, 'if you go into hospital when you're OK, not during a bad time, they can do it so you just have this pouch thing, like a new bottom. You won't have to have a bag at all. But when you're in remission, when you're better, we can discuss it then. It's the only way to stop all the pain, Juliette.'

That was the last thing he said to me before picking up his little test tubes full of my blood and heading back to the surgery. I really liked him. He actually listened, and he didn't patronise me, or make me feel as though I had wasted his time. I lay back down on the sofa and drifted in and out of some kind of sleep, waking only with stomach cramps so bad I was doubled up as though I'd been stabbed. I then thought, 'hang on, why didn't he call an ambulance out?'

The cramps were a sign that more blood was on its way out of my body. I was exhausted. The phone rang and woke me from my sleep. It was my doctor. He'd got me a bed at the hospital. 'I don't see the point in you going to A&E,' he said, 'you'll end up being left on a trolley for two days. You might as well be at home until you know there's a bed.'

He'd told them I needed to be admitted, that I was in a bad way. I rang Dad. We arranged that they would come and pick me up - an hour or so drive for them straight down the motorway - and take me into hospital on Thursday morning. When I look back on this, it's incredible that I was so calm, that I didn't say, 'right, please come uh, now.' I told them I was so weak I might need to be shoved in a wheelchair.

'We'll worry about that when we get there,' said Mum.

I rang Rolie and told him I'd be going into hospital on Thursday, could he come round tomorrow night, and did he mind making his own dinner because I felt terrible. I didn't even ask him to come over that night. I didn't want to be a burden, even though I wanted him there. It was my coping mechanism kicking in, as usual. I had a sip of water, pulled my warm socks on, picked up Panda - the teddy I'd slept next to every night since I got him for my first Christmas - climbed back into bed and tried to sleep but a part of me was saying, 'ring an ambulance, you massive idiot.'

Wednesday went something like this: go to the bathroom, pass out, wake up, get up, sip some water, go to the bathroom, pass out, wake up, ring home, ring the doctors, pass out, swallow some more painkillers, go to bed, throw up the sip of water, lay on the sofa, wait for Rolie to turn up, somehow get up and shove a pizza in the oven for him whilst apologising for not cooking proper dinner, go to bed, cry, have a cuddle, get up, go to the bathroom, pass out, get back to bed, say goodbye to him just after seven, realise it's Thursday, tell him not to worry, get up, have a bath, lie on the settee, wait for them, lose consciousness, regain it an hour later as they buzz the door, take almost 10 minutes to let them in because I had to get down the stairs.

I got in the car. No sooner was I in than I had to tell Dad to open the door again because I had to go to the toilet. I staggered back up three flights of stairs and sat on the toilet. I came back downstairs and climbed in the car. We arrived at the hospital. I got in a wheelchair. I cried with the pain while we waited to see the consultant. He told me they would only admit me if it's an emergency. Mum tells told them that it was. Dad reminded them that it was my doctor who had booked the bed.

People in the waiting room looked alarmed or sympathetic or both. They said they hadn't got a bed. The consultant examined me and asked me what I want him to do.

'What?' I whispered, confused and delirious.

'What do you want me to do?' he repeated, curtly.

'Make me better, maybe?' I responded, incredulously. My parents brought up the subject of surgery.

'She was told she should think about it sometime in the future, if things don't improve,' said Mum.

'There's no need to even think about that,' said the consultant, 'that's years away, if at all. We really don't need to discuss that now. We'll get her on a steroid drip and see how it goes. She should be better soon.'

Then we waited in the corridor for the bed which was meant to have been booked but wasn't. A nurse came over and gasped when she saw my face. I'd seen her before.

'Oh Juliette,' she said, softly, tucking my hair behind my ear and tilting my face so I could focus on her, 'we'll get you a bed, don't worry.'

She took one look at Mum's face and shook her head, touching her on the shoulder as she left. Dad got up, put his hands in his pockets, counted out some change and went off to put some more money in the meter. Mum helped me to the toilet when I doubled up in agony. Dad came back and busied himself arranging our coats on the backs of the chairs, occasionally wandering out to reception and coming back to tell us that he'd seen the consultant and that he waved Dad away as though he was a beggar, saying, 'there aren't any beds, don't ask.'

I don't know how long went by, a couple of hours maybe, me drifting in an out of consciousness, Mum saying she wished there was something she could do, Dad trying his hardest to fight back the tears at the sight of his daughter, crumpled in a wheelchair, tears rolling down my cheeks, head hung, the occasional sigh of exhaustion passing my lips, cups of tea being waved away for fear that they would bring on more stomach cramps. Food and water were now my poison and I didn't want them anywhere near me.

It was 5pm when the nurse came back having at last secured a bed.

'I've done it,' she beamed, releasing the brake on the chair, 'I've got you a bed on the digestive diseases ward, let's go.' I thought she said she'd got me a bed and some digestive biscuits. I was both excited and confused. She was rushed off her feet, answering questions fired at her from consultants and receptionists as she wheeled me down the corridor.

Mum helped me into my pyjamas and I got into bed, crisp cotton sheets pulled so tightly across the bed I hadn't got the strength to lift them so that I could climb inside. Dad loosened the sheets and propped me up, Mum started unpacking my bag. I'd brought some more clothes with me, slippers, a nightie, some snacks - caramel rice crackers, non-dairy yoghurt, even some crisps although I hadn't eaten anything solid for three days. I'd imagined sitting in the chair beside my hospital bed, flicking through magazines, reading books I'd always meant to read, occasionally being allowed outside with my drip stand to get a breath of fresh air, or even cigarette smoke when my nicotine-riddled friends turned up. I couldn't have been further from reality.

I don't remember much about that night. Mum and Dad left at around eight. They were tired, emotionally and physically. It was as though they had aged ten years in a day.

'I had no idea you were this ill,' said Mum before they left my bedside, 'you should have said. We'd have come sooner.'

'I didn't like to make a fuss,' I told her, 'you know I hate that. But I wish I had, I really wish I had. I feel like I'm dying,' I said, turning my head so she wouldn't see me cry. She squeezed my hand. They both kissed me on the forehead and told me they'd be back tomorrow. I tried to wave goodbye but I could only lift my hand a couple of inches. Dad winced and unable to hold himself together any longer, let out a sob as he reached the door. I lay in a half asleep, mostly awake stupor, getting up every hour or more to go to the bathroom and pass blood.

Rolie visited that evening, and was clearly shocked at how sick I was. By soldiering on around him, I'd let him think I had a grip on it. I hadn't, obviously. He was visibly shaken, but it was so good to see him. He gave me a kiss on the cheek before he left, and told me he loved me. I really wished he could have hidden under the bed until lights out and not had to have gone home. By this time, my veins were so weak the doctor couldn't get the needle into the back of my hand. It kept wobbling about, spiking my flesh as it moved. Whilst he was fighting a losing battle of his own, I was being told by a nurse to drink fruity milk based drinks that contained about as many vitamins and minerals as you probably get in the whole of Holland & Barrett. I was asked if I wanted dinner.

'No, I don't,' I said. The doctor gave up.

'Your veins are shot to bits,' he told me, cheerily, and disappeared.

The dietician was back. My parents had brought in some soya milk. Mum had spoken at length to the dietician before they left, explaining that I didn't eat wheat or dairy, and still nobody was taking any notice of anything I said.

'We can get simple meals made up for you,' the dietician had said, 'chicken, pasta...'

'I don't eat wheat,' I explained,' but chicken and vegetables or rice or baked potato is fine. Even just vegetables. Or one vegetable. An egg. Just not pasta or mince, really. Or lamb. Or pork.' The dietician sighed. I sighed, too, because I knew that if I didn't eat pasta for religious reasons (imagine!) then there'd be no problem. It was crazy.

The menu for the evening meal was being read out from a piece of card by a young Nigerian man.

'Lamb jalfrezi,' he said, slowly, stumbling across the second word. 'Fish cakes!' he boomed excitedly, looking around the room in anticipation, as if he was reading out nominations for the Oscars. He continued with gusto.

'Shepherd's pie, ham sandwich, and for dessert, ice-cream, jelly or cheese and biscuits!' I liked his enthusiasm and thought he'd make a great game show host, but I didn't think much of the menu.

'Why am I being offered a curry?' I said to the dietician, 'I'm on the digestive diseases ward, shitting blood. Seriously. A curry? That's the last thing I need.' I turned away, exasperated. When it came to meat, if I didn't know it was free range, I didn't eat it. I didn't need to ask about hospital meat. The very idea of it made my stomach churn.

The dietician sighed, and picked up her clipboard.

'I'll have a word with the kitchen,' she whispered.

I busied myself getting in and out of bed and going to the bathroom, a pattern I would repeat for the next five days. That night, I didn't eat, as nothing that I could eat was offered to me, and I didn't sleep a wink. I was scared. I was in pain. There was so much noise coming from all directions, from patients, from nurses, doctors, machines, even the blinding fluorescent light buzzing above my head. The breakfast trolley slammed through the doors at 6.45am.

'We've got porridge, Weetabix or cornflakes,' said the girl beside the trolley, one hand on her hip, the other adjusting her glasses.

'I've got some soya milk in the fridge,' I explained, 'can you please put that on the porridge instead of proper milk, please?'

'No can do, love,' she replied, already pushing the trolley towards the next patient, 'haven't got time for that.'

The girl handed a plate of toast to the woman in the bed opposite me. It smelled delicious. The woman, who must have been warming up for a national complaining competition, prodded the toast and barked: 'This is brown toast,' she said, 'I wanted white. I can't eat this muck.'

A nurse took the toast away and went off to the kitchen, saying 'don't worry, I'll get you some white.' I wondered why none of the nurses took any notice of me. I lay there for hours until one of them walked past and actually looked at me. I hadn't had anything to eat, because there was nobody to put some soya milk on some porridge.

'Could I have my bed changed, please?' I asked, drenched in my own sweat from the plastic sheets and pillowcases.

'We'll do it in a bit,' she said, and off she went. Everyone else's bed had been changed. I didn't understand why I didn't matter. I sat in the chair while they did the bed, an hour later, wondering why I wasn't being given blood instead of them taking it from me and it spilling out of me. Then I went to the bathroom to wash my face. I managed to have a sit down shower, but was so weak I couldn't stand up afterwards and had to ring for a nurse to lift me out of the chair and wrap me in my towel. I put on a clean hospital gown - I didn't want to wear any of my own because I would get so hot and sweaty and it would have meant Mum having to wash one every time she came to see me, which would make me feel like even more of a burden than I already was, so I flopped about in a one-size-fits-all-if-you're-size-20 gown, my bottom peeking out from the gap in the back. I was losing my insides, my mind and now my dignity. I couldn't read. I tried, but the words on the page just swam in front of my eyes. Mum and Dad arrived at lunchtime, and were pretty aghast to see that I was clearly getting worse, not better, and that I hadn't been put on the drip yet. They felt helpless, and were clearly worried sick. I told them to take a break and come back on Sunday. I cried forever when they left.

I was so tired, yet my brain was fully alert and in panic mode. I couldn't sleep, but that's all I wanted to do. I just stared at the end of the bed for hours and was wide awake when a different doctor came round at 4am to have another go at getting a drip into my hand. It wasn't easy, he said, but he got the needle in.

'You should be much better in a few days,' he reassured me, 'just let the steroids do their stuff,' he said.

What else could I do? I wondered, pulling the plug and heading for the bathroom, the cramps starting up again.

I had more visitors on the Saturday. In fact, it was like Piccadilly Circus around my bed. Emma, an actress and brand new friend I'd met a couple of times through Leo came in, despite the fact that we barely knew each other. She lived just around the corner in Laurence Olivier's old house, no less! Later on, I had a visit from Alice and her husband, Ryan. I'd met Alice at the internet company I had struggled to get to in London. She also lived in Brighton and we got on like a house on fire. Again, we weren't close friends - I'd only just met them both - but here they were visiting me in hospital like long-lost siblings armed with flowers. I had six vases around the bed. Sometimes the flowers got in the way of the nurses when they came to administer my drugs and so they'd move them out of the way. I'd find I couldn't see them because I couldn't turn my head to look, I was so weak. I kept meaning to ask them to move them on to the other table, but I only ever remembered once they'd gone. They were so busy that I don't think they'd have had time to actually hear the question. I still hadn't eaten anything.

Rolie had looked terrible when he came in that evening armed with a bunch of red roses. He told me he wasn't sleeping without me.

'I'm worried about you, baby,' he'd said, stroking my arm, moving his chair as close to the bed as he could.

'I'm a bit worried about me too,' I whispered, trying to force a smile. He kissed me on the forehead, then the lips, then on my cheek. He just sat and stared at me. He was staying at my flat, just five minutes' drive from the hospital. He told me he was sleeping on the sofa as he couldn't bear to be in the bed without me. That made me feel so sad I started to cry. I wished he could have stayed next to me all night. I looked forward to his visits so much, and he always gave me a big smile, even when I knew that he was terrified of what he was watching unfold in front of him. He left at 9pm, kissing me goodnight and just like Dad, got as far as the door before I saw him raise the back of his hand to his face and heard him let out a sob.

At regular intervals, amidst the chatter from the nurses, the bright lights above each bed which they would insist on keeping on throughout the night, the shouts from the elderly patients, the snoring and the deafening sound of the nebulisers, I would slide from under the covers, unplug the machine, put my feet into my slippers and stagger to the bathroom. I'd push the drip stand through the door first, somehow keeping the lead and plug balancing over my shoulder so I didn't have to bend to pick it up again on the way out, and there, upon the toilet, I would sit, in agony, shoulders hunched, my head between my knees, shivering and shaking with cold until I had passed another few millilitres of thick, red blood. I would wait a few minutes before getting up, because if I rose too quickly I would pass out. It had happened before and I had told a nurse how dizzy I'd felt but she'd just smiled an 'oh well!' kind of smile and that was that. I don't know if she didn't hear me properly or she just didn't care. I would stagger to the washbasin, run my hands under the hot tap - well, just the fingers of my right hand because the needle took up most of my hand - dry them on a paper towel which would scratch my hands and go back to bed, plugging the machine back in so it could continue to pump my body full of steroids which were slowly reducing my bone density, wasting my muscles and clearly not doing what they were supposed to be doing - making me better.

Opposite and beside me, propped up in their beds by a bundle of pillows, old women chatted away amongst themselves. Their husbands, daughters, sons and grandchildren would drop in with flowers, sandwiches, chocolates, crackers, new nightgowns and magazines, some with crosswords on the front; one lady read a lot of gardening magazines and instructed her husband which bulbs to purchase so that she could see them come up in spring. I lay uncomfortably in bed, my back stuck to the pillow with sweat, my hands freezing cold outside the sheet reaching for some water which I would slowly sip, frightened to consume anything which might cause my stomach to spasm and force me out of bed to the bathroom. I'd become frightened of my own body.

At one point I was connected like an overloaded extension socket to three drip stands. One contained blood - at last doctors had decided it would be a good idea to pump some back into me instead of just taking it out - the others a concoction of potassium, vitamins and nutrients and hydro cortisone steroids. I was not getting better, I was getting significantly worse. I lay there all day, just staring in front of me, wondering why nobody seemed to care. I may as well have been at home on my own than in a hospital. It didn't make sense. It was as if I was on a ward after having my appendix out or something, like I was OK and would go home soon. This was back when you weren't allowed to have a mobile phone in hospital, so I had no way of calling my parents or Rolie, and it didn't occur to me to ask for a TV, either.

My parents arrived on Sunday afternoon and pointed out, a bit too politely for my liking, that I seemed to be getting worse rather than better, and asked if I had seen a doctor over the weekend. The nurse replied that she had paged a doctor twice on Saturday evening because I was deteriorating but none of them had responded because 'they were backed up in A&E.' Mum was clearly shocked at her answer, but in her current state of mind, didn't push it. She regrets not making more of a fuss, but at the time, I think she wanted to trust that the doctors knew what they were doing. I felt completely invisible. I thought I would just slowly die and nobody would notice, then they would come in and say, 'um, she appears to be dead,' and they'd just say, 'oh dear!'

On Monday morning the doctors did their rounds. One, who I'd not seen before, decided that I didn't look 'very well'. I summoned enough energy to sarcastically reply with 'Really? Are you sure?' and raise one eyebrow. He started me on a drug called Cyclosporin, a stronger version of the intravenous steroids. He looked a bit worried, but that was it.

'You'll be better in a couple of days,' he said, pulling the curtain open again and ushering his sidekick out of the cubicle.

'That's what they said on Friday,' I muttered. He disappeared. I wished people would leave my curtain closed, so that at least if the nurses weren't going to acknowledge me, I might as well have some privacy.

Rolie came in to see me on Monday night after work, just as he did every night. I had nothing to do but anticipate his arrival and he'd pretty much turn up like clockwork at 7pm, after he'd had his shower and some dinner. I'd watch that clock like my life depended on it, which it did, I suppose. I heard him arrive when I was in the bathroom. He'd obviously gone to my bed, and when I wasn't there, he said to the lady opposite my bed, 'Where's my beautiful girl disappeared to? She's not done a runner, has she?'

I tried to call out to him as I heard him walk past the door but I don't think I managed it. The back of my head hurt. I must have passed out. My hospital gown was bunched up around my thighs and my drip stand, miraculously, was still standing. Finally I managed to lift my arm high enough to press the help button. It rang and rang. I heard his voice outside the bathroom.

'Are you OK, baby?' he enquired, sounding worried.

He called the nurse. They unlocked the door.

'Shit, baby' said Rolie when he saw me on the floor. He knelt down next to me, cradled my head in his arms, and picked me up under both arms until I was on my feet. He said later that my eyes 'were in the back of your head, all wonky'. He scooped me up and cradled me to his chest, asking the nurse to walk behind him with the drip stand.

'I've got you,' he whispered. He carried me back to bed.

As he leant over and kissed me on the forehead I felt a tear hit my cheek. I thought it was mine but I wasn't crying and I looked up and his whole body was shaking and the tears were pouring down his face as he tried to hold himself together. I reached out for his hand and took it, told him to sit down. He took my hand in both of his. He has strong hands, workman's hands.

'Hands that graft,' he always said.

He leaned on the bed, his head resting on top of my hand on top of his. His head shook slowly from side to side. He sat up.

'I love you so much,' he said. 'What are they doing to you? Why aren't they making you better?'

'I think I'm some kind of experiment,' I whispered, each word sapping what little strength I had, 'I think they've got wagers on how long I'll live when I'm not eating or drinking a thing but something keeps on coming out from me. I think I'm caving in. It's my insides. They're disintegrating. That's what's coming out,' I said, turning my head away from him, letting the tears fall. He sat there for an hour, stroking my arm, dodging the tubes and plasters and needles, telling me he'd cleaned my flat, had his dinner, and had a good day at work. That Sainsbury's was so busy he left without buying anything. That he couldn't remember what he needed anyway. He said he'd ring my folks when he got back to my place and let them know that I was getting worse.

'I'll tell them to come in tomorrow,' he said.

At 9pm he got up to leave.

'OK, baby,' he smiled, putting on a brave face. 'I'd best be off. It's closing time. Last orders for a kiss,' he laughed, and held my hand to his lips. He stroked my cheek, traced my lips with his thumb. One of the old ladies watched from the other side of the room. He kissed my lips. They were starting to feel sore. The skin was cracking. I was falling apart. 'I'm falling apart,' I said, 'you'll have to make me into dog food.'

He bit his lip. 'I'll see you tomorrow night, my angel,' he whispered.

On his way out he said goodnight to the old ladies.

'Goodnight, Rolie,' they said in unison. They liked him too. 'He makes me feel young,' said one of them to me as he left. 'It's his hair. Reminds me of Elvis,' she giggled, nodding at me.

'I know,' I whispered, but she didn't hear me.

Occasionally I would meet the gaze of one of the ladies and sometimes they would smile at me, other times look straight through me. They would whisper about me, wondering why I was on the same ward as them when they were all seventy or eighty years of age, riddled with unexplained lumps and bumps, digestive disorders which come with old age. What's wrong with her? Have you seen her boyfriend? He's always here. Doesn't she have a lot of flowers? That must be her mum. Her dad looks tired. On and on the whispers would go, and I would be too tired to satisfy their curiosity or even look in their direction.

Sometimes I would hear the nice, uncomplaining lady in the bed opposite the bathroom tell the nurse that I had been in the toilet for some time and that she was a bit concerned. Would she check that I was OK? Then there would be a knock on the door. 'Juliette? Are you OK?' the nurse would ask, and I would reply, barely audibly, 'Not really,' doubled up on the floor, shivering on the cold tiles, my head in my hands, and then she would wait a second or two. 'Press the button if you need me,' she'd say, before tending to another patient who wanted more butter on her toast, or a pillow fluffed up. There was no clock in the bathroom but sometimes I would look at the clock at the end of the ward as I set off to the bathroom and I would often not make it back to bed within half an hour. On the worst days, just as I would be climbing back into bed, teeth chattering, hands shaking, I would be gripped with the sudden, overwhelming pain in my stomach and know that it would start all over again.

When the now familiar sound of the tea trolley being shunted through the ward door startled me at 6.45am, I thought I might have been asleep. I hadn't been. I'd last looked at the clock at 6.20am. Before that I looked at 5.45am. Before that, I remembered, I'd stared at the ceiling for a while, been to the bathroom and had begun to write down on a chart how many times I was passing blood. I leaned towards the end of the bed and picked up the piece of paper, the pen dropping to the floor as I pulled up the covers. I'd started writing it down at 11pm. Almost exactly on the hour, every hour, sometimes on the half hour as well, I'd gone to the bathroom. My last entry was made at 5.45am. The description of what left my body ranged from 'thick, dark red blood' to 'a lot of horrible green stuff' and at one point I'd simply written 'Dead stuff. Is anyone reading this?'

It was Tuesday morning, 7.15am. I'd been in this bed since Thursday. I hadn't eaten for five days. Nobody seemed very concerned about my health. Nurses were still ignoring me, still leaving me in sweat-ridden unchanged sheets, not asking if I'd eaten anything, not bringing me fresh water. All they did was take my blood pressure, in silence, then walk away. If I asked for something – my bed to be changed, to have some help going to the bathroom so I could wash myself, they said, 'We'll do that in a minute,' but never reappeared.

I so badly wanted a bath, but the room with the bath in it was really for disabled people, and despite me saying that I'm sure Mum would give me a bath when she came in, the nurse said no. Apparently I could have a shower if I wanted to, but I could only use one hand to grab the soap or shampoo my hair as the other was attached to the drip stand, so doing this on my own, when going to the toilet was so difficult, wasn't going to be fun. With the tube snaking its way around me, and the needle dragging underneath my skin, it was painful just to move my right hand. I slipped off my gown, sat on the plastic chair in the shower and turned it on to warm. I managed to put the shampoo bottle between my knees and get the lid off, and pour it into my hand, kind of with my knees. Don't ask. I rubbed it in my hair as best as I could and then rinsed it out by simply sitting there for another couple of minutes. It took all my strength to stand up and dry myself - all with one hand - and then get the towel to my head. I was so exhausted I couldn't brush it, so it clung to the back of my neck in wet knots. I was in tears by the end.

By the time I'd got myself back into bed, the other patients' sheets had been changed and I could smell the beginnings of lunch, a pungent mixture of lamb curry, macaroni cheese and the sickly sweet aroma of rice pudding, all with the ever present smell of disinfectant and used disposable toilet trays which gathered in the bathroom. They were never cleared away, just left on the floor. I had to step around them to go to the toilet. It was as disgusting and unhygienic as it sounds. No wonder the hospital had a horrendous outbreak of MRSA just months later. I'm surprised the bathroom alone didn't finish me off.

The doctors did their rounds at 11am. I asked if they would care to look at my distended stomach, pulling the sheets down to my thighs and saying, 'it's a bit big, don't you think?'

There were a few worried looks. After much prodding, one suggested I have an X-ray. I looked eight months pregnant. He prodded me again. It hurt. I told him I felt as though I was going to burst.

He told me they'd send me down to X-ray soon. I went back to the bathroom, barely able to drag myself out of bed. I wobbled on my feet, and slowly made my way to the toilet. I closed the door behind me, pulling my drip stand in and sat on the toilet. I was so thin now that sitting on the toilet actually hurt. I closed my eyes, and just waited for the inevitable cramps and blood. A few moments later I heard Mum's voice as she walked past the door. This was beginning to be a habit, people turning up and me being busy.

'She's not in bed, Charlie,' I heard her say, 'she's probably in the bathroom.'

My head was spinning. Eventually, supporting myself with my arms, I slowly lifted myself off the toilet, pulled up my knickers and pulled down my nightgown and opened the door. As it swung open I fell to my hands and knees. I actually crawled towards my bed, dragging the drip stand behind me. Mum took one look at me and ran towards me to help me up. Dad took my other arm and they got me back onto bed. I couldn't even speak. My head fell to one side and I struggled to focus on them as everything became a blur.

I could feel the tears rolling down my cheeks. I just sat on the bed, slumped forward, too weak to sit up.

I don't think they knew what to do. The nurse passed by them, and according to Mum, 'glanced at you and kept walking.' Mum went over to her and interrupted her with another patient. She told her I was in a dreadful state, and asked why nobody was doing anything to help me.

'They've seen Juliette,' she replied, 'she's going to X-ray in a while,' she said, smiling that fixed smile that a newsreader does just after they've reported an earthquake which has killed millions. She clearly wasn't even going to speak to them, nor check on me. I was dying. I knew it. My parents knew it. I'm sure the nurse would have known it too if she'd bothered to look at me.

The porter arrived with a wheelchair to take me down to X-ray at 4.30pm. Mum made sure the yellow blanket covered my bare legs and Dad pushed the wheelchair, before soon realising that he had more control if he pulled it behind him. My head lolled from side to side whenever we went over a slight bump.

'She's so ill she can't hold her head up,' whispered Mum, as though I wasn't there. 'I know,' replied Dad, 'I know.'

After some difficulty in actually getting on to the X-ray table, I was zapped.

'Is there any chance you might be pregnant?' asked the radiologist.

'Yeah, with an alien baby or the son of Beelzebub,' I said.

We waited outside for 20 minutes until the films were handed to me by the radiologist.

'Just take it straight up to the ward, Juliette,' she said, giving me a sympathetic smile, 'one of the nurses will give it to the doctor.'

I nodded and off we went, back out into the bowels of the hospital, along an outdoor walkway – it was November, so it was freezing – and back in to the Millenium Wing where the Digestive Diseases ward was situated. It was a fair old trot, so I had time to peek inside the envelope. As Dad pushed my wheelchair through the swing doors I took the sheet out of the envelope and held it up to the light with both hands.

'I think that's my colon,' I said, turning to look at Mum, 'or else I've eaten a pillow.' I said, and as I put it back inside the envelope I yelped in pain. It felt like something was exploding inside me.

'Mum, it's not good,' I said, trying to turn my head to look at her, 'it feels like I'm about to burst.'

Dad helped me back into bed. Mum held my hand. Alice and Ryan came in at that moment with more flowers, and Dad went to the kitchen to get a vase. I don't remember when Alice and Ryan left I'd, and I'd barely given them a wave when the next thing I knew, the curtain was pulled around my bed by The Nurse Who Wouldn't Look At Me and in came a doctor, someone in surgical scrubs and a very tall man in a pinstriped suit and red silk tie who looked like a cross between the British actors Peter Bowles and Basil Fawlty.

He sat down on the edge of the bed, took my hand and said, quite simply: 'Juliette, darling, you're going to need surgery'.

'Her doctor mentioned that,' interjected Mum, 'but the consultant said she didn't need it when we brought her in.' Said consultant was standing next to my bed, looking like he wished the ground would swallow him up. I wished the same.

'No, no,' said the surgeon, shaking his head, 'Juliette needs surgery urgently. She needs to have her bowel removed.'

Nobody said anything for a moment. Mum gasped. Dad put his head in his hands. I just sat there, and I think I might have laughed. Not because I thought it was funny, but because I laugh when I'm nervous. And I suppose it's normal to feel nervous if you are dying. The surgeon explained that if my entire bowel wasn't removed within the next few hours I would die. Well. For once I was lost for words. I don't think I blinked for a full minute. I might not, he said, preceding his statement with the phrase, 'in all honesty', make it through the night.

CHAPTER EIGHT
'THE NIGHT IS SO LONELY'
GENE VINCENT

The surgeon wanted to operate there and then - it was 6.30pm, Tuesday 6th November 2001 - but he was just on his way home after a hard day with other people's insides when he was shown my X-ray. He assured us that a surgical team would be on hand should I need them, and that he would be called in if necessary. He then paused, before adding, 'we'll get you down to theatre as soon as we can tomorrow. Try and get some sleep, darling.'

He squeezed my hand, gave me a smile, shook Dad's hand and left.

'My little girl,' Dad sobbed, tears streaming down his face, holding my hand so tightly I had to tell him to let go because it hurt. Mum was stunned. We all were. Alice and Ryan came back in and Mum told them the news. Alice started to cry and came over to give me a gentle hug, and stroked my hair, kissing me on the cheek. She pressed her lips to my face and really gave me a kiss. I didn't think about it at the time but it was clearly going through her mind that this might be the last time she'd see me. Obviously I didn't feel much like chatting about the weather so they left pretty swiftly, promising to come back in as soon as I was back.

Rolie came in later and Dad told him what was going on. Mum was holding us all together as she always does. I don't know how she does it, but she does.

Mum was the calm one when they drove me to hospital just before Christmas, and it was she who somehow stayed calm 20 years ago, when our cat, Whizzy, had leapt at me from my lap and scratched my eyes. I had flung the cat off me and run screaming up the stairs to the bathroom. Mum was in there bathing my brother who was six months old at the time. She opened the door upon hearing my blood-curdling scream, just as I had reached the top of the stairs. There I was, holding my hands over my face, blood pouring down through my fingers. What a nice surprise that must have been. Mum took a sharp intake of breath then simply asked me what happened.

'Whizzy scratched my eyes!' I wailed, stamping up and down.

Mum had hauled me into the bathroom, got Dad to get Jonathan out of the bath and into his little play suit and considering what a sight I must have been, calmly prised my trembling, bloody hands from my face, grabbed my flannel and gently wiped my eyes. Fortunately, the blood was coming from underneath my eyes, but Whizzy had scratched the surface of the eye as well. Mum cleaned the blood from my face and hands and lay me on the bed - I recall I was wearing a mustard coloured jumper and brown dungarees (it was 1981 after all) - and she put my duvet around me as I was in shock, and shaking like crazy, while she got Jonathan into his cot and found the car keys for Dad. See? My eyes are bleeding and we don't call an ambulance (this is probably why I never bothered calling one all these years later either).

Dad and I set off for the hospital. I had a gauze pad squashed against my eyes on the way to A&E and was too afraid to open them in case I was blind. I was terrified. It turns out that once we got to the hospital, I was sort of OK. Dad was about to park in a No Parking Tow Zone and I had just tried opening my eyes. They still worked. I saw the sign and helpfully said 'You can't park there!' and that was when we both knew I wasn't blind. Hoorah! It turned out that after a tetanus jab in the backside I was able to go home. A thorough investigation showed that Whizzy had scratched my cornea and had she ploughed her pesky claws into me another thousandth of a millimetre or something equally ridiculous like that to the left, I would indeed have been blind in my right eye. I remember coming home, having some biscuits and a glass of milk and getting into my pyjamas. I wore a patch across my right eye.

I went to school two days later with the still patch on and despite continuous mickey-taking, felt pretty cool, like a pirate. Whizzy was given less chicken than usual that weekend, which for her must have been punishment enough. I was thinking about all that as I drifted off.

At 10pm, I took a deep breath and told them to go home. They hugged what was left of me, with Mum whispering, 'you're so thin, Juliette, you're so thin,' and drove the 60 miles back to Orpington to break the news to Jonathan. Mum, of course, did some washing and ironing. I've inherited the same bizarre 'domestic control' obsession. When something major is out of your control, such as your daughter dying, there's only one thing to do - seize control of something else. I do exactly the same, cleaning, washing clothes, tidying sock drawers. It's a bit weird, but it gets stuff done. A year or so after this night, Mum would say that she couldn't believe that they drove home in the first place. Neither could I.

'I don't know why we didn't stay at the hospital,' she said, 'or go back to your flat. I can't believe we were so far away. You could have died.'

She says that neither of them slept that night, and I'm not surprised. 'We were waiting for the phone to ring,' she said, 'ready to go at a moment's notice.'

The night staff came on duty and took more blood samples.

'Jesus wept,' I said, 'I haven't got much more left.'

They changed the intravenous drip bags, watched me swallow a couple of paracetamol and swig my mouthwash. I'd had a severe reaction to the antibiotics and developed terrible thrush in my throat and mouth. They took my blood pressure, my temperature and scribbled on my chart. They left the light on above the bed. Even when I closed my eyes it was still bright. My curtain was pulled open, exposing me to the stares of the other patients. I sat up in bed and cried, very quietly, until I started to drift off to sleep. I'd finally been given a shot of something that knocked me out, and not before time. It might well have been a smack around the head with a frying pan, I don't know. With hindsight, I'm guessing the surgeon recommended something fairly strong so that I might get a bit of rest before surgery, as it was pretty obvious that I hadn't been prepared for what was going to happen, and that I was in a state shock.

The nurses came and went on the hour every hour. I didn't say a word. Just went through the motions. Only one of them spoke to me. It was just after 5am. It said 'Lorraine' on her badge.

'You OK, sweetheart?' she asked.

'Not really,' I said, 'I'm pretty sure I'm dying.'

'You'll be alright,' she said, patting my hand. I asked her to pull the curtain over but she didn't hear me, and then it was time for breakfast but now I wasn't allowed to eat even if I'd wanted to.

As I waited for my parents to arrive or for a nurse to tell me what was happening the old ladies started chatting about their Weetabix and their toast while I just stared at the veins in the back of my hands. My skin looked and felt like tissue paper. I was almost sure I'd see the bones if I concentrated hard enough.

What I wanted most of all was a bath and to be able to wash my hair before going into theatre. If I was going to die, I wanted to be clean. If I wasn't going to die, I wanted to be clean now because I wouldn't have much chance of doing it afterwards. I really didn't know what to think. I was so ill I just thought logically, and I wanted to be clean. I hated being in that bed with its plastic sheets and pillowcases sticking to my back and my legs, my hair getting sweaty and entwining itself around the tie-ups at the back of my stupid hospital gown. A Chinese nurse pointed at the red varnish on my toes and shook her head.

'You should take off before operation', she scolded, waving her pen at my feet.

'That's the least of your worries,' I said, lifting up my gown and showing her my belly-button that I'd had pierced in Soho in a moment of madness five years before.

She looked horrified.

'Can't do surgery with pin!' she exclaimed.

'I know. I forgot it was there, I'll take it out,' I whispered, wondering exactly how I'd manage.

She then tutted at my earring, a steel one on the top of my ear which I'd actually forgotten about I'd had it so long, but I couldn't take that out without pliers and frankly, didn't want to, so she clumsily taped it up along with most of my hair and walked off. I thought it was just as well that the nose piercing I'd had a few years earlier had closed up one night of its own accord so she didn't have that to contend with as well.

I asked for some nail scissors to prise open the steel ring on the belly button piercing, and the tiny ball that held it together pinged across the bed and rolled on to the floor. It disappeared under the cupboard and I forgot all about it. I put the ring on the table and stared at my bare navel. 'Now what will I fiddle with when I'm bored or nervous?' I thought.

The nurse told me she wasn't sure what time I would be going to theatre but that it would be around lunch time as I 'hadn't got any worse', and that the surgeon was in theatre removing bits of someone else who'd been rushed in that morning first. OK, she didn't quite word it like that but it was along those lines. I laughed at the irony. Lunch time. Dinner time. It had no relevance for me; I hadn't eaten lunch or dinner in days. Where were Mum and Dad? It was gone 11.30am and they were meant to be here at 11am. I started to imagine that they'd been killed in a car crash and that I might actually die and then if they'd died, only my brother and Pebble the cat would be left. Jonathan couldn't cook, so Pebble would have to look after him. It wasn't good. By midday I was absolutely frantic. When they walked through the door at 12.06pm, I almost cried with joy, but I didn't have the energy. I hugged them.

'Where've you been?' I asked, relieved but also a bit annoyed that today of all days, they were late.

'Traffic was terrible on the M25,' Mum said by way of explanation, sighing and putting her bag on the floor. I pulled the covers back.

'I took out my belly button ring,' I explained, 'it looks crap.'

Mum looked pleased.

'About time.'

She took my hand. Dad got me some fresh water and pulled the curtain across. Mum went off to find out when I would be going down to theatre. Then all of a sudden it hit me - I wasn't just going to have an operation, I was going to have life-saving surgery. Which might not save me. This could be the last time I saw my parents. I wanted to see Rolie, but he was at work. I'd told him not to come. Now I couldn't understand why he wasn't there. Mum and Dad had been through this all before during my heart surgery in 1976 and my odds weren't stacked particularly high that day, so they'd had some practice at this.

They went off for some lunch while I slept. I awoke soon after they'd gone, and sat there contemplating what was going to happen to me. Well, I tried to contemplate what was going to happen to me, but in reality, my head was spinning. I was on a morphine drip by now, clicking the dosage up myself to try and relieve the stabbing pains in my stomach.

The stoma nurse came round while my parents were out and showed me some ileostomy bags. I'd not had to think too much about the difference between a colostomy and an ileostomy at any point in my life until now because I hadn't really been that ill. Even the consultant had rubbished the idea of me needing surgery only five days earlier. It was something I didn't want to think about, but now I had to.

If I was completely honest with myself, I didn't really know what an ileostomy was and hadn't even considered what would happen once my bowel was removed. I wasn't really of sound mind, so it was hardly surprising I had a lapse of logic. Although I had joined a support group for ulcerative colitis sufferers, I skipped over the depressing, horrific side of surgery and other people's problems, never thinking that I'd get this sick. I preferred not to categorise myself as a 'diseased person' and instead as a person who happened to have a disease. Had I started worrying about having surgery or dying, or reading other people's surgery stories, I'd never have got on with my life as I had been. I wanted to think it would never happen to me. That I would just coast through it, sometimes having bad days, sometimes good, and that would be as bad as it got. For a lot of people, that *is* as bad as it gets. For 20% of sufferers, it gets much worse. Now, I was one of 'them'. As I'd not had any real symptoms until this week, I didn't think that it was normal that I should end up in hospital having emergency surgery. It didn't make sense and if anyone with UC is reading this, please don't panic, because it still doesn't. It's *not* normal. You'll find out why I ended up in that state a bit later on.

I later learned that the correct term for my condition was 'toxic mega colon', which means the colon has become dilated. Without surgery, the colon will perforate. The mortality rate in toxic mega colon is 20%, which is high enough to get worked up about. I think 'toxic mega colon' sounds like an autobot enemy in *Transformers*. I imagined Optimus Prime and Bumblebee fighting him and his evil friend, Megatron.

'I'm ill and not prepared,' I said to the stoma nurse, 'which I think translates as ill-prepared. This is mental, I feel sick.'

She explained what would happen. I caught half of it, as I was drifting in and out of a morphine daze. I hated morphine – it didn't make me high as a kite; instead it made me paranoid, panicky and nauseous. I'd close my eyes and see demonic faces, I'd open my eyes and they'd still be there. And I'm not talking about the nurses. Still, the panic was mildly preferable to the agony I would be in without it.

'An ileostomy is formed from an opening in the tummy to one side of the belly button, about an inch lower. You will be having a total colectomy, which means that your entire colon is being removed and thrown in a bin rather than merely a section of it.'

OK, I think I added a bit to that, but that was the general gist of it. When people have a colostomy bag it means they have had a section of their large bowel (colon) removed. This is usually in cases of bowel cancer, or a blockage. When the entire colon is yanked out, like a long string of sausages, the insides which poke out of your outsides is actually the tip of your small intestine (ileum), the one which goes straight from your stomach to your colon. The difference is pretty vast – an ileostomy means food goes into your stomach, and then almost whizzes straight out of your side because it's not compacted in the colon after it's digested. You're actually getting rid of water, stomach acid and bits of food rather than pooh. With a colostomy, it's formed from whatever is left of your colon (large intestine), so you are actually churning out pooh, but from your tummy. Either way, it wasn't good news. And I only knew all this afterwards, not at the time, which didn't really help matters.

'I don't get how your insides can sit on your outsides. I don't want to see it, I don't want it on me,' I whispered, panicking.

'It'll be OK,' said the nurse, 'we just have to get the site correct so that when they do the surgery, it's in the right place for you.' I glanced at the bed, at the bags.

The bags. My God, they were a horrific sight. Because nobody had been prepared for this, least of all me, the stoma nurse (who incidentally didn't have a stoma, but should have, because then she might have understood the horror and shock of it better) hadn't brought along any 'girl sized' bags. I had what I would call 'fat old men's size'. And they were big, ugly, typical NHS constructions, like deflated, flesh-coloured balloons. Some were so big they would have covered my entire stomach I had lost so much weight. They were the same size as my head. I almost retched when I saw them. The stoma nurse asked me where I wore my jeans so that she could determine where the stoma should be formed.

'I haven't really got a waist,' I explained, 'I wear jeans on my hips.'

She winced and looked away quickly, but I knew what she was thinking. 'You'll still be able to wear those things,' she said, avoiding eye contact, and pulling aside my gown to mark a black cross in marker pen just to the right of my belly button so that the surgeon could see where to position the stoma.

'It looks a bit low,' I said, rubbing the cross.

'It's difficult to position,' the nurse explained, 'because normally we'd visit you at home before the operation and talk you through everything. We'd get you to wear your normal clothes so that we could work out where it should be so that you could do things up around it. In fact, you'd even have some counselling to talk it through so that psychologically you're prepared for what will happen. Like this, with you lying down and in hospital gowns, and having lost so much weight, it's more difficult.'

'You've got that right,' I said, staring at the ominous black cross on my stomach. I felt like I was being marked with the sign of the bubonic plague. That's what my disease had become - a plague. It was destroying my life and the lives of others around me.

I felt a tear slide down my cheek as the nurse handed me a pamphlet with pictures of an old couple laughing their heads off as they cycled along a leafy lane. Inside the pamphlet they continued to jump for joy as they walked their golden retriever. They appeared to be ecstatic at having half their insides removed and the opportunity to empty a bag from their stomach each day. Hallelujah!

'You'll be free of all the rushing to the toilet,' said the nurse, folding the bags and standing up to leave, 'and you'll be able to live a normal life, do everything you did before,' she explained.

'But I didn't have my insides poking out of my stomach before. I didn't have to imagine a life like this before. In fact, I never had to rush to the toilet until this week,' I said, turning away, wondering how on earth it had come to this. 'I was managing just fine, so I'm sorry to be on a downer, but I'm not getting any positives out of the fact that I'm dying.'

If you broke your arm and some bone was poking out, it'd get put back in, right? Nobody would expect to see bones poking out of someone's arms or legs, so how come I was going to have my intestines poking out of my stomach? I was horrified, and working up to a real panic yet all the while, so exhausted and dreadfully sick that I wasn't sure I even cared what happened anymore. Did I even want to live, with this monstrosity constructed upon my body? With something that everyone thinks only happens to old people? I wasn't sure if I did. Here's   an extract from the pamphlet. Don't read it if you're about to eat your dinner.

'An ileostomy is part of you. Your bowel needs to be diverted away from its usual route and out onto your abdomen. This means you will no longer sit on the toilet to open your bowels as your bowel motions and any wind will pass into the bag. The consistency of the motion will be a mixture of bowel liquid and semi-solid motion with some wind (still keeping up?). However, you will still be able to pass urine in the normal way. Your ileostomy will be on your abdomen, usually on the right of your belly button. Its size and shape will vary, but within a month or two it should be about the size of a 50p piece or smaller. Its normal colour is pinkish red and it may not be round. It is usually referred to as a stoma - it will always be moist and may bleed if touched, and is similar to the inside of your mouth. It will protrude a few centimetres from your abdomen.'

Sounds great, doesn't it?

Mum and Dad came back in to find me in tears. I'd put the pamphlet on the chair. Dad picked it up and raised his eyebrows.

'See how nice it is to have a stoma?' I said, pointing at the leaflet, 'if I was two hundred years old, I might be as delighted as the people on the front of the leaflet. As I'm 29, I'm less thrilled.'

Mum put the leaflet in her bag. They exchanged glances but ignored me. They'd been to a cafe in Kemp Town, a lovely little spot in Brighton just down the road from the hospital.

'The eggs and bacon were lovely. We told the waitress what we were doing there and she wished you well. You'll have to come and have your favourite there when you're better.'

'Egg, beans, chips, a slice of bread and butter and a cup of tea,' I whispered, smiling at Dad. He took my hand. A few seconds later the nurse came in to tell me they were ready for me in theatre. Emma then appeared unexpectedly, popping in with more beautiful and extravagant flowers. It looked like she'd gone to Hawaii to pick them herself.

'What's going on, Willsy?' she said, plonking herself down on the bed, 'you look bloody awful. What's happening?'

Dad told her she was just in time to say goodbye before I went to theatre. Emma was an actress.

'Not your kind of theatre,' I joked, 'hospital kind of theatre.'

'Eh? What for?'

'I'm about to pop,' I told her, fighting back the tears and giving her hand a feeble squeeze, 'and I might not come back, so give me a cuddle now'. She started to cry. I didn't know what to do any more.

'We'll be here when you get back,' said Dad.

'If I don't make it,' I said to Emma, 'take the flowers back and get a refund.'

Dad wiped his eyes with the cuff of his blue shirt. He looked exhausted. All this driving wasn't doing him any good and I knew full well that nobody would be helping him out at work. He was in a new job as a stock controller at a local engineering firm, and while they understood he had to take some time off to come to the hospital and were hugely understanding and sympathetic, on the days they didn't come to see me he didn't get the chance to relax or take stock of what was happening, he had to go to work. It was an endless round of work and hospital - much like it was when I was having my heart surgery in 1976. It was all too familiar, and it scared the hell out of me. But I made it then, and I hoped I'd make it now. I don't give up without a fight, but at the same time I didn't think I had anything left to fight with. Or, more to the point, the thought which was firmly in my mind right now was that I wasn't sure I wanted to fight for a life I didn't want.

'Mum,' I said, taking her hand, as she reached into her bag for a tissue, 'promise me you won't wait in this place all afternoon. Go out, do something nice then come back. Sit on the beach and have a sandwich. Go and have a glass of wine in the pub. Anything. Just come back and keep a look out for Rolie around seven.'

I got Mum to take me to the bathroom. I didn't have time to have the shower I so desperately wanted before surgery, but then I was hardly well enough to have one anyway. I was so weak I could hardly stand at the sink. Mum held my hips as I bent down to clean my teeth and wash my face. I rinsed the basin - how typical, like cleaning matters at this point - and had one last look at myself in the mirror. I was shaking, both with fear and because I was so hungry and weak. In theatre I reminded the anaesthetist that I needed an extra needle full to put me to sleep.

'I see from your notes that you have problems with anaesthetic,' he said, raising his eyebrows.

'I woke up too early once,' I explained, 'and had to have another dose. It was less than pleasant.'

This had occurred during laser treatment for endometriosis in 1997. I came round with a blood-soaked arm from where they'd panicked and swiftly given me another shot to put me back under while they carried on burning the flesh away from around my womb and bowel. How lovely. I'd actually started to wonder if my colitis had been kicked off by this surgery. I wouldn't have been surprised. I had heard what was going on but nobody believed me then, even when I recounted a conversation back in the ward.

'So what I'm saying is I seem to be a bit resistant. I really don't want to wake up early from this.'

He smiled, patted my hand and moments later, the cold fluid wormed its way into my bloodstream, around my body, and I was out.

I had been born with a hole in the heart which doctors discovered when I was 18 months old. I had to wait until I was four to undergo the surgery to correct it, as it was too risky a procedure to operate any earlier. It was a case of getting on with it, and trying not to do anything too nuts to exacerbate it. Of course, as a toddler, I had no idea what was wrong with me and when I couldn't keep up in races with other kids, or got tired walking with my parents, I just became frustrated.

I had the operation at the Royal Brompton hospital in South West London in 1976, and I was foul to the nurses and screamed at the doctors. I was in for two weeks, was given a 70/30 chance of coming through the operation and scared my parents half to death. I pulled through, of course, or I'd not be writing this; straight after the operation, I defiantly yanked the tubes out of my chest and throat in a rage.

'Get these things off me!' I screamed, pulling at the tubes in my neck and on my chest like some little Hulk child. I remember the room, too. I had to have my arms taped down to the bed to keep me still. I'd pulled a chest drain out, and was quite simply going nuts.

'I know everyone says their kid is a fighter, mainly because nobody wants to say their child is rubbish,' Dad would tell me, 'but they don't come much more of a fighter than that!'

The day after my surgery I was begging to be allowed on a tricycle. The day after that, I was on it, whizzing up and down the hospital corridor as if I'd just popped in to have a mole removed. The day I left hospital it was a crisp November morning. There was something about November I was starting to not like. Dad tells the story now, as I wait to be wheeled down to theatre.

'You dragged me across the road to the park,' he said, 'and insisted on going down the slide. Not the little slide, the big slide. Your mum said, 'But Juliette, you've just had an operation, you can't do that!'

I picked it up from there.

'And I said that I didn't care, that I want to go down the slide.'

And so I did. At the top I remember changing my mind. It looked such a long way down, but it had taken so much effort to climb up it that I couldn't back out and admit defeat, so down I slid, my red coat flapping in the wind behind me, Dad catching me at the bottom. I didn't do it again, but that's clearly the point at which I decided that I had something to prove. I had already registered failure or what I perceived then as weakness just not being an option. What a weird kid.

Mum and Dad went to the canteen for a cup of tea once I'd gone down to theatre. Rolie turned up when I was still in there and the three of them sat in the appropriately entitled waiting room and waited. And waited. I was meant to come back to the ward at around 7.30pm. By 9pm, they were getting worried. I finally got up to the ward at 9.43pm. I knew it was later than it should have been because it was pitch dark and all the lights were on. I could vaguely make out their faces as they stood by the bed, Dad to my right, Rolie at the foot of the bed and Mum on my left. Dad stepped forward and I could see the tears in his eyes. He looked terrible. He held my hand and I squeezed it so hard it hurt my stomach. He laughed.

'Ouch! She's just squeezed my hand really hard,' he said. I tried to speak but I had an oxygen mask on and tubes down my throat and in my nose. My mouth was so dry I couldn't say a word. I motioned for a pen.

'She wants a pen, Charlie,' said Mum, fishing in her handbag. She pulled one out along with a Post-It note. She passed it over the bed to Dad. Trust Mum to have every useful item on earth in her bag. I certainly haven't inherited that trait, unfortunately, and never have anything. No tissues, no pens, nothing.

Dad gave me the pen and held the paper. I couldn't see what I was doing but I wrote, 'they messed up the epidural,' in joined-up, albeit messy handwriting. Dad took one look at the note and shook his head. He told Mum and Rolie what I'd written.

'Oh baby,' said Mum, coming round to hold my right hand. Rolie held my other hand. I took off the mask and tried to speak.

'Don't try and talk now,' she said, 'just relax.'

Dad could see that I wanted to say something. No change there, then. There was a plastic cup with water in it and a lollipop sponge that could be dipped in the water and pressed to my mouth to relieve some of the dryness. Dad did just that with it.

'It hurt,' I whispered.

Mum was crying now, and so was Rolie. I think I was too but I don't remember. Right there and then I just wanted to die. That's why I was so late back up to the ward, but of course, nobody had told them what was happening, that the epidural hadn't been in right, so I had no pain relief, that my blood pressure had gone through the floor and that it had almost killed me right after they'd just saved my life.

My entire colon had been removed, and the ileostomy formed from part of my small intestine. This is what poked out from the right hand side of my belly button, encased in its huge, clear bag. I had a 10-inch scar that started from my pubic bone, and snaked its way around my belly button, finishing at the top of my rib cage. I was left, inside, with what is charmingly known as a 'rectal stump', which means your actual bottom hole (I know there's a medical term for that but it's such a vile word I won't use it) and the inch or so of my back passage just above it. They staple this bit shut, and this is where the most vile fluid ever known to man would escape from four or five times a day – it was post-operative muck, basically. Dead stuff.

I slept that night, on and off, but the next day was horrendous. I couldn't move. I was stuck to the sheets and pillows with sweat. If they didn't put plastic sheets on the bed, I wouldn't sweat so much. If I didn't sweat so much, they wouldn't need to keep changing the sheets! My hair was matted. I had dried blood on my hands around the drips and could feel dried blood and matted hair underneath the plaster that held the tube in my neck.

I had a tube up one nostril and down my throat and an oxygen tube in my nose. I couldn't see properly because I didn't have my glasses on, which made things even worse. I was terrified of looking at what lay on my stomach, but I had to see for myself, had to come to terms with it as quickly as possible, to get used to it. After all, I was stuck with it. I lifted up my gown to see my stomach swollen and bruised, just black and blue from my chest to my groin. I gasped. On the right hand side of my stomach, a few inches from my now most definitely not pierced belly-button, lay the clear plastic bag. In the middle of this bag, which lay flat against my hot, damp skin, I could see a lump of angry red flesh the size of a peeled plum tomato moving around of its own accord. I cannot to this day express how repulsed I was by my own body. My insides on my outside, in a bag, surrounded by black, tar like mucus. It was like a mutant goldfish in a plastic bag at the fairground. I felt like a circus freak. It was indescribably horrifying.

I put the covers back down and let the tears roll down my cheeks. I was too tired to wipe them away.

By midday, visitors were coming in to see other patients. I thought I was in intensive care.

'You are in intensive care,' a nurse told me, 'but on a ward. We can't leave you on your own because we need to monitor you every hour; we need to be able to see you.'

'But it's so noisy,' I croaked.

'Don't worry, they'll be gone soon,' she said. Visiting time on the ward was from midday to 3pm and 4pm to 7pm. Between 3pm and 4pm was supposed to be a 'rest' time, when the nurses did their paperwork and patients had a nap. Fat chance. The old woman opposite me kept shouting about how uncomfortable she was, the other old woman next to me kept complaining about the height of her bed or the temperature of her water and asking what the time was every five minutes.

I was fixed in one position - half up, half down, slightly on one side. I wasn't allowed to lie on my back as apparently it was likely I'd end up with a chest infection through not filling my lungs properly when I breathed. This was easier said than done - I had a tube in my neck on the right side, the ileostomy and its hideous see through bag on the right of my tummy, two drips in my right hand of which the needles dug in whenever my hand was anything other than flat and a container under the bed sheets which drained my stomach fluid on the left hand side, as well as a catheter between my legs which snaked its way under my body and out of one side of the bed, and the fluids drip in my left hand. Oh, and the epidural still in my back so I couldn't lean against that. Getting comfortable was impossible. I couldn't feel anything from my chest to my knees, and my legs were swollen to three times their normal size.

Mum and Dad came in that afternoon. Jonathan came with them this time. I could see that he was horrified at the state of me, terrified by the whole situation and angry at being so powerless to help me. Mum and Dad told me long after that he found it too difficult to see me like that; he really couldn't cope with it and refused to talk about it at home. Meanwhile, I felt guilty for causing him so much stress during his exams. I knew it wasn't my fault, but I couldn't help how I felt, that I was just a burden to everyone.

I'd been here a week. I felt like I was going mad. All the time, visitors came and went. There were kids running about and strangers staring at me. I was right by the door; my curtains pulled open so that visitors keep looking over at me while I blankly stared into space, hour after hour.

All night the old ladies snored grotesquely like walruses and when they did wake up, they would buzz for the nurse at any given moment. I didn't get given my tablets until half past ten so I had to try and stay awake for that and then the nurse comes round to get my bloods done while the *really* old women need oxygen machines to help them breathe which sound like drills going into concrete. I was the only patient under 75. After that it's time for me to have my steroid treatment fed into the tube in my neck, the cold liquid passing through my veins, and all the lights are on all the time, even right over the bed. Then it's bloody breakfast at 6.45am, but I'm still not able to eat. I'm pretty sure sleep deprivation through continuous noise and light along with starvation is a punishable offence. Even the FBI isn't allowed to do that to terrorists, yet the NHS has no problem with it. Then, when you are permitted to eat, they feed you inedible muck with zero nutritional value. How the hell are you meant to heal when your body is on high alert 24/7 and you're being fed worse food than prisoners are being given? It makes no sense at all, but it does need a major re-think. It's insane.

I watch the clock for half the night - the other half I'm turned on my other side where I can't see the clock. None of the nurses or doctors thought to prescribe me sleeping tablets. I had asked for some Diazepam to calm me down as I felt as though I was in a permanent state of panic. I described the feeling to Emma, when she came to visit.

'You know when you step out in front of a car and just miss getting hit and you get that split second of panic?' I said.

'Yeah, I know what you mean.'

'Well I feel like that, except that split second is constant. My heart is going nine to the dozen, whatever that means. I feel like I'm going to explode.'

People turned up to see me with flowers and chocolates. The flowers were nice but I thought bringing me chocolates was a bit daft. I still wasn't even allowed a sip of water. Mum took the chocolates home and looked for more vases. Someone had left a copy of *Glamour* magazine on the bed. Days later I'd flick through it, all I could see were photos of bare midriffs, perfectly toned and bronzed, celebrities with their perfect bodies, how if you weren't already perfect, you could be if you followed their advice. I gave it to Mum to take home. It had no relevance to my life and I suddenly thought how shallow and superficial and pathetic fashion and beauty magazines were. I didn't want to look at another one as long as I lived. A headline screamed 'Bags to die for!' and I didn't know whether to laugh or cry. I'd certainly got one of those.

That evening Alice turned up. She was still working in London and had left early to see me, all wrapped up in scarves and gloves and carrying a load of work with her as she'd jumped in a cab straight from the train station. I was so pleased to see her. Her visits meant so much to me. She always managed to say the right thing, or not say anything when she didn't know what to say. I told her God had sent her to me so that she'd be here when all this was going on. I don't know what I'd have done without her.

She held my hand and kissed me on the cheek.

'Hello baby,' she said softly, 'how are you doing?'

Mum and Dad came back from the cafeteria at that moment. Dad took Alice to the kitchen along the corridor to get a vase for the tulips she'd brought in. She would tell me weeks later that as Dad was filling the vase with water, he'd broken down in tears.

'I wish I could take her pain,' he told her, 'I just wish I could make her better.' Alice had given him a hug and she too was crying. I was in such as state of shock - but an almost calm, eerie, 'so what?' kind of shock that it hadn't hit home yet how close I'd come to dying. Rolie came in that night. He looked terrible.

'Blimey, you look as bad as me,' I said, 'have you had any sleep?'

'Nah, not really,' he said, putting on a big smile and squeezing my fingers, rubbing the back of them to warm them up. 'I've been on the settee in my house. I don't like sleeping in my bed without you just like I couldn't sleep in your bed without you. I can't stop thinking about it all. I wish there was something I could do to help you, baby.'

'Me too,' I said, 'although you do look very handsome so that's good. Things are bad enough without having an ugly boyfriend.'

He gave a hearty chuckle, throwing his head back and smiling at me. He moved all the tubes out of the way as best as he could and gave me a kiss on the cheek. He pulled his chair closer to the bed and held me.

'How can you bear to come near me? I'm hideous, like a soggy worm.'

'Don't be daft,' he whispered, 'you're not a soggy worm. I love you. You'll always be my beautiful baby.' What a trooper, eh?

That was when I decided to see if he really could take it. I'd not shown him my stomach, the bag, all the blood stained dressings. I'd had the covers pulled up to my chest all the time, almost as if I was trying to hide it all from myself, that if I couldn't see it, it didn't exist. As I lifted my gown, the bed covers caught the tube in the back of my right hand, the needle dug into my flesh and I gasped in pain. Rolie lifted up my gown ever so slowly, moving the tube that came out of the side of my stomach at the same time, and looked at my tummy. The bag sat clumsily on the right side of my stomach, the clear plastic holding what was left of my stomach contents and old, dead blood. It wasn't a pretty sight.

My abdomen was so purple and swollen I looked as though my body had been dragged from a river where it'd been rotting for a fortnight. There were bandages and dressings and stitches everywhere. Dried blood was caked around the tube protruding from my left side. He winced, but he didn't throw up all over me, which I took as a good sign.

'It's old stomach lining, I informed him, 'how disgusting is that?'

He flinched, rubbing his face with his hand, then put his forehead on the back of my hand so I couldn't see his expression. I didn't really want to. I pulled the covers back up and he lifted his head and kissed my hand.

'Don't think about it. I'd best be off,' he said, stroking my hair and leaning over to kiss me on the cheek once more.

'I'll see you later, baby.' He rubbed his chin again. He only ever rubbed his chin like that when he was worried. All I could think of as I lay there, staring at the clock, was that he'd be better off without me.

CHAPTER NINE
'WAKE UP ALONE'
AMY WINEHOUSE

By Sunday I was feeling worse, not better. I had been out of theatre for three days but was still only allowed to sip water, enough to moisten my mouth, but I couldn't gulp it and I was so thirsty. All I felt was despair, and the most desperate longing to be out of there. I still hadn't slept a wink, either. I was being offered breakfast by the kitchen staff even though I wasn't allowed to eat anything, which drove me mad. I still had to watch old ladies eat their toast and drink their tea, had to endure the waft of both nice kitchen smells (breakfast) and awful kitchen smells (anything else) while I hadn't eaten a meal for two weeks, since my soup at Rolie's that Sunday. I was now being fed through a tube, just pure vitamins and minerals but it's not exactly the same as sitting down to dinner, believe me.

The tubes up my nose and down my throat made me feel as though I was choking on a pencil. Constantly. I sounded like a cat with a hairball. Every gulp I took made me wince. I had to ask the nurses to change my catheter bag so many times because somehow, despite the fact that I wasn't drinking anything, I was weeing for England and scared that the bag by my bed would burst and my pee would go everywhere, particularly all over my visitors' shoes. The container which was shaped like an accordion at the end of the drip attached to my stomach was full of green bile, and rested against my side exactly where I would have put Panda. He'd been through it all before when I had my heart operation, so he was used to seeing me filled with tubes and covered in weird hospital stuff. He had to sleep on the pillow on the chair next to the bed and I'd just lie there for hours, propped up by the pillows and their plastic covers that brought me out in a sweat within seconds, whispering to him.

'Panda,' I whispered, 'tell your nanny and granddad that you want a few nights off. Go home with them, watch some TV.'

I swear he said 'No! I have to stay here with you!' and I reached out and touched his little arm. I'd had enough. I couldn't do this anymore.

I didn't know how to just let go, to not pretend I was OK. I'd never given in to anything before, never let anything beat me, but this was getting the better of me. I was exhausted. I've always thought that vulnerability is a sign of weakness, and I can't bear weak people. 'I can't' is just not in my nature, so I simply didn't know how to deal with my emotions, to say that it wasn't fine, it was awful; to admit that I wanted to die because I didn't have the strength or the desire to live. I honestly didn't know how to do it, so the easiest thing to do was to not have to do

103

it, and that meant not seeing anyone who cared about me, anyone I loved enough to spill out my thoughts to. It seemed quite simple at the time, but in retrospect, it was an odd, if not troubling, decision. I don't think anyone expected me to be anything but horrified, afraid and terribly sick.

My parents had the onerous task of calling friends and family and telling them what had happened. Some had found out through other friends and wanted to visit, but I'd told Mum and Dad that I didn't want them to see me.

'It doesn't matter what you look like,' Mum told me, 'they'll be able to cheer you up. Helen is desperate to see you. So is Charlie. She's your best friend. They're very upset you don't want to see them.'

'I can't,' I said, 'I just can't. They can come and see me once I get home, if I ever do. Tell them that. Please. I don't want anyone else to come. You and Dad, Jon, Emma. Rolie. And Alice. That's it. They've all seen me already, they know. Nobody else.'

Mum was exasperated. Jon came in and told me Helen was upset that I wouldn't see her.

'Why will you see me, Willsy, but not Helen or Charlie?' asked Jon.

'I don't know,' I said, and I didn't.

I shut them out because I didn't know how to let them in. I also felt as though I had to entertain people. Seriously. It's kind of what I do normally, but under these circumstances I don't think anyone was expecting my usual jokes and supercilious conversation. I didn't know how to admit I needed support, emotionally and physically. I didn't want to put them through any trouble. I didn't want to upset them or scare them. They'd also have to pay quite a lot for the train and they both lived in London and I thought it was too far to come all this way just to see me. I was trying to protect them, I guess, or at least save them money. I do this all the time. I tell people the complete opposite of what I actually want if I think they'll be better off.

Years later I realised that perhaps I couldn't bear to see them because they were a stark reminder of what I was missing. I should have been going out to parties and gigs with them, wondering what shade of lipstick to wear not wondering how to survive. Seeing them would only slam home exactly how bad things were. I would have been jealous, I suppose. I can't really explain it. I would never be the same again, and I couldn't expect them to understand that, because *I* didn't. I wasn't ready to face up to what had happened – who would be? Does it make any sense? Not really, but I was in such as state I couldn't think straight at all. I felt humiliated, in a way, I think that was it. I was such a wreck, physically and mentally that I was almost embarrassed by it. I felt so vulnerable, so exposed, my emotions as raw as the scars on my stomach. I simply couldn't bear to be seen like that.

That day a couple of the nurses said I should sit in the chair beside the bed. They helped me put my feet on the floor, gathered all my tubes, and sat me on the chair. I flopped down, unable to hold myself up properly. My stomach felt like a ton of bricks was strapped to it. It was so heavy, so swollen. The epidural helped to numb the pain, but I couldn't bear the fact that I couldn't feel anything at all. I couldn't sit up straight, or lie down, or stand up. I didn't know what to do with myself. I just tried to sit up, not fall off the chair and not cry at the sight of my puffed up legs.

I begged one of the nurses to give me another bed bath. She duly wiped me down with my flannel and soapy water, and dried me off. Tubes were moved in all directions as she gently stroked my flannel along my arms, up my legs, and then on my feet. It felt pretty good to be clean in the limbs, if nothing else.

It occurred to me that I hadn't remembered to put my glasses on all this time, so I hadn't been able to see anything properly, which can't have helped my mindset. Still, there was nothing to see anyway. If anyone was coming to talk to me or visit I'd see them by the time they got to the bed and make out whom it was before they sat down. Just. I wondered how straggly my eyebrows had become. For an hour I sat propped up in bed or in the chair, just staring into space. Mum and Dad came in and this time I didn't have much to report.

'I've hardly got anything exciting to tell you. I've not really been out much,' I quipped.

Mum couldn't believe that she'd not reminded me to wear my glasses. She hadn't even noticed, she said. I know now this was perfectly normal for someone who's going through a trauma like that - there is no more 'normal', and habits are broken. They stayed for an hour or so then headed off on their long journey back up the motorway. I missed them so much and couldn't bear the fact that I couldn't go with them. I wished I could have managed without them so that they didn't have to drive 60 miles to see me and 60 miles back. It seemed like such a waste of their time, and such a waste of petrol, but the idea of them not coming in again was unbearable.

It took me back to when I was in hospital for my heart operation. Dad was working all hours at Sainsbury's depot in Charlton, South London, driving after a night shift across London to visit, parking about two miles away from the hospital, coming to see his four-year-old daughter who did nothing but scream blue murder at him for no particular reason then he'd leave, go back home, sleep a while - maybe - and go to work again.

Mum, meanwhile stayed at the hospital for the best part of two weeks and hardly left my side. I can clearly remember the ward and the other patients and I have a picture in my mind of me in this bed, which felt huge and so high up because I was tiny, sitting up in my pyjamas and

Mum telling me she had to go and get some lunch. I started crying, and she gave me her watch. She said that when the big hand got to the six, she'd be back. Half an hour, she said, that's all. It was midday. She gave me a kiss and left the ward and true to her word, was back at 12.30pm. I don't know how she managed to eat anything in that time or even get to the canteen and back, but she did that for two weeks and I still feel guilty to this day that I wouldn't let her leave me. I was a total brat, and Mum says it's hardly surprising because I'd just had major surgery and was cross because I wasn't allowed to ride the tricycle up and down the corridors like the other kids who'd had minor operations. I couldn't bear to be in bed, watching the world pass me by, even at that age.

Now, 25 years later, the same panic would flood through me the minute they stood up to go. I was still their little girl, except this time I had to get through the nights on my own.

Rolie came in later, and I moaned about how annoying the woman in the bed next to me was.

'When the lights go out - or rather one of the lights goes out and all the ones above the bed stay on - she starts banging on about her tablets, like she's the only patient there. Nurse, I need to take my tablets. Nurse, I need some fresh water. Nurse, I need you to make my pillows more comfortable. Nurse, what time do I take these tablets? Nurse, are you coming? Nurse, could you pull my curtain. Nurse, I am going to get out of bed and go to the toilet. Nurse, could you pick up that magazine I've just dropped?

'It's driving me mad. I can't stand it. The woman opposite shouts and screams at her daughter and her grand children run riot around the ward every day, then she shouts some more at the nurses and anyone who'll listen, which unfortunately is all of us as we can't *not* listen. I get left until last every night for tablets and blood pressure and every morning and I don't know why. I get the bloody bed right next to the door so I can hear the doctors and nurses chatting all night and trolleys bumping into walls and hitting doors and just about every noise you can imagine. I have to get out of here. I just want to get out of here.'

I want to cry but there are no tears. I just hold his hand and he kisses me on the cheek. I tell him I had a sort of wash. He looks at me with a mixture of pity and fake excitement.

'Amazing, huh? I mean, at home, I only have, like two baths a day and wash my hair all the time and clean my teeth a million times and paint my toenails and put lotion everywhere, now I'm ecstatic because I had a bed bath. I feel so disgusting. I feel like I'm just rotting away. My hair must be like a wet birds' nest.'

'Baby, calm down. I think you're beautiful. You don't look well, but I still fancy you.' He winked at me. He was doing his best.

'As if! I've got tubes in my side, in my bladder, up my nose, down my throat, a whacking great needle in my spine, a needle in my neck, in my hands, arms like sticks, matted hair, a stomach which looks like it's been savaged by wolves after I've swallowed an air bag and a plastic sack on my stomach with crap in it and a big lump of my insides wobbling around like a lump of jelly.'

'Yeah,' he said, 'and I still think you're lovely.'

He really was something else.

The next morning one of my favourite nurses, Tracey, came over and asked if I'd like to have my hair washed. I thought I'd gone to heaven. Well, hospital heaven. Mum and Dad were bringing my godparents in that day. They'd flown over from Spain. I was obsessed with being clean when people came in and as the clock neared 11am, I started to panic.

'They'll be here soon, Tracey,' I pleaded, 'please can we get me clean?'

'Course we can,' she said.

I couldn't imagine how I would get to the bathroom. It was to my left, about 10 metres away. I'd not had any need or been able to go to the bathroom since the operation. I had a catheter, an ileostomy and I hadn't eaten or drunk anything for over a week. Somehow, Tracey gathered all my drip stands and tubes and unplugged me from the ones she could take out for a little while, and helped me swing my legs out of bed. I couldn't move them myself because they were so heavy and numb due to the epidural. It took forever but somehow she walked me, and all my tubes, to the bathroom. I was sweating like mad with the effort it took just to stand up, and I was doubled over, my stomach so heavy and numb where the muscles had been cut. I had no way of standing straight. I couldn't breathe; I was sweating and shaking.

'Shit,' I whispered, trying to hold my ground, clutching the edge of the basin, 'it feels... it feels like massive wolf has got its claws in my tummy and he's hanging off me.'

'You're strange,' she said, laughing, 'but I know what you mean.'

She decided that the best method for this would be to sit me in a chair at the sink and tip my head forward. I hadn't got the strength to hold it up, so it just kind of flopped into the basin anyway. When the warm water ran through my hair I almost cried with joy. Well, I would have if I hadn't been in such pain where I was doubled over.

'I can't believe I'm having my hair washed,' I mumbled, 'I'm so grateful. I know how busy you are. It's so horrible being all hot and stinky. I'm so happy that I'll have clean hair. Thank you so much.'

She talked about her little girl to distract me from the pain of sitting hunched in the chair, my neck aching as much as my stomach from leaning over the sink.

She poured the conditioner into her hands and rubbed it through my hair. My neck was absolutely killing me by now and my tummy felt as though a whole *pack* of wolves were hanging off it, not just one. I have never been so uncomfortable in all my life, but hey, I had clean hair.

She wrapped the towel around my head and I looked into the mirror, for the first time since my operation. My head was wobbling with the weight of the towel. Tracey took off the towel, patted my hair and left it around my shoulders.

I gasped. I knew I wouldn't look too good, but I was horrified at my reflection. She put her arm around my waist.

'No doubt you've looked better,' she said.

'Just a bit. I look like the girl in *The Exorcist*.'

'No you don't,' she said, 'you look fine.'

She was a terrible liar. I stared into the mirror. The thing staring back at me had black eyes. They were mad eyes, completely devoid of expression, eyes that stared blankly, unblinking, totally still. Dead eyes. I looked like a government warning for the perils of heroin addiction. It was a look of emptiness. I knew that I wouldn't look too clever, but I had no idea I looked as frightful as this. I didn't recognise myself.

My skin was deathly white, but I have to admit, it was so clear, like porcelain. I had cheekbones for the first time in my life. My collarbone protruded from my chest as though it would burst through the skin at any time and my boobs had completely disappeared. You could see my ribs when I turned to the side; my hip bones could have cut cheese.

She helped me back to bed. For the first time since I came in to hospital, I picked up my book and read a couple of pages, but I couldn't concentrate for more than two minutes. The words just swam in front of my eyes. None of what I read mattered. It wasn't real. This was real. And I hated it. I put on a fairly brave face for my godparents, but it was all smoke and mirrors, people, smoke and mirrors.

At night the nurses would move me on to my side, bringing tubes and bags and containers around the bed, tucking tubes behind my ear and the oxygen tube up around my pillow so that I could lay my head down properly. Once I was settled, squashed in between two pillows because I couldn't support my own weight and would roll backwards, I couldn't move again. At all. Only my toes, arms and head. I lay there, sweating against the plastic under sheets and pillowcases, listening to all the noise around me, and then it happened. I felt this hot liquid between my legs. It burned. Something was leaking. I called for a nurse. Her name badge said Lindsay.

'It's alright,' she said, 'it's just fluid from your bottom. It's not much. It happens. Don't worry.'

'I can't lie in it. I'm sorry. I'm sorry, Lindsay,' I said, wondering if I'd ever be able to claw back any dignity. She wiped my bottom and put some paper towels underneath me. I wanted to cry - I mean really, *really* cry - but I couldn't even seem to do that.

It was the following Monday night when I was told I could move to a private room. My own room. My own bathroom. No more cardboard 'potties' full of indescribably vile bodily fluids left on the floor for hours, rotting. A toilet that, if it got dirty, was only dirty with my own dirt. That I could live with. Just. There was even a view of Brighton Pier. It was amazing. I still felt terrible, still couldn't walk, couldn't get out of bed on my own, but I would no longer have strangers staring at me, wouldn't have to worry about not being able to get in the bathroom, would be able to put my things on chairs and around the sink, eventually, without having to move anything. I could even get a proper kiss from Rolie once I had some tubes removed!

Well, the kissing would have to be put on hold. I'd developed an allergic reaction again to the huge volume of antibiotics I was being fed. My tongue was swollen. I had ulcers all over the inside of my mouth and huge, gaping sores on either side of my tongue. It was absolutely revolting, and incredibly painful. My lips became cracked and sore, and blisters lined the outside of my mouth. They would bleed if I so much as smiled, which, I must admit, I didn't feel like doing very often. I could hardly speak. Mum cried when she saw me. I looked mental. I had a green mouth and a crazy, thousand-yard look on my face.

One morning, after I'd had a whole 20-minute snooze, I woke up at 6.30am unable to breathe properly. I felt as though my throat was closing. I couldn't swallow or draw breath. I buzzed for the nurse. Around 10 minutes later someone came in and asked what was wrong. I pointed to my mouth, and tried to say that I couldn't breathe, but I couldn't, probably because I couldn't speak. He broke up some paracetamol and handed me a glass of water. I started to cry, because I couldn't open my mouth to get the tablets down without my lips bleeding and cracking, blisters bursting open. Holding the glass to my lips was agony. I threw the tablets as far down my throat as I could but they sat there. I coughed them back up. The nurse shrugged his shoulders and suggested I try and take them again later.

I sat up in bed, bewildered, struggling for breath as he left the room. I don't know what was happening, maybe it was a panic attack, but I had every reason to panic. Perhaps, because I hadn't slept or rested my brain in so long, my body went into some kind of weird state that when I wake up, it was way behind me and still asleep. Who knows? Even now I can't explain what kind of mental state I was in, other than one of complete shock. All I would do, for hours on end, was stare out of the window, or move the glass of water and tissues around on the tray in front of me. I had several books and a newspaper to read but I never once looked at them, and I love reading. I read cereal packets for fun, I really do. It was as though I didn't even know how to read. I had no interest in anything outside of the room, yet all I wanted to do was get out of it, to escape this hell. But how?

I couldn't comprehend that things were going on around me, outside of the hospital. I was completely focused on those four walls and the thought of anything else happening seemed impossible. It was as though all life had stopped, not just mine. The only sounds I heard were the cars going over the ramp on their way to the hospital car park. Whenever my parents were due in, the sound seemed to intensify, and with each noise, I wondered if it was them. When, 10 minutes later, they hadn't appeared, I knew it hadn't been them, and so it started again. As you can imagine, this went on for some time.

I just wanted it to stop. I needed to sleep. I hadn't slept in almost a fortnight and I wasn't sleeping more than a couple of hours a night before I came into hospital as it was, and now I was on my 12th day. I knew I was going crazy. I wasn't even oblivious to it. It might have been more fun if I had been.

'I feel like I'm in *One Flew over the Cuckoo's Nest*,' I told Rolie that night, even though he had no idea what I was on about. He gave me a kiss on the cheek, between tubes, winced at the sight of my mouth, stroked my hair, which oddly enough looked really great - shiny and lustrous and as straight as though I had ironed it.

'My hair's gone mad,' I said to him as he got up from the bed, 'it's never looked better. Look how shiny it is. It must be because I'm being fed nutrients straight into my blood. I'll have to try that at home.'

He waved goodbye. It was 9.15pm and I felt tired, but I still didn't sleep. I was amazed at how quiet it was. The nurses on the night shift came in occasionally, administered the hydro cortisone steroids through the tube in my neck, the familiar feeling of the cold fluid racing down my neck, then took my temperature, my blood pressure, gave me painkillers. At last I lay in darkness, no fluorescent light beaming down from above the bed. Just the light from the corridor filtering through the room helped me to see where I was, just in case I forgot. The lights on Brighton's Palace Pier flashed in the distance. I stared at the helter skelter. It was so enchanting.

I was, however, so disillusioned and in such a strange mental state that I thought the view was, in fact, a poster. I would watch the lights flashing on and off all night, just my head turned to the right, the rest of my body completely still, numb everywhere else from the epidural. I'd had that feeling now for five days; my legs had swollen up like the legs of an obese old lady. It was a strange sight - a distended, swollen and bruised abdomen, thighs like sticks and legs like a hippopotamus from the knee downwards. My feet were puffy, my toes looked tiny. My arms were so thin that the bones in my wrists stuck out, my shoulder blades could have been classed weapons. My mouth was bleeding, cracked and sore. I couldn't have felt worse. Not a single part of my body was without some kind of problem. It was constantly uncomfortable, painful and exhausting.

As I stared out of the window, I would see the sun come up behind the pier, a beautiful array of reds, pinks and yellows which would turn to a clear blue sky, despite the fact that it was November. The room would become quite warm after a while, and I'd have to ask a nurse to pull the window down an inch or two. At around 2pm I would start to feel the cold. This was my routine. I would then ask someone to shut the window for me when they had a minute and most days, I'd then wait for whoever was coming to visit. I always wanted it to be Mum and Dad; when they couldn't make it Mum always made sure somebody came to see me, ringing my friends the night before and trying to get someone to go in for a while. I could always rely on Rolie in the evening and don't know what I'd have done without him. He coped amazingly well considering we'd only known each other two months when it all happened. He took it all in his stride - some things went over his head completely which might have made it a bit easier - and reassured me constantly that he still loved me.

I'd insist he stayed at home at weekends and go out to the rock 'n' roll clubs and have a drink or six for me, but I knew it wasn't the same without me as for a start, he didn't have me to dance with. I developed a guilt complex about how much time I took up in Mum and Dad's and Rolie's life and would tell them to stay home and not visit, but deep down I would just lie there wishing that they could be there every second of the day and every time they left, I felt utterly abandoned, and terrified.

On the Thursday evening, two weeks after I had come into hospital, Emma walked in the room followed by Leo, laden with all sorts of potions: moisturisers, shampoos, cooling leg gels, cleansers. She asked if I wanted her to rub my legs, if they were sore.

'They're just swollen and horrible,' I said. 'My feet are a mess. Everything's overgrown. I need a gardener.'

She lifted my legs on to her lap, one at a time, and gave me a foot rub and a massage for the next half an hour.

'You should be getting physio, shouldn't you?' she asked.

'You'd think so considering I'm now getting bed sores I've been lying here so long and I can hardly move.'

Emma sat in the corner and we chatted about anything other than what was happening. She asked if I'd been able to sleep. I didn't answer her. Instead I looked away and started to cry.

'I've had enough, Em.'

'What do you mean?' said Emma, while Leo rubbed my foot as though her life depended on it.

'I've had enough. Of this,' I gestured, waving my arm in the air, 'I can't pretend to everyone that I'm OK and that I feel positive and I'm lucky to be alive and isn't it great that someday I might actually get out of this bed and have a shower and stand up on my own and be able to walk and go home and feel like I want to be alive, which at the moment I don't.'

Leo and Emma exchanged worried glances. I would have bitten my lip and tried not to cry but I couldn't bite it because it was covered in blisters. Instead I turned my head to the wall and one measly tear slid down my cheek. It ran cold down my neck.

'Would you like us to tell someone how you feel, get someone to talk to?' said Emma.

'I don't want to make a fuss,' I said.

'It's hardly a fuss,' said Leo, 'we'll go and speak to someone now.'

She and Emma left the room, Leo giving my foot a little squeeze on the way out. Five minutes later they were back, putting their coats on, gathering their belongings, talking about when they'd next come in.

'We spoke to one of the nurses who said they'd talk to the sister,' said Emma, a 'don't-mess-with-me' look on her face. She is very bolshy, in a good way. Leo, too. A short while after they'd gone, the sister came in to talk to me. I was still crying. She held my hand and sat down beside my bed.

'What's wrong, poppet?' she asked.

'What's right?' I said, kind of half laughing, half sobbing.

I explained how I wanted someone to inject me with something to send me to sleep, forever. That every moment was absolutely wretched, that I still hadn't slept, that I watch the sun go down and the sun come up and I don't move in between, I just sat there, unable to turn over or move my own pillows which I'm always stuck to with sweat. That if I were a cat or a dog, I'd be put to sleep and buried in the garden in a cardboard box.

'I wouldn't even mind that. I could rot next to Whizzy, our old cat. She'd look after me.'

She smiled and patted my hands.

'Believe me, Juliette, it will get better. It will. It just takes time. You will get out of here, you know. I've seen people like this, and I've seen them walk out of here a week later. You'll be back to see us in a few weeks and you won't believe how much better you are. Trust me. I know you can't imagine that now but it will happen. You've got so many friends and family and your boyfriend love you very much. They're all here to support you. I'll come and see you tomorrow night, love. I'll send the psychiatrist down on Monday to have a proper chat. Let's get you sorted out with something to help you sleep tomorrow.'

I felt as though an enormous weight had been lifted off my shoulders. I'd finally admitted that I wasn't coping, that the 'good old Juliette' who always pulled through, always laughed about everything, had gone. I was sick of being poked about, prodded, of having my blood taken out of me every day, of being pumped full of shitty medicines and steroids through my neck, sick of having my temperature taken, sick of being handed tablets I couldn't swallow and really, really, sick of doctors bringing round hordes of medical students to gawp at me in the mornings. I felt like a living experiment, and the way doctors treated their patients as 'cases' rather than people is shocking.

'She's a very interesting case,' one of them had said the day before, tipping his clipboard in my direction, pulling back the curtain when I was in the middle of picking my nose and taking a peek under the covers at my stomach. A group of students and this doctor all stood at the foot of my bed, staring at me.

'How are you today?' said the doctor his students surrounding the end of the bed, all false smiles and awkwardness, beaming like they'd just won a two-week all-inclusive trip to Florida.

'Top of the world,' I said, sarcastically.

'Well, nobody wants to be in hospital,' he chuckled.

'I'd rather be put down than be stuck here like this any longer. Can you arrange that? Stick me outside with the clinical waste bags or some laundry?'

He raised his eyebrows. His students took a step backwards away from the bed.

'I'm sick of being 'an interesting case,' I said, mimicking what he'd said. 'I'm not a case, I'm *me*. Actually, I'm not me. That's even worse.' He looked at the other students, his eyebrows raised.

'I see you've managed to lose the catheter,' he said.

'I didn't lose it,' I said, trying to irritate him on purpose, 'someone took it out.'

He talked about me having the epidural out. I said I'd like to get rid of it as soon as possible, that I hated being numb.

'I think I'd rather be in pain - at least it would remind me that I'm alive and maybe my legs wouldn't look like they belong on a baby elephant.'

'Well...' he paused, waving his clipboard, 'I'll speak to the surgeon and see if we can take that out tomorrow. You might be able to get rid of another tube in a day or two. See if we can get you eating some food,' he finished, seemingly oblivious to the fact that my mouth was falling apart.

'Great,' I said, looking out of the window, almost retching at the thought of eating, 'I can't even sip water. Whatever.'

Finally, the epidural came out and my pain was controlled, instead, by codeine and paracetamol. My mouth, however, had still not healed. In fact, it was getting worse. The pharmacist paid a visit and prescribed steroid tablets (oh joy!) that I was told to place on the ulcer.

'*The* ulcer?' I said, incredulously, 'I've got a mouth full of the things.

Where exactly am I meant to put them?'

'Just roll it around your mouth, put one on the outside. Try it.'

She left the room. I'd been given a mouthwash two days earlier which wasn't working, it just stung like hell. I put a tablet in my mouth and rolled it about as best as I could. It tasted vile. I stumbled to the bathroom – now that I'd had the catheter taken out I didn't have a choice as to whether I could get out of bed or not, but at least it gave me something to do. It took around 10 minutes to get out of bed and into the bathroom, and another 10 to get back into bed. I looked in the mirror, and pushed one on to my lip, covered already in Vaseline so it stuck a treat. It kind of foamed up a bit then dribbled down my chin. Lovely. I looked like I had rabies. I couldn't feel it because my lips were so swollen they'd gone numb.

I was sent down to X-ray for an ultrasound a few minutes later. I'd not been out of my room since I was moved and I felt panicky about leaving. A porter wheeled me down, asking if I'd like a blanket to keep my legs warm.

I declined. That was a big mistake. As he propelled me down the corridors of the hospital I felt the breeze from outside, a crisp, cold late November afternoon. I was suddenly terrified, shaking and almost in tears at being taken out of my room. I shivered and pulled my dressing gown around me, praying that he wouldn't trip over a bump and let my wheelchair go. I was, after all, on the top of a very steep hill. The ultrasound was uneventful, thankfully. I never heard any more about it.

It was Friday night when Sam, my favourite nurse, asked me if I'd slept.

'Nope,' I said, 'nor the night before'.

'What? At all?'

'Not a bit. I've shut my eyes for a while, but nothing happens.'

'What's keeping you awake?'

'House prices?' I smiled, 'I don't know, I just feel so panicky all the time, I forget to breathe.'

She considered things for a moment and then said the magic words.

'We need to calm you down, Juliette. You've had a terrible, terrible shock, and it sounds to me as though you're still in shock. Am I right?'

'I suppose that's what it is. I feel bewildered by it all, like I'm watching myself in a film but I don't understand what's going on. I get that a lot with films, though.' I am still making jokes. It's quite incredible.

'I'll be back in a minute,' she said, and she was. With a sleeping tablet.

It was so quiet. I closed my eyes. On my chart, Sam wrote that she had spoken to the psychiatric nurse, and the over the phone prognosis was 'post-reactive depression'.

I took the pill and closed my eyes. Guess what? I still didn't sleep.

CHAPTER TEN
'KNEE DEEP IN THE BLUES'
THE DERAILERS

It was Saturday morning when I finally had the tube I hated the most removed, the one which went up my right nostril and down the back of my throat to my stomach to feed me. Getting the thing out wasn't much fun - I had to take a great big deep breath while the nurse yanked it up through my throat and out of my nostril in about five seconds. It hurt like hell, scraping my throat as it came out, but the relief was amazing.

I no longer had to endure the tube taped to my neck, the plaster across my nose, the tube stretching across my face 24 hours a day. It felt wonderful. Well, as wonderful as I could have felt at the time. I recognised it as a big step to getting out of here. I *had* to get out of here.

I was told I'd have to start eating proper food despite the fact that my mouth was even more covered in ulcers and sores than it was two days before. The staff nurse, Paula, brought in some jelly and ice-cream.

'Is it someone's birthday?' I joked, touching my fingers to my lips to try and keep them from bleeding, whilst pushing the spoon around the bowl. 'Are we playing musical chairs after, because if we are I reckon you'll win. I'm a bit slow these days, Paula.' She shook her head and tutted at me, but she was smiling.

'Eat what you can,' she said, 'it'll do you good.'

I wasn't sure how jelly and sugary dairy would do me good, it wasn't exactly nutritious, but I managed a spoonful, in several stages. I will never understand why hospitals feed their patients such awful food. It's not even food. Firstly, I needed protein to build up my strength and carbohydrates – rice or pasta or potatoes, or even a banana - to give me some energy. Secondly, I had given up dairy, so introducing a food which I was known to have a problem with made even less sense. It was exasperating, but I went with it, because I wanted to get the hell home where I could eat actual nutrients. If I stayed here any longer I'd end up with malnutrition. How the Government doesn't have the sense to look into what patients are fed is beyond belief. If they want people to get better, if they want more beds, feed them what they need, and what they want to eat. It's not difficult. I'd sooner have paid £5 a day for something decent to eat than be given the crap I was faced with.

Each time I put the spoon to my mouth I gasped in pain, and each tiny bit that I swallowed I held my stomach with my left hand because I couldn't imagine where it was going and how my insides would cope with it. I thought of little men inside me, all shouting 'No! Not food!' and it dripping on their heads as they crouched in a corner in my stomach. I put my hand to my throat and followed the ice-cream down to my tummy, holding both hands across myself, convinced it was going to pour out of my skin.

Tottenham were playing Arsenal that afternoon. I asked Paula if she'd help me into the TV room so that I could watch the pre-match coverage. She helped me out of bed, slowly and not without some difficulty, and into the room. The room was about 10 metres away, but it took 15 minutes to get there. I was holding her arm and kind of moon-walking but forwards, as I couldn't actually lift my feet up to walk properly. My drip was in Paula's hand, being wheeled along beside me, and she had my dressing gown over her arm. My feet slid clumsily across the hospital floor. Even my slippers seemed embarrassed to be seen with me.

Once the door was open Paula came around the other side of me and sat me in a chair, switching on the television with the remote that she then put in my lap. She gave me a smile, put the dressing gown over my shoulders and shut the door. The minute I tried to lift my head up to look at the television I broke out into a sweat, my back soaking wet within seconds. I began to panic. My dressing gown was so heavy on me - it was only a towelling one but if felt like a suit of armour - and I couldn't get it off. It felt like a lead weight pushing down on me, and with my legs as swollen as an elephant's, I couldn't move any part of me other than my hands. I was slumped forward, remote in my right hand, my left hand on my left knee, trying to steady myself. The room began to spin, and I closed my eyes.

I was nowhere near the call button. I tried to focus on the television, but I felt dizzy and I was being dragged down by my own body, my tummy so heavy I couldn't keep my head up. It was no surprise that I couldn't sit up, as the muscles had been cut when my colon was taken out (I later found out that it's cut away from the muscle with a laser, so it's basically burnt away from the body - nice.) I was fighting for breath, in a state of total panic, sweating like crazy. It was like being drunk, but as if I had a weight pulling my head down to my chest. I literally didn't have the strength or the energy to hold my head up. I leaned on the arms of the chairs and lifted myself up, ooh, for about a nanosecond before I slumped back down. The pain was excruciating. It felt as though I was trying to move 20 stone. The door opened and a nurse walked in.

'I can't sit here, I'm sorry,' I told her, all flustered, 'I can't sit up.'

I started to cry. I felt pathetic, but I knew it wasn't really my fault. Everything just felt so weird, as though I had no control over my body. In truth, I didn't. My legs were so heavy I couldn't put one in front of the other without the nurse doing it for me. I finally got back to bed, shuffling along the corridor and wondering why my feet felt like lead and how I would ever get any better if I couldn't even sit in a chair. After all that, for the first time since I could remember, I didn't even care if Spurs won the game. I also couldn't remember who our manager was, and that was really weird. I knew then that I'd suffered massive psychological damage as well as the physical damage I had endured. It's just that one was far more obvious to the casual observer than the other and nobody in the NHS has time to notice mental stuff.

Paula popped in to my room a few minutes later and I explained what had happened. She looked puzzled.

'I just flipped out,' I said, 'I couldn't sit up, I kept flopping down and it felt horrible. It's as though someone's put an invisible rope in my belly button and they're pulling it down all the time. It's dragging me. My head just falls down. It's so horrible. I don't seem to have the strength to hold myself up at all.'

I was back in bed, my back soaked in sweat and sticking to the pillow, propped up like an old lady and wondering how I would ever get better. I was so glad to have my own room, a place where I could stare at the wall for two hours straight and not be stared at back. I didn't think about anything. My mind was blank.

I still couldn't sleep, but I closed my eyes and listened to the sounds around me; cars driving over the ramps leading up to the hospital, nurses talking outside the room and the voice in my head that just repeated, over and over again, 'I want my mum, I want my mum, I want my mum.' I drifted off for a few minutes, and then woke up to Paula asking if I'd like anything to drink.

'Gin and tonic, please,' I whispered.

'Seriously, Juliette,' she said, 'how about a cup of tea?'

'That's mad,' I said, 'I'm allowed a cup of tea? That's such a *normal* thing.' It was really peculiar. I hadn't done 'normal' for a while.

I said yes, and a few minutes later she came back with one. I let it cool down, just staring at the cup for 10 minutes. This is how weird things had become. I'd get obsessed with one silly little thing and concentrate on it as though my life depended on it. I think, in a way, that it did. You know when someone says, 'Can you watch my bag?' when they need the loo? Well, I could have done that all day to a very high standard. As it was, I tried to take a sip of tea and cried out in pain as the cup touched my lips. Blood was on the rim. I put the cup back down, pressed a tissue to my mouth and then cried out again when it got stuck and I had to tear it off, along with half the skin from my lower lip.

I'd already been told that if I couldn't eat or drink, I'd have to have another tube put in, and be fed again intravenously. I'd only had the tube removed that morning.

'We can't have you not eating,' said Paula, 'you need to get your energy levels up and put some weight on you.'

One of the doctors who were hovering outside the room asked me why I wasn't eating. I pointed to my mouth.

'Yes, but you have to eat,' he said, as if I didn't know that.

'I know,' I said, the words barely forming because it hurt so much to speak, 'but it's too painful and it's all inside my mouth as well.'

He nodded, walked to the end of the bed and wrote 'possibly anorexic' on my chart. I know that because I had a look at it a bit later. Did I tell you doctors never listen?

I had the tube put back in, much against my will. Talk about one step forward and two steps back. I wasn't anorexic, but obviously I didn't exactly have much of an appetite either. Who would, for hospital food, with a mouthful of ulcers? Later that day I asked Paula if I could have a sedative.

'I need to relax a bit, I'm no good like this. Maybe I'll get some sleep. Don't worry, I'm not going to start dealing prescription drugs.'

That night I started a new routine. Paula gave me a Diazepam at 6pm while she changed my nutrition drip, adding another bag to the stand. Then, when the next shift clocked on at 9.30pm Sam came to me first and gave me my medication, took my blood pressure, my temperature, gave me a sleeping pill, wrote it all down, then went and took care of the other patients. I was so happy that I would be left alone and not have to sit waiting for them to jolt me out of my stupor and start poking about and feeding me drugs. A couple of hours later, when Sam came back to check on me again, I told the her how grateful I was, that it meant a lot to me that she had not only listened but done something to help.

'Don't be daft,' she said, 'I wish I could do more. I mean, you've had a Diazepam and a sleeping tablet, enough to knock anyone else out, and here you are, wide awake, at midnight. What are we going to do?'

'Sam,' I said, 'you're my favourite nurse. Can you just shoot me and feed me to the seagulls?' I meant it, too. She gave my hand a little squeeze and suggested that when my parents came in the next day they should take me out of the hospital, go for a drive or something.

'What, am I allowed to do that?' I asked, my eyes wide open in disbelief.

'Probably not,' she said, 'but I think it'd do you good.'

'What if I don't come back?' I whispered, winking at her.

'You'd better,' she laughed, 'or I'm out of a job.'

'Well in that case I promise I'll come back,' I said.

I lay awake all night - just for a change - not quite believing that I would be allowed to leave this place. It couldn't possibly be as simple as my parents taking me out for a drive. It just couldn't. When I think about it now, it was as exciting a prospect as winning Euro Millions, growing C-cup boobs overnight, finding out that cheese isn't fattening or made from cows and that Brad Pitt had a massive crush on me and was about to leave his 348 children and Angelina Jolie to set up home with me in the helter skelter (of course, years later they did divorce, but he hasn't called me. Yet).

Morning came, a baby pink and tangerine sun rising behind the Palace Pier. It looked like a postcard. A clear blue sky melted into the sea, and I followed a boat, a tiny white speck in the distance, across the waves, until it disappeared from view. I thought I was watching a film. It was Sunday November 18th, 2001. I looked at the clock. It was 7.10am so I must have actually been asleep. Blimey!

There wasn't a cloud in the sky, and as I lay awkwardly and uncomfortably in bed, plastic covered pillows either side of my body to keep me from turning on my back; my heart was beating so hard and fast I thought I would explode. I felt like I was choking. I was shaking, drenched in sweat, my stupid, huge hospital gown stuck to my back. I managed to twist my body around so that I could get out of bed. I got hold of the drip stand, and knew that I could unplug it for a few minutes. It wasn't like I was having a blood transfusion, it was liquid food. I wheeled the stand closer until I could reach it.

I needed the toilet. I was also incredibly hungry, although I wasn't sure what I was feeling when my stomach rumbled because it had been so long since I'd eaten. It took me almost 30 minutes to get out of bed. As I pulled the covers back and pushed myself up with my left arm, I gasped. My legs weren't swollen now that the epidural had come out, but I was left with these two deathly white, stick-like legs, the red nail varnish looking macabre on my toes.

My legs were so thin I could join the thumb and forefingers of both hands around the top of my thighs. The skin was baggy, almost translucent, and it felt dry and thin, like parchment paper. I had a few very fine hairs on my legs, but they were soft, not prickly. I didn't realise at the time (oddly enough) but it was 'new' hair, like baby hair, because my body had shut down and my hair follicles had given up. These were my hair follicles coming alive again. It was well weird. I swung my legs over the side of the bed and just looked at them for a few minutes. I couldn't believe how thin they were. I lifted up my nightgown and looked down at my stomach, a protruding mess. An ugly scar, red and raised, ran from just underneath my breastbone to my pubic bone. It ran around the side of my belly button. To the right lay the ileostomy. I gagged.

I dropped my gown back down and made my way across the room - all four feet of it - and went to the toilet, using all my strength to bring the drip stand with me and steady myself with that, then slowly lower myself on to the toilet to have a wee, and somehow finding a little more in my reserve to get me back up again. I needed to empty the bag. Although I wasn't eating as such, I was still producing waste, and I couldn't bear the hot, gluey liquid sitting in the bag and weighing heavily on my skin, dragging the lump of flesh downwards with it. It was such an unnatural feeling, like tar being poured on my stomach while this lump, this thing, wriggled around trying to set itself free. Even the stoma itself wanted to get away from me.

I lifted up my hospital gown, tucked the bottom of it into the neck, like a giant napkin, took hold of the bottom of the bag, hanging clumsily off my right side, to relieve my tummy of the pressure of the weight of the contents, and sort of leaned as low as I could over the toilet bowl. It wasn't very low at all, as I couldn't bend, so I just hoped it didn't splash everywhere, because I'd have to be the one to clean it.

I undid the plastic clip at the end of the bag and opened it, emptying out the vile dark green gloop, the result of yesterday's mouthful of ice-cream and god only knows what else. It was like squeezing out the lung of a 200 year-old, 60-a-day smoker. It hung off the end of the bag like slime and stank like Dad's compost bin in the garden. I'm surprised I wasn't covered in flies. I wiped the end of the bag with toilet paper, flushed the loo and did up the bag by folding over the end with the plastic clip - which, I might add, constantly scratched at my skin. I smoothed my gown back down and tried to forget about it but the lump started moving again and I thought I was going to be sick. I walked around the room, my slippers shuffling along the cold linoleum floor, the slow, purposeful steps you associate with the elderly.

My mouth wasn't any better, but I felt like I needed to eat, rather than absorb. I asked for some toast, which was typical - I don't go the easy route and have porridge or soup, but toast. I hadn't eaten anything wheat-based for almost two years and I could hardly wait. I stared at the clock, wondering if one of the nurses would have time to help me have a shower and wash my hair before Mum and Dad turned up. I started thinking about getting out of the hospital, deciding that I would ask Dad to drive us along the seafront to Rottingdean where I could watch the waves smash against the rocks from above.

I nibbled at the cheap white toast with its thin layer of margarine on it like a mouse. I knew I wouldn't be allowed out of here until I was eating properly. I couldn't even imagine sitting at the table, or at home on the sofa, eating three meals a day. Where would it go? I didn't even know, at this stage, whether everything would even work. Neither did the doctors. I was terrified, yet totally indifferent all at the same time.

After my toast – I managed a whole quarter triangle - I asked the nurse if she could help me wash my hair. She said she'd be back in a while, that I should get started and she'd come back and see how I was doing. I later realised that it was a ploy to get me to do something on my own. She knew that if I put my mind to it I'd do it.

I undid the tape on the gown, and it fell to the floor. I stood in front of the mirror and looked at myself. My elbows and shoulders stuck out. My ribs were protruding, and I noticed for the first time that the bottom rib on my left side was way lower than the one on the right. My shoulders dipped. I was completely wonky. That would be evidence of the scoliosis taking its toll. My hair was long, falling below my shoulders, shiny and lustrous, like it had never been, almost black against my deathly white skin. I was gaunt, deathly pale and didn't look anything like the person I'd been before. My mouth was open, because I couldn't close it, covered in ulcers and sores, green stuff, blood and cracked skin. I couldn't register that it was myself staring back; I looked like the girl from 'The Ring'.

I staggered to the shower, turned on the taps and sat on the chair, my bony backside aching as soon as I sat. I still had a lot of dressing on the scar but I was told that I could take it off in the shower and get a new one put on afterwards, that the water might do it good and clean the wound. I was alarmed when I pulled it back, starting at the top and working my way to the bottom to discover that somebody had shaved off almost all of my pubic hair! I know I didn't have time to book a bikini wax, what with being rushed into hospital and all, but that was quite a surprise. I wondered they had taken my photo unbeknown to me and sent to a porn magazine, possibly entitled *Ileostomy Wives*. The bag flopped on to my lap. I hated it. Because I was so thin and the bag an unsightly post-op bag, it took up so much space on my body, like having a deflated orange football taped to me. I reached for the shower gel and slowly began to wash myself. It felt wonderful. I couldn't bend down to wash my feet nor lift them on to my lap to do it, so I let the soapy water trickle between my toes. I sat for a while, my eyes closed under the water, and when the nurse knocked on the door, I told her I was OK.

I picked up my shampoo and started washing my hair. I had a big grin on my face. I was washing my hair. Well, to be honest it was more a case of me having a dollop of shampoo on my head that was now washing away under the shower, but it was a start.

The strength it took just to sit upright was unbelievable, and as fast as I was getting clean I would break out into a sweat and spoil it all, but I had to do it. I wanted to go home. My stomach was aching so much I was crying, my arms raised to my head, stretching every part of me. I rinsed the shampoo out and managed to slap a dollop of conditioner on my hair. I was so exhausted that I couldn't wait the minute for it to work, and rinsed it off straight away. I sat for a few minutes, breathing rapidly, my heart pounding, trying to calm down enough to get up. I wobbled and fell down again, luckily landing on the seat. I let my head drop and tried to breathe deeply and slowly before attempting to get up again. I was beginning to shiver. I stood up very slowly, one hand holding the rail, and wrapped myself in a big white towel. I felt dizzy again, and held on to the rail for support. I went to wrap a towel around my head but it was too heavy, my head lolling around as though I'd broken my neck. I shuffled back to the bed and sat down. I could already feel myself getting hotter, my heart racing, my wet hair dripping down my back.

I was absolutely shattered from the shower but mouth was so sore I couldn't contemplate even a sip of water. The nurse came back in and dried my hair for me, saying how well I'd done. I believed her. I had done well. I'd done it all on my own, and now I just wanted to climb back into my clean bed and sleep. Instead, the stoma nurse popped in with an array of bags for me to look at.

I sat on the edge of the bed, two pairs of thick pink socks on to keep my feet warm, and stared down at the chair where she was arranging the bags. I can't say as I was overly excited at the prospect of attaching any of them to myself, particularly when she held up one the size of a small island. It wasn't exactly the kind of personal shopping experience you'd get in Selfridges. I was reassured that the bags came in smaller sizes, and stopped panicking, although I don't know why I stopped - after all, it wasn't as if being told that they were smaller made it alright, just better.

I was told I'd have to change the bag myself today, with her help, before they'd think about letting me go home. I shuddered. I couldn't bear the thought of it. Up until a couple of days ago, when I could get out of bed myself, nurses had emptied the bag for me into a cardboard bowl. How anyone could do that was beyond me. I couldn't do it for all the money in the world. I'd always had the utmost respect for nurses, particularly since giving them such a hard time when I had my heart operation, but I couldn't believe the things they had to do. I know it was because I couldn't do it myself, but what an amazing job they did. I never once felt as though I was a nuisance, and although having to ask for my bottom to be wiped clean of hot, acidic post-op mucus at 4am or for someone to squeeze the mess out of my stoma bag goes down as the most undignified time of my life, they tried their hardest to make me feel as though it wasn't a problem. Post-op, they were great. Pre-op, terrible. I do think I had a bit of a bond with a couple of the nurses just because I wasn't far off their age. They were in their early twenties and here I was, only five years older than them and in this state. I think they were all too aware that they could count themselves lucky that they were looking after me, rather than actually *being* me.

So. This was the big moment, except I was so weak that I couldn't even lift my head up or sit up straight enough to do it. The shower had wiped me out, as if I'd been on a 50-mile run. I'm not one for failing before I've even tried something, but on this occasion, I simply couldn't do it. Instead I sat in the hard plastic chair just inside the bathroom door, completely naked, slumped forward, all skin and bone with this clumsy thing hanging from my side waiting to be peeled off and dumped in the special little blue bags, scented to mask the odour from the stoma bag. I was too exhausted even to worry about how awful I looked, and that I was completely naked in front of someone I didn't know. I didn't care anymore. My body wasn't mine.

I told the nurse I couldn't do it. I think she realised that it was 50% fear and 50% exhaustion, so she didn't force me. Instead I cried a little, quietly, as I looked down and watched her do it instead - a complex operation involving little pots of warm water, scissors, wipes, plastic backing, soft tissues, creams and sprays. She sprayed something around the plastic base of the bag. It stung like hell. I cried out, my hands gripping the side of the chair.

'It stings, I know,' she said, 'but it melts the glue.'

She gently pulled the plastic away from my skin. The base of the bag is plastic, and you have to cut a hole in it to match the circumference of your stoma. All stomas differ in size depending on the size of the person. Mine was about two inches in diameter, raised an inch from my skin. Can you even begin to imagine that? I doubt it. The bag was attached to the plastic disc, so you peel off the backing to the disc after cutting your hole, and press it to your skin, so the stoma itself is popping out of the middle, with the bag over the stoma. It's basically like a Hoover bag.

The nurse was cutting the new disc to size, explaining what she was doing as she was going along. I looked down for a moment and as I saw the stoma uncovered, I threw up. By that I mean I would have thrown up had anything been in my stomach. It was revolting. It was bright red, protruding from my side like something out of *Alien*. I was shaking uncontrollably, trying not to scream.

'I can't do this,' I sobbed, 'I can't do this.'

I just sat, shaking and shivering with cold. The nurse put a towel around my shoulders to try and keep me warm.

'You'll catch your death like that,' she said.

'Good,' I said quietly, turning my head so that I couldn't see what she was doing. I felt a hot, wet tear run down my cheek.

The stoma had to be cleaned before the new bag could be put on. There was glue, stitches, blood and waste all around the stoma. It was utterly revolting. The nurse dipped a soft wipe into the plastic cup of warm water, and wiped around the stoma. It hurt. A lot. The stoma responded by moving around, like a cat rubbing up against its owner's legs for attention.

'You have to get all the bits off,' she explained, 'all the glue, all the waste, or it'll go septic.'

'Excellent,' I said, my sarcasm knowing no bounds.

'Juliette, I know this is hard, but you will get used to it. It'll get easier. It'll just become part of your life.'

'That's why I'm so horrified,' I said, 'because I don't want this as part of my life. It's hideous.'

She sighed, and took another wipe from the packet to dry the skin, careful not to snag her nails on my stitches. Next, she peeled the backing off the plastic disc, and stuck it over the stoma, pressing down on my stomach. It was a gentle pressing, but it still hurt like hell. The new bag was on. It felt better - at least I was clean, and because it was a flesh-coloured bag, rather than a clear bag, I couldn't see anything inside, which was preferable to seeing your insides *and* the contents of your stomach. The nurse wiped dry the water that had dribbled down to my thighs, and held my hand.

'I promise you it will get easier,' she said, 'but you have to do this on your own before you can go home.'

I'm not great when it comes to accidents and injuries when they're in real life, and I have a very strong phobia about snakes. I can't see one on the TV without almost passing out, so to me, this was like a red snake. 'Like one whose face has peeled off,' I told Mum later.

I vowed then that I would never let anyone see it. I don't want to see it. It's disgusting. And it's on me. It's a muscle, so it moves of its own accord. That can't be right, can it?

This is how I explained it to my parents when they came in:

'It's right there, all the time, like it's fighting to get out and slither along the floor. It's so horrible and it's on me and I want to flick it off but I can't. I just want to get it off,' I cried, having my first proper hug in weeks now that Mum could get her arms around me without the threat of detaching me from tubes and machines.

'My poor little girl,' she said, stroking my clean, shiny hair and planting a kiss on the top of my head, 'let's take you out, then. Where shall we go?' She went off to find Paula, who reassured her that it'd do me good to go out, and that I'd just have to be back in two hours to be re-attached to my drip stand.

'Two hours it is,' said Dad, looking more worried than I've ever seen him look in his life, even more than when we got lost in the dark in London's East End on the way to football once. Even more than when I made him dinner with garlic in it. And even more than when I dated an Arsenal fan. Actually, maybe not as worried as that.

I took a walk along the corridor with one of the nurses to prove to that I could walk a bit, taking about four days to go 10 yards, and although I struggled to put one foot in front of the other, I made it all the way to reception and back to my room. I could finally see a light at the end of the tunnel. Now, of course, I know that the idea of going out had been more of a psychological treatment than anything else. The nurses knew that I would want Mum and Dad to see that I was progressing. I didn't feel like I was, at all.

The surgeon had come in that morning to see how I was doing. He'd been in every day, sitting on the bed, holding my hand or even my foot if it was out of the covers, talking to me like I was a real person, not a 'case study' or a walking disease. He told me that if I ate lunch and dinner he'd think about letting me go home in a couple of days. I didn't believe him.

'You're teasing me. I know you're going to keep me in here, experimenting on me and testing potions and stuff in my food.'

'You eat your lunch and have some dinner and we'll see about you getting out of here,' he said, smiling, 'when would you like to go home?'

'It's Sunday today. Can I go home on Tuesday?' I asked, 'not Wednesday, not tomorrow. Tuesday.'

'Tuesday it is then,' he said, smiling, 'if you're eating properly and it's all working, and you've changed the bag yourself, then you can go home.'

He gave me a playful tap on the hip with his clipboard and headed home. I winced as he caught me right on the bone that was protruding rather nicely from my gown, but I didn't say 'ouch' in case he made me stay in for another week.

I was walking, albeit slowly and with difficulty, putting magazines and papers in one place, trying to bend down and pick up my wash bag - impossible - and clutching my stomach with one hand at all times because it still felt as though it was hanging off me and that if I didn't keep hold of it, it would fall to the floor. At one point I bent down and couldn't get up again, and had to call the nurse, the panic washing over me in hot floods as I crouched rooted to the spot, pain shooting through my whole body.

'I've got some bother with the bend down, get up stuff,' I said, screwing up my face in pain.

'You're not supposed to be able to do everything just because you can go home in two days, Juliette,' said Paula, 'you have to take it easy. You've only just started walking!'

'The surgeon says I can go home on Tuesday if I behave myself and eat my dinner. Can you come and get me if he lets me out?' I said, grinning at Dad.

'You betcha,' he laughed, while Mum looked horrified. She wasn't prepared for me to come home that quickly, and I knew it. She averted her gaze, clasped her hands together and said, 'Right, OK, fine, OK...' and busied herself tidying up my pile of tissues, unread newspaper and cups of water.

'As if we wouldn't come and get you,' said Dad, brightly, 'and Paula tells us you're allowed out of here for a couple of hours. Where do you want to go?'

'I'll show you,' I said, 'just turn left out of this hell-hole and keep going and I'll tell you when to stop.'

'As long as it's not when we get to Dover,' said Dad, 'I haven't got that much petrol.' Mum helped me put on my dressing gown and Dad picked up the blanket from the bed. They held an arm each and asked if I wanted a wheelchair. I said no, even though I had no idea how I would walk as far as the exit.

'You have to walk really slowly,' I said, my breathing getting heavier as we walked along the corridor, 'I can't go any faster. I'm about the same speed as a seal, dragging itself along the beach on its tummy.'

'Yes, dear,' said Mum, rolling her eyes, 'just take your time.'

Dad went to get the car while Mum sat me down in reception, covering my pathetic little legs with the blanket. I must have been shaking because she held my hands and told me not to worry.

'I think I'm scared of going outside,' I said, looking out for Dad. 'I don't know why. I'm sorry. I want to go, I just feel frightened.'

'I can see that by the way you're shaking,' said Mum, 'but if you don't like it we can come back. Here's your dad.'

Mum helped me into the car and got in the back with me. I leant against her, wrapped in her coat and the blanket and my dressing gown. It was only then that it occurred to me that I was going out without getting dressed.

Dad drove turned left out of the hospital and kept driving, right along the seafront as instructed. I could see the sea on the right, crashing against the rocks at Rottingdean. I told Dad to park in the car park of the big pub which is right on the top of the cliffs, but once we'd stopped I could only see anything from there if I got out of the car and sat on the wall. Instead I wound down the window, breathed in the fresh sea air and told them I couldn't wait to come home.

'You'll have to tell us what you want from the flat to take back on Tuesday,' said Mum, 'you'll need your clothes, your phone, your nice leopard print blanket and CDs and books and all sorts. Your dad and I can get some things on Tuesday then come and pick you up.'

'No,' I said, shaking my head and sitting up, 'let's go there now. Let's go to the flat and I'll sort it out now, then it's done.'

'You won't be able to get up all those stairs, Juliette,' said Mum. 'Don't even think about it. You've only managed a few steps in three weeks. You can wait in the car and tell us where things are.'

'Mum, I can't even remember what my bedroom looks like let alone where anything is or what I even want. I don't know. Let me try and get up the stairs and do it myself.'

I couldn't quite believe I was doing this. I had three flights of stairs to climb, an arduous task at the best of times, but I was determined to do it. I think I was born mental.

I don't know why I always think I've got something to prove, even like I did on that slide at four years old - what is it with me and climbing steps after life-saving surgery?

We pulled up outside the flat, high on a hill overlooking the sea. Mum helped me get out, putting the blanket over my shoulders. It was cold out. My teeth started to chatter.

'You'll catch a cold and then the doctors will be really happy,' said Mum, sarcastically, 'just stay in the car and let us get your things.'

'No! I'm coming in,' I answered, 'just help me up the stairs.'

Looking back now I can see how unfair I was being. If something had gone wrong, if I had fallen or collapsed or pulled a muscle, I would have been in serious trouble. At the time, though, I was determined to get up those stairs myself whatever the cost. Just like the slide episode, I have no idea why I did it, nor why my parents didn't absolutely insist on my not doing it, but I suppose it doesn't matter now. I did do it, and it didn't kill me, I just don't know *how* it didn't. I really am an idiot.

With my parents either side of me I walked to the gate. Dad went on ahead and opened the front door. I went to lift my foot up the step on the path and almost fell over. I'd not lifted my foot up, gone up a step or done anything like that for three weeks. My leg didn't know what I wanted it to do. I had to lift it with my hands. God knows what the neighbours must have thought. I made it to the bottom of the stairs and stopped to catch my breath.

Mum held one arm while the banister supported the other. I sort of slumped and slid my way up. It took 25 minutes. We only had another half an hour before I had to be back at the hospital to reacquaint myself with my drip stands. It nearly finished me off but they knew even then that I had to do it. Slowly but surely I lifted my legs up at the back of my knees with one hand and plonked my feet down on the stairs. It was clumsy and slow and I thought I'd never make it but I did, resting every four steps or so. Finally I got up the next flight inside my flat, and Mum tried to make me sit down on the sofa while she got my things together.

I knew that if I sat down it'd be even harder to stand when I wanted to get up, that I had to keep moving or I'd stop altogether. My flat looked so bright, and so untidy! I picked up my mobile phone and listened for messages. I had 14, mainly from people wondering why I wasn't home and offers of work which I'd obviously missed. I picked up my charger, my bank cards (why I did that I don't know, it wasn't like I was going on a shopping spree any time soon), and Dad gathered my post. I wandered to my bedroom and looked longingly at my bed, its crisp white cotton sheets luring me in.

'This is mad, I have to go back to that hospital room when I could stay here.'

'You can't stay here,' she said, 'you've got to go back on your drip in a bit. We've got half an hour to get you back, Juliette. You're not meant to be at the flat. It's ridiculous and you look as white as a sheet. Come on.'

I went through my wardrobe and picked out a few clothes, not knowing that I wouldn't be able to wear most of them either because they would fall off me - I'd lost almost two stone and I was only eight stone five to begin with - or I couldn't do them up around my stoma.

Dad put everything in a bag as I pulled random things out of the drawers, and I sat on the bed for a few minutes, swaying a bit and feeling like I was going to pass out, but too scared to mention it. I directed Mum to my moisturisers, make-up and body lotions and then sort of waved a 'whatever' wave and said I couldn't sit there anymore. I started to panic, as I was finding it hard to breathe and my stomach hurt like hell. I had a burning pain that was getting worse by the second. I had completely overdone it, and now I was panicking, and quite rightly. My head was spinning. Time to go.

We picked up my leopard print blanket and began the slow descent down to ground level. Several times I thought I was going to faint with the effort of it all but I stayed on my feet, albeit unsteadily, and made it back to the car, and eventually, with the aid of a wheelchair once we arrived at the hospital, back to my bed. Mum was busy telling the nurses what I'd done whilst they connected me back to all my tubes. They were horrified.

'We didn't say you could go home or climb stairs, Juliette!' said Paula, tucking me back into bed.

'She won't listen,' said Dad, 'she's always been the same. But then if she wasn't a fighter she wouldn't be here at all, would she?' He squeezed my hand and I gave it a kiss.

'How grim is that? I just kissed your hand and left a blister behind on it from my ulcerated mouth as a token of my love.'

I was awake, of course, throughout the night. Sam was on her last night shift and came to say goodbye. She'd been wonderful; she'd seen me at my lowest, in terrible pain, ready to give up. Not only was she a great nurse, she was compassionate, understanding and sympathetic. She did all she could to make me comfortable, she took me to the toilet, she emptied my ileostomy bag, she wiped my backside when it leaked horrible mucus and she came in to see me first every night in the vain hope that I might get to sleep if I was left alone after all that. It didn't work, but she did her best and I'm eternally grateful to her for that. I've no complaint about the after care from the nurses, they were all fantastic, it was the doctors who made me angry, who treated me not as if I was a person but an experiment, something for them to try different drugs out on. I felt like a mouse being batted around by a cat, slowly losing the will to live and wishing someone would put me out of my misery. I told her I'd miss her and she gave me a hug.

'You're being really brave,' she said, 'and I promise you, you'll come back here in a few weeks and you'll be so much better.' She gave my hand a squeeze.

'I'm off in a minute so I'm saying goodbye before you go to sleep.'

'Sleep? What's that? I've heard about it, other people tell me of this natural wonder.'

'Oh, you,' she laughed, 'I suppose you'll be wide awake when I come back in to take your blood pressure. I'll try to be quiet and not wake you if you are out of it.'

She gave me a sleeping tablet and shut the door, turning out the light as she went. I had no need for earplugs or an eye mask in here. It was dark, quiet and I was on my own. I lay on my side, arranged all my tubes above my head on the pillow and - get this - I must have dropped off because the next thing I knew it was 1am and I had just woken up, needing the toilet. I felt pretty drowsy and got out of bed slowly, still having to lift my legs out of bed. I stood up too quickly, and swayed to the right. I couldn't hold my balance because I couldn't feel my legs, and I fell against the door, hitting my head on the wall, my back on the industrial bin and grazing my elbow on the floor. I had fallen straight onto my right hip, unable to react quickly enough to put my hands down. It hurt like hell, and as I crashed to the floor I cried out in pain.

Sam came rushing in.

'What happened?' she asked, lifting me up by my arms.

'I just got out of bed, stood up, and boom, over I went. I'm well dizzy.' She asked where it hurt and told me I should see the doctor.

'Sam, I can't be bothered. It hurts but I'm OK.'

She had a look. My hip bone was grazed and bright red. There was a definite bump but there were no bones poking out. Well, not right out. Sam helped me to the bathroom, waited while I had a wee then hauled me back on to the bed and pulled the covers up.

'I really should get the doctor. You've had quite a fall.'

'No, I'm OK,' I insisted, 'you go and have a cup of tea. Take some of my biscuits, I can't eat them.' She picked up a couple of custard creams, squeezed my hand and left the room.

'I really hope you get back to sleep,' she whispered.

I did, for another couple of hours. I awoke at 4.15am and that was that. I watched the sun come up and waited for my breakfast. Today I was going to eat a slice of toast and some porridge, despite having to get it past my sore mouth and down my sore throat.

By 8.30am I'd eaten the lot and washed it down with a cup of fruit tea with manuka honey I'd asked mum to bring in to ward off the infection. The sticky oats were literally like glue on my lips. I must have looked like a baby, with white, lumpy, wet food all over my mouth. I forced myself to swallow. It was Monday morning. One more day to go.

CHAPTER ELEVEN
'I'M COMING HOME'
ELVIS PRESLEY

I wanted to get in the shower and freshen up before any visitors turned up. Emma was bound to pop in and Mum had said that Alice was going to try and get in. I sat up in bed and waited for the doctor.

I was feeling much, much better today. It must have been the knowledge that I would be in the car and out of here this time tomorrow. I couldn't wait. But at the same time, I was starting to wonder how on earth I would manage. I'd only been eating for half a day. I hadn't eaten for three weeks before yesterday. I couldn't walk properly (after yesterday's day trip my legs had gone into some kind of aching spasm and I wobbled whenever I got out of bed to go to the loo). I couldn't sit, stand or do anything for myself and I knew that the things I achieved the day before were a one-off. Adrenalin and determination got me to my flat, but my body wouldn't be able to cope with that again in a hurry. In fact, I'd probably made things worse by going nuts.

Added to that, I couldn't even look at the stoma. My mind was racing. 'How can they send me home?' I suddenly panicked, 'I'm not ready!' At the same time, I just wanted to get out. I was terrified of going, but even more terrified of staying. He asked me a few questions - what had I eaten for breakfast, was I capable of changing the bag.

'Since you ask, I had kippers, freshly squeezed orange juice and a selection of jams and preserves with toast and a pot of coffee. And to the second question, I haven't done that on my own yet.'

He had the grace to laugh. 'I don't know how you think up these things on the spot like that, Juliette. Dear me. Well, you can't go home until you can change the bag by yourself so I'll send the stoma nurse round and she can show you how it's done. If you do that this afternoon we'll see. Still want to go home tomorrow?'

'Just a bit,' I nodded.

'Well, as long as you're still eating OK - and I mean three meals - and you can do the bag, then you can. OK?'

I nodded. The stoma nurse came in a few minutes later and ordered me into the bathroom. This time, I stood at the sink and did it myself. It took 45 minutes. I cried, I shook, and I just about managed to stop myself from throwing up. I was naked, shaking with cold, a towel over my shoulders again to keep them warm. My hair hung limply, obscuring my view of my stomach. I felt repulsed not only by the stoma, but at the sight of myself in the mirror. I looked like a zombie. When I wiped the stoma clean, picking up the 'waste' and the glue from the old bag, it moved. I yelped. 'It does that,' said the nurse, 'and it might start emptying out while you clean it, too. Best to do it in the morning before you eat.'

Let's just get this straight. Surgeons can pick up a foetus from the womb, operate on it and put it back. They can make big boobs small, small boobs big and turn men into really tall women with big hands and feet and even transplant pig organs into humans and create a penis from a vagina. So how come this is the best they can do for me? Leave me with my insides on my outside, wobbling around, pulsating? It's like they've just forgotten to finish the job and left the last bit out, like a builder going home and leaving all his tools on site.

I finished cleaning the area around the stoma, and put the tissues into the special blue waste bag that was hanging from the tap. I was shaking and crying so much as I emptied the warm water out of the pot where I put the wipes that the water went all over the floor. I couldn't bend down to wipe it up. The nurse cut out the disc in the new bag, and handed it to me. The skin around the stoma had dried, so I put some calamine lotion on. It was already blistered and I wondered how I was going to cope with the soreness, apart from everything else. I stuck the bag over the stoma, pressed down and folded up the end. I sealed the opening with the clip and slumped over the sink, exhausted.

'Can I sit down?' I whispered, trying to catch my breath.

'Of course,' she said, helping me to the bed, putting my nightshirt over my head and lifting my legs up and under the covers.

'You've changed the bag,' she said, tucking the covers around me, 'so you've done very well. Once more change tomorrow morning and you can go home.'

The television I'd forgotten that I'd requested four days previously turned up. Someone plugged it in. I sat in awe as it came to life. I don't know what was on, it was just great to have some noise in the otherwise silent room. I knew that if I'd had a television in the room a few days earlier, in the weirdest way I can't really explain, it would have speeded up my recovery. I think the fact that I had gone from constant noise to complete silence was too much of a contrast. I knew I was getting better because I got cross at *The Weakest Link*.

I had put on a clean nightshirt – this time it was a grey one Mum had bought me, with a cat on the front. Not an actual cat, of course, a picture of one. It was a bit twee, but it was soft and smelled nice and it wasn't a hospital gown. I had refused all offers of underwear and even my own towel because it would mean Mum having to wash it all, not that she would have minded in the slightest. On the contrary, she might have felt more useful if she'd been bringing me clean things to wear and seeing that I had a nice fluffy towel to use instead of the scratchy, thin hospital towels. The thing is, I didn't feel as if I deserved anything nice until I had reached my goal of going home. How stupid is that? I'd reached it now, so I could feel more human again by wearing something 'non-hospital'. I was punishing myself for something that wasn't my fault, and rewarding myself for good behaviour. How nuts is that? If I'd actually *seen* the psychiatrist, he'd have had a field day. I'm sure I'd have had a Government-issue straitjacket in no time.

I sat in the chair next to my bed, holding my faithful Panda bear and reading some of my book. It was still an effort just to sit in the chair, but wiggling my toes helped my circulation and I was so excited at the prospect of going home that I had a big grin on my ulcerated face.

'I'm reading a book,' I said to Panda, 'so that means I'm getting better, and we're going to go home.' I swear he gave me the thumbs up, even though he hasn't got any thumbs.

I watched TV for a minute then got back onto the bed as it was softer on my bones than the chair, perched somewhat awkwardly in the middle of the bed, changing position every few minutes to try and get comfortable. I had thick socks on my feet to keep them warm. I rubbed lotion into my bony arms and legs, took a sleeping pill when the nurse came in at 9.45pm and - at last - fell asleep at 11pm.

At 2am I woke up to go to the toilet. At 4am I woke up and went to the toilet again. This time I stayed awake, but I didn't mind, I was going home today. I got out of bed and stood at the window. I read some cards. I laughed at a letter that my friend Kit, who played football for Fulham at the time, had sent. It was hysterical. Dad had called him and told him what had happened. He sent a get well card but also wrote a load of old nonsense and told me how the season was going at the club. It was the first time I'd laughed in weeks.

As I gazed out towards the pier, the sunrise seemed more vibrant than it had before. I still wanted to talk to someone, but the psychiatrist never came. They had forgotten. I felt let down, invisible, and alone. I guess I had to just get on with it on my own. Again.

Mum and Dad arrived mid-morning. They had brought down my Converse trainers, a T-shirt and a sweatshirt, and some tracksuit bottoms, all of which I'd given Mum at the flat in preparation for me coming home. I hadn't had anything on my skin that had a waistband since the operation - I wasn't even wearing knickers yet because the elastic pressed against my scar - so it was quite a job to get dressed. Mum helped me while Dad gathered my things. I had to ask Mum to help me put my Converse on, and when I tried to take a step, I almost fell over. I should have just worn thick socks to the car, as I didn't have the strength to put one foot in front of the other.

Dad went to get the car, and Mum helped me to the exit. I was grinning like mad, so happy to be leaving. I'd said goodbye to the nurses and they all wished me luck. I was cold again, but Mum had told me that she'd brought my leopard print blanket down in the car, so I could snuggle up in that on the way home. They helped me into the car so that I was sort of sitting up, but along the back seats. I had a pillow (Mum really does think of everything!) and had taken my Converse off. I was in too much pain to sit up, so before we reached the motorway I asked Dad to pull over so Mum could help me lie down a bit more. I felt nauseous all the way home (this is when I discovered I suffered from travel sickness), and Mum had to remind Dad to go slowly when we hit roads with speed bumps.

Just over an hour later we pulled up outside the house. Mum got out first and helped me into the house. Dad brought all my things indoors. As soon as the front door was shut, I insisted on unpacking everything there and then. For once, Mum said no. I was actually relieved. The journey had wiped me out and I wanted to rest. Dad helped me upstairs. Mum came up with a cup of tea for her, green tea for me, and unpacked for me. Pebble was asleep on the bed. I was so pleased to see her but I couldn't bend down to kiss her. Mum picked her up for me and I kissed her soft tummy, then let her go back to sleep. She was, as usual, unimpressed by the whole event.

While I'd been in hospital, Mum and Dad had been looking after my hamster, Babylegs. Mum had mentioned a few days earlier that she'd gone off her food - the hamster, not Mum - and was looking fed up.

'She's depressed, I expect. She misses her mum. She doesn't even want a pumpkin seed or a cornflake. She didn't eat her banana this morning at breakfast. She wouldn't come out and play last night. Come and see her.'

She looked ill. Her sparkle had gone, if a hamster ever has such a thing. A piece of banana and some seeds lay untouched in her bowl. She poked her little face out of her house, sniffed the air, opened her eyes for a moment and saw me, then went back inside, nestling under her bedding, a luxurious combination of soft wood chippings and dried out, ripped up baby wipes.

She looked sad. I told her I'd get her out to play later on and that I wanted her to eat her food or she'd be as ill as me. I waved at her then I went downstairs, wondering if I could get her fixed up to a nutrition drip like I'd had.

For two days I hardly spoke. I was in some kind of catatonic state. I was home. I had to get better. It would take a long time. I could hardly make it up the stairs. I couldn't sit in the chair, upright, to eat my dinner. I was slumped on the settee, half up, half lying down, covered in blankets because I was so cold all the time. Mum had been shopping and bought me a couple of pairs of tracksuit bottoms which she'd had to take in, I had nice thick socks borrowed from my brother, and because I was still so weak too many clothes were heavy on me so I wore vest tops and covered up with the blankets. Pebble kept me company. I didn't know what to do with myself, and I felt useless, hopeless, a waste of space. I started to wish that I hadn't woken up from the operation, but I kept my thoughts to myself. I didn't want to make things harder for my parents than it already was.

I ate snacks rather than proper meals, or had a child sized portion of dinner. I was still afraid that something would become blocked, or that the bag would explode or fall off. I slept fitfully during the day, on the sofa, and not much at all at night in bed. I couldn't get comfortable. The bag would flop to my right if I lay on my right, and I couldn't anyway because my hip hurt from the fall. I felt anxious as soon as I'd turn out the light, so I had to have a nightlight on. The Diazepam I'd come home with relieved a little of the panic, but sometimes I'd wake suddenly in a real state, crying and drenched in a cold sweat. I wasn't sure I would ever feel 'normal' again.

I had to figure out what I could wear - everything hung off me now. I didn't know what I was supposed to do. I sat on the sofa, legs outstretched, my old Tottenham Hotspur duvet over me which my brother had donated, albeit temporarily. Mum brought me cheese on toast and Marmite drinks, both of which I craved like mad because everything was passing through me so fast I was dehydrated, and my body craved salt. I tried to avoid changing my bag and would sometimes not get in the shower until midnight, putting it off as long as possible. The district nurse came round and checked my scar, which was weeping at the bottom. She told Mum to get me some Savlon spray. I used it after a shower and it stung like hell. I read the instructions that said that it wasn't to be used on wounds or new scars. Great. I tried good old-fashioned salt water compresses and it cleared up.

I was sorting out my tablets for the day. I was still on steroids as I had to be weaned off them gradually, and was also taking painkillers, vitamin supplements, anti-histamines, a mouth wash and a horrid gunk I had to put on my sore lips several times a day. In my medical bag I found the half empty packet of tablets that the doctor had given me shortly before I went into hospital. Something clicked. I sat down to read the leaflet that was enclosed with the tablets.

Patient Information Leaflet: Brexidol Tablets

Brexidol is used to reduce inflammation and pain in conditions such as rheumatism, rheumatoid arthritis and osteoarthritis.

Before Taking Your Medicine

Do you have, or have you ever had, a stomach ulcer or bleeding? (yes)

Do you suffer from Crohn's disease or any other disease of the bowel or intestine? (yes)

Are you taking any other medicines including corticosteroids such as prednisolone? (yes)

Hmm. These were included in a great long list of questions. Answering yes to three of them set alarm bells ringing. My doctor knew my history, so why did he prescribe these tablets for me? I continued reading.

After Taking Your Medicine

Like all medicines, Brexidol may occasionally cause side-effects in some people. These side effects are usually rare and mild, such as: mild gastric upset (discomfort, nausea, constipation, wind, and diarrhea), mild skin rashes, swollen or irritated eyes or blurred vision, headache or dizziness, drowsiness or insomnia.

And the clincher:

If you experience any of the following side-effects, stop taking the tablets and tell your doctor as soon as possible: severe or continuous stomach upset, pain or indigestion, vomiting blood or passing black stools, wheeziness, persistent sore throat or high temperature

'These tablets are what put me in hospital,' I shouted to Mum who was in the living room watching the lunchtime edition of *Neighbours*, my head inside the kitchen cupboard. I showed her the leaflet.

'This is what did it,' I explained, 'do not take if you have bowel disease. I can't believe I was given these. They got rid of the pain but I think it's a bit more than a coincidence that a week later I'm almost dead.'

I sat down and had a hug. Someone in *Neighbours* was in a hospital bed. I laughed because the room was lovely, there were no tubes poking out of her neck and her hair and make-up were perfect.

'She's clearly not in Brighton,' I said to Dad, pointing at the television. 'I don't remember looking like that. I can't believe nobody thought to pluck my eyebrows or put a bit of lip balm on me. Honest to God – I think my face must have looked worse than my stomach.'

When I felt able to, I read the leaflet I was given as I was leaving hospital. I had to understand more about what had happened, and more importantly, what was likely to happen. You don't get told anything, you have to read it. So, I read it. It did not cheer me up.

Q. What should my stoma look like?

A. At first, a pinkish red blob protruding a few centimetres from the abdomen, which after 1-2 months should shrink to about the size of a 50p piece or smaller. It may not be exactly round, it will always be moist, and it may occasionally bleed slightly if touched.

Q. Will it smell?

A. Having a stoma does not increase odour. Modern stoma bags are odour-proof. You can gain extra confidence and reassurance if you wish by using one of the deodorizing products available nowadays. You can also take care with what you eat as some foods cause more odour than others – eg. eggs and fish.

Q. What can I eat and drink?

A. It is important to take plenty of fluid in order to prevent dehydration. Some extra salt should be taken as more salt is lost through a stoma than usual. You can help prevent wind by chewing food well (thus taking less air into the digestive system) and by taking care which foods you eat as some create extra wind in the gut (eg. beans, cabbage). Alcoholic drinks (wine and spirit) can be taken in moderation, as can beer and lager, however the latter may produce extra wind.

Q. Will I get food blockages?

A. Blockages can sometimes be caused by eating certain high-fibre or less digestible foods such as nuts, sweetcorn, celery, or mushrooms. You will know if you have a blockage by experiencing colicky pain, and stoma output will either cease or become watery. If a blockage occurs, stop taking solid food but try to continue taking fluids.

Q. How should I empty my drainable ileostomy bag?

A. Whilst a few people prefer to stand or kneel in front of the toilet bowl, the majority of men and women sit just down in the usual way.

Q. How should I dispose of my used stoma bags?

A. Drainable ileostomy bags should first be emptied in the usual way, and then after removal from the abdomen wrapped in a paper or plastic bag and placed in the household waste.

Q. Can I go back to work?

A. In the vast majority of cases, yes. However do not try to do too much too quickly – although stoma surgery is more routine nowadays in many hospitals, the formation of an ileostomy or internal pouch still represents major surgery, and you should pace yourself in your recovery accordingly. If possible, return on a part-time basis, or with lighter than usual duties, as this will help the recovery process. The same rule of thumb applies to performing housework, sports, or hobbies.

The phone never stopped ringing, but I didn't want to talk to anyone. A week after being discharged I still wasn't sleeping. I couldn't get comfortable despite the fact that I no longer went to bed with a load of plastic tubing. Where I had fallen on my hip in hospital, I couldn't sleep on that side. In fact, I couldn't lie on my side at all as it hurt my hip bones. I was six stone seven pounds. I'd lost almost two stone and put back half, and I was only a size 4, wearing children's underwear from M&S. My knees were the same width as my thighs. I think Mum was waiting for me to cry, but it didn't happen. I didn't feel anything. I felt completely devoid of any emotion at all. It was as though I was watching everything happen to someone else, almost like an out of body experience. Looking back, I'd say the diagnosis of post-traumatic depression was spot on. It's just a shame nobody thought to do anything about it.

Rolie had been calling each night to see how I was. I spoke to him, and to a couple of friends but three nights later, when the phone had rung seven times already, and Mum had come in and told me someone else wanted to talk to me to see how I was, I shook my head. Poor Mum was answering the phone non-stop, and I didn't have the energy to talk. I also didn't know what to say. I wasn't well, I wasn't fine and I didn't feel I could say otherwise. I was too tired to go through it more than once or twice a day.

Friends came to see me at home who hadn't seen me in hospital and hugged my bony frame. Some brought flowers, some sent flowers. At the end of the week, four bouquets turned up within half an hour of each other, and Mum had actually run out of vases.

My happiness was short lived, and sort of superfluous, as it was only receiving flowers that perked me up and gave me something to be excited about. That afternoon, Babylegs, my beloved little cinnamon hamster, passed away. A few days before I came out of hospital, Mum had taken her to the vet as she 'wasn't herself'. The vet said she probably had a kidney infection. Antibiotics didn't work. She wouldn't even come out of her little house within her house. I knelt on the floor and took the lid of the cage, reached in to pick her up and tell her I loved her, and she bit me. I let her be. Later on I took off the roof of the plastic house she slept in and there she lay, in a ball, shivering. She was getting worse, and I wished that she would just let her little self go and be in peace.

'She's like you,' said Dad, 'a tough little girl. She won't go without a fight.' We all had tears in our eyes. Dad thought she was great, calling her his little granddaughter whenever I brought her home for the weekend. We put more bedding around her, a blanket over the cage and left her to sleep.

The next morning, I reached in and found her all curled up in a tight little ball. She was stone cold, and didn't wake up when I stroked my little finger along her side. I cried so much, had a big hug from Mum, and put Babylegs in a Christmas wrapping box on some clean bedding. Dad dug a hole in the garden the next day beside our cat Whizzy's burial place. Two pets together. I said a prayer for her and put a homemade biscuit in on top for her to eat when she got to heaven. It was getting cold so I went back inside.

CHAPTER TWELVE
'DO ME NO WRONG'
PAT CUPP

On the Saturday, four days after I came home, Rolie drove up from Eastbourne to see me. I'd been a bit rubbish on the phone with him because he'd been saying things which wound me up like, 'you'll be OK in a couple of weeks, then', when I knew I'd never be OK as long as I had this thing attached to me, and that just because I was home didn't mean it was all over and everything was OK.

I didn't want him there all weekend. We'd never had anything to talk about. We were good at going out dancing and that was it. We didn't like the same films (he liked old black and white ones, I liked *Free Willy* and modern war films), he didn't read and he never opened the curtains in his house so it was always really dark and dingy. I couldn't imagine spending a whole weekend with him now that we wouldn't be dancing. I asked him to come up on Saturday lunchtime, and stay for tea, then go back to Eastbourne, rather than stay over until Sunday. It was harsh, but I just needed some space after the constant poking, touching, investigating and fiddling with me that had gone on in hospital. I'd had no privacy for weeks and didn't feel as though I was up to resuming my role of girlfriend. I needed my space more than ever.

My GP had suggested that I join a local support group – the Brighton branch of The National Association of Crohn's and Colitis, so I did. When I got the newsletter through, however, I felt worse. I didn't want to read about other people's stomas or other people's problems, nor was I cheered up by tales of how most of their lives had improved following surgery. I'd never had the symptoms that other people were having, so there was no relief for me to have a bag. I still didn't understand how I could have been diagnosed with colitis but never needed the loo, lost weight, or had any pain until that last week. I also felt like I was being defined by my disease by belonging to a group. I'm not really a 'group' person. At all. I had no desire to talk to anyone other than my mum about it, and certainly didn't want to share stories of surgery or stomas or bags or hospital trips. I know their support is invaluable to most patients, but I'm not most patients. It's just not for me. With hindsight, perhaps I was still in denial. I was still pretending that I wasn't a sick person, or at least that I wasn't defined by it. It was part of me, but it wasn't all encompassing and I didn't read any more pamphlets ever again.

At last, my mouth had healed and Rolie was delighted because it meant he could kiss me. The last thing I wanted, though, was a kiss. I was repulsed by my own body, but I'd put some make-up on and plaited my hair, put on my decent tracksuit bottoms and put some perfume on. Mum and Dad were delighted that I was making the effort.

He kissed me on the lips and looked so happy to see me it almost broke my heart. I just felt nothing. It was like having a total stranger in the room. I couldn't wait for him to go home. He left at 9.00pm, driving down to the coast to go to a gig. I shut the front door, leant against it for a few minutes, and went up to bed. He'd expected nothing from me, but I felt like that was still too much. I was too tired to even speak to him. I left a message on his answer phone apologising for the way I'd behaved, but asking him to back off a bit, let me call him when I felt ready, in a few days. I called him on the Monday, but he didn't return my call. I tried on Tuesday; nothing. On Wednesday, nothing.

On Thursday evening, right after my dinner, I burst into tears. I was sitting on the settee in my dressing gown, and it just happened. Mum and Dad came over and sort of collectively hugged and stroked me like you would a pet until I stopped. I couldn't believe that Rolie hadn't called me back, that he'd just deserted me. I was absolutely heartbroken. I'd just wanted some time to get my head around what had happened.

I was exhausted as I still wasn't sleeping and when I did finally get to sleep, I'd get up three times in the night to empty the bag. I just didn't have the energy to be in a relationship, particularly one that I knew didn't have a future, but I wasn't ready to cut off from him yet. I felt abandoned - as if he'd supported me for nothing all this time. I didn't understand how he could just disappear. Was it because of my bag? Maybe it was. He'd put a brave face on but perhaps he'd had a change of heart. After all, I'd only known him a few months. I convinced myself that this was the reason. I was revolting. Who would want to be with me?

On the Saturday, I decided to call him. Just once more. He picked up. We had a row immediately, him saying he didn't call because he was angry with how I had been the previous Saturday, telling me I was happy to see my friends but not him. I told that I really didn't need anyone shouting at me, making me cry, that my friends stayed for an hour then went home, and that he wanted to be there all weekend and that it was completely different. We'd never even slept together, and he was talking about 'when you're better we can finally, well, you know,' and I couldn't even imagine kissing anyone again or why on earth he'd want to come anywhere near me. We left it that he'd call every other day.

I developed a routine, a focus. I had to. I would get up around 9am, make my way into the bathroom and downstairs, and have my breakfast. Mum would prepare it for me - usually cereal with soya milk or toast and Marmite as I was still too weak to stand without holding on to something. After a week or so I felt able to do it myself; before that I couldn't guarantee that I wouldn't spill milk everywhere or drop the bowl. I'd have a cup of green tea or two - I was still not drinking milk -

then pluck up the courage to have my shower. I should really have done that first thing, but I've always had a cup of tea and breakfast before anything else, and I didn't want to change the habit of a lifetime. I need some semblance of normality in amongst all this mess.

Every other day I'd strip off my clothes, get in the shower and wash and condition my hair. I would then wash around the bag, rinse off then get out and sit on two towels (I was still so thin that I couldn't sit on the toilet without my bones aching) and dry myself. I'd dress the top half of me - my bras didn't fit anymore so I didn't wear one. I wore a thermal vest, as it was so cold, and a long-sleeved T-shirt. The rest of me would stay naked. I'd have all my equipment ready, lined up behind the sink. There was a little blue tub of warm water, dry wipes, a spray to remove the glue, the bag and scissors. I'd start by cutting out the stoma hole in the plastic disc on the back of the new bag with the nail scissors. This was cut to a 4cm circumference. I'd put that back on the side and taking a deep breath, begin the ritual. The bag sat on my right side, hanging down between my legs. To get it off, first I'd have to spray around the plastic backing which held the bag on to my tummy with the 'glue exterminator'. It stung like hell.

Once that was dripping down my legs I could slowly peel the bag off, inch by inch, exposing the sore, red skin beneath. As the backing base peeled away, I'd hold the bag itself and pull it all off in one go, then throw it into the blue plastic disposal bags, fragranced to mask the smell. Then, whilst praying that the stoma wouldn't churn anything out, I'd have to wipe around the stoma with a warm wet cloth which I'd dipped in the blue bowl of warm water - later I'd find using fragrance-free baby wipes a lot easier - until I'd removed all traces of glue, waste and sometimes blood. I nicked the stoma once with my nail and it bled like mad, it was hideous. Then I'd dry the area with another disposable cloth, and apply calamine lotion around the stoma to try and stop the soreness and itching. Usually just as I'd applied it, standing waving my hands back and forth to help it dry out, the stoma would start to pulsate and I'd end up with a mixture of calamine and hot, acidic green liquid snaking down the inside of my thigh.

While that burned its way down my legs, I'd grab the cut-out plastic disc with bag attached and stick that over the stoma so that it poked out of the hole I'd cut, making sure it stuck down properly, with no bumps. The bag was attached to the base - only later would I have to learn how to wrestle with a more complex two-piece kit - and with any luck, it'd stick firm and I'd roll up the end of the bag into the clip, tuck it away and get dressed. As I was so thin it didn't show beneath my clothes and anyway, I was still wearing delightful tie-waist tracksuit pants so at least I was comfortable. I felt so much cleaner but hated changing it.

One day, when I'd changed the bag four or five times over a fortnight or so, I decided to get in the shower without the bag on to give my skin a breather. I'd decided that it couldn't be helping the skin around the bag if it had something permanently glued to it. Feeling hot running water on the stoma was really weird, but I just tipped my head back and washed my hair and tried not to look down. It was like intestine-induced vertigo.

All of a sudden, I felt a little wriggle on my side. The stoma was starting to 'perform' as I showered. Runny green gloop plopped to the shower floor and disappeared among the bubbles and down the drain. This happened on a number of occasions, with me having to tell Mum that I'm sorry, but I sort of did a mess in the shower. Nice. When the consistency was thick, after I'd eaten potatoes or bread, it felt like a worm was pushing itself out of my tummy. Can you even begin to imagine what that is like?

The warm water on my skin felt great, but I noticed that small red welts, like little blisters, were appearing in patches around the stoma where the bag would stick. Worse still, it really itched under the bag. The skin was sore and broken. It looked terrible. The stoma nurse arrived with a barrier cream, but it didn't make any difference. I tried all sorts of different manufacturer's bags - cutting the back off, sticking the discs to my skin on my stomach around the bag, working out which ones hurt more than others. One I could hardly peel off at all and subsequently took the top layer of skin with it. I binned the lot and, literally, stuck with what I had.

Once I'd mastered showering, changing the bag in less than 15 minutes and drying my own hair, I had nothing much to do except remark on how quickly my nails were growing.

'At this rate,' I muttered to Mum over my third cup of Marmite, 'I'll soon be like that old man in India who sits with his right hand in the air all day showing off his curly old fingernail.'

I had a visitor almost every day, but I still had no desire to read, to listen to music, to do anything normal. I felt useless and I missed working. I flicked through magazines, watched television without really watching it, because nothing held my interest for more than a couple of minutes. I couldn't work out why. I just felt fazed by everything. By the end of the week, was eating as much as Dad at dinner. I was snacking on biscuits between meals. After three weeks my weight was up to seven stone three. I looked better. I was still too small for size eight knickers and living in tracksuit bottoms that Mum had doctored so that the waistband was loose on my stomach, and still in vest tops and sweatshirts. I looked a state, to be honest. I was desperate to get dressed in jeans and boots; all the things I hadn't worn since October. I hadn't left the house, either, save for little walks around the garden.

My friend Kirsty visited from London one evening; she phoned the day before and asked me if there was anything she could bring me.

'Yes, Warm Bear,' I said, excitedly.

'What's a Warm Bear?' she asked, a bit confused and probably ready to commit me to a mental institution.

'It's a bear I saw in Topshop a little while ago. He might not still be for sale. He has a hot water bottle in his back. He can keep me warm.'

Kirsty duly arrived via Topshop and there he was - a lovely golden bear with a hot water bottle in his back. He kept me company on the sofa all day long and sat on the bed with me all night. I suppose I could have asked for something more normal, like fancy cheese or some flowers, but I wanted Warm Bear. Needless to say he's been around ever since. Also needless to say, I cooked dinner. Seriously. I could barely stand at the kitchen worktop but I insisted. What's the point? Nobody expects me to cook, I've just come out of hospital. I don't know why I do it, I really don't.

In the third week, I asked Mum to take me to Bromley so I could do some shopping. None of my clothes fitted me, and I wanted to be prepared for when I was ready to go out. I was still very weak, so didn't want to go on my own. We took the bus and even that was exhausting. Of course, I pretended everything was fine but in reality, I couldn't sit down on the bus (sitting was so painful) and standing up meant holding on to the pole, which in turn meant straining my stomach muscles to stay on my feet.

When I tried things on, I could see how thin I still was. There was no bump once I'd got the clothes on, because my stomach was still concave. There was nothing of me. Size eight jeans were too big, and the shop assistants whispered about me, trying not to stare but failing miserably.

I felt like doing some work. I'd been home for three weeks. I wasn't ready, by any means, to go back to Brighton yet. I still couldn't get up and downstairs in one go, I couldn't drive, I couldn't carry anything heavier than a piece of paper (well, that's what Mum would have you believe) and mentally I wasn't ready to be on my own. I was toying with the idea of selling up or renting out the flat and staying at home again forever. It was safe, I had Pebble there, the neighbours were nice and I could park my car. I could have, and with hindsight, should have given in and done just that. However, as usual, my determination to overcome everything, even to the point of punishing myself by not letting myself have what I really wanted, pushed me into going back. Just as I had pushed myself to go there in the first place, when I really didn't want to, I was now pushing myself to return. What an idiot.

It was almost Christmas. I wanted to go and do some Christmas shopping. Mum thought I was mental, and of course, she was right. She dropped me off at the bus stop so I could catch the bus to the town centre. I'd insisted on going alone even though I suspected that I really wasn't ready. Again, I didn't think of the position this put her in. It was so unfair of me. I was exhausted just from catching the bus. I managed to go to three shops before I had to admit defeat. I can't remember what I bought, but I had also forgotten that I didn't have the strength to carry anything. I think I got Dad a book, Mum some perfume and Jonathan some aftershave. I couldn't walk any further nor carry anything else. Every movement hurt more than the last one and I was starting to panic that my bag would need emptying. Fortunately I got a bus almost straight away, rang Mum to tell her I was on it and she picked me up where she'd dropped me off a couple of hours earlier. I was freezing cold, deathly pale and I could see how relieved she was that I was in one piece and I hadn't had to call her to come and rescue me from a shop floor. I apologised for being an idiot. That set me back about a week, rather than propelling me forward.

On Christmas Day we all breathed a sigh of relief that I was actually sitting at the table rather than being remembered.

'At least Dad would have had more turkey if I hadn't have pulled through,' I quipped.

'Not true,' he said, raising a glass and an eyebrow simultaneously, 'I'd have just made Mum buy a smaller one and saved some money.'

January 2002

I moved back to Brighton mid-January. I was getting restless, and felt as though I could tackle the stairs and drive my car now. My scar was healing nicely and my muscles were getting stronger. I was still short of breath and didn't have much energy, but I felt a lot stronger than I had before Christmas. Dad drove me down, with Mum looking over her shoulder at me on the back seat, asking if I was OK every now and then. I think she meant 'OK' as in emotionally whereas I thought she meant physically. I said 'Yeah, fine' when deep down, I wanted him to turn around and take me back to their house again.

Rolie and I had started talking again on the phone, and he'd agreed to come and put a shower in my bathroom, as I only had a bath. A bath was useless with a stoma as the hot water melted the glue and the bag would come off in the water. I couldn't change it every day and I felt so horribly unclean with this thing on me that I wanted to shower every day. Dad had to beg him, mind you, to do it. He came over that weekend and duly tiled the bathroom and put the shower up. We were tentatively moving around the flat, scared to bump into each other. It was tense, to say the least, but he seemed in good spirits. I made him a coffee and a bacon sandwich, and he then said it:

'Me and you, baby, are we back together?

'I don't know,' I replied. 'I think so. I've missed you. I'd like to be.'

With that he gave me a big smacker, an even bigger grin and said, 'I'm gonna finish them tiles, my little darlin', then be right back for a cuddle.'

He finished the bathroom and got his cuddle. It felt right, being back in his strong arms. I felt safe with him. I knew he loved me and I knew then that I really did love him. I couldn't see a future for us as far as marriage went, but for now, it was everything I wanted - security, and someone I could trust. Imagine my surprise, then, when he called me following night and told me he'd changed his mind and that he didn't want to see me again.

I really couldn't keep up with it all - emotionally I was so drained, physically I was only just able to do normal things like clean and cook without falling over. I put down the phone without even saying anything in response, and just sat on the floor with Pantouf (Panda wanted me to change his name to something more exotic than, well, 'Panda'. We'd been to the cinema one afternoon to see *Chocolat*, where the little girl's imaginary wallaby was called Pantouf, and he liked it, so it kind of stuck). This was it now. Once again, I was on my own.

A couple of months later it was The Rockabilly Rave weekender at Pontins holiday camp in Rye, East Sussex. It was a 90-minute drive, and I felt able to do it on my own, only once I'd arrived I wished that I wasn't there. This weekender, as with all rockabilly events, is all about how you look. A lot of the girls would go through three different outfits in one day, with perfect pin curls, flawless make-up, dainty Lucite handbags and original 1950s dresses and shoes which meant they looked a million dollars (and cost about the same). I'd never been one for bothering with all that - no real surprise given I was working on football magazines rather than women's magazines - but now, standing in front of the mirror, I felt an overwhelming lack of confidence in myself and my appearance. I wished I'd had a wardrobe full of vintage dresses, anything to distract from the reality of what my body had become.

I was embarrassed, frightened and a bit panicky. In the end, I just wore jeans (no belt) and a black vest top over them. It was clingy, but you still couldn't see the bag unless you were trying very hard to. It turns out that nobody had any idea other than Aaron, and he just had to remember not to shove me in the tummy on that side as he spun me around during a dance. I had a couple of dances all night, and didn't dance with anyone other than him because I couldn't be sure they wouldn't grab me around the waist and recoil in horror, or worse, just really hurt me.

Rolie was there, of course. He nodded a hello as he walked past at the bar. A few hours later, I went to talk to him, and asked him if he still wanted to not speak to me. He turned his back on me. I walked off, tears welling in my eyes, and sat down next to Charlie.

'He can't even look at me,' I said, shaking my head and finishing my drink. We stayed up until the end (7am, would you believe) and headed back to the chalet. Hilariously, we had bunk beds in our room, and I was on the top - really practical just after surgery, but of course, I'd insisted because I loved top bunk!

The next morning Charlie slept soundly whilst I was enjoying a cup of coffee and a custard cream in the sunshine, sitting on the doorstep of the chalet in my stupid teddy bear pyjamas, hair on end, no make-up, not a care. Whose voice should I hear in the next chalet? You've got it, of 3,000 or so people, Rolie was booked in next door. He came outside, and looked quite surprised to see me sitting there.

'I'm not following you,' I said, smiling and shielding my eyes from the sun with my packet of biscuits, 'I'm in this chalet. How mad is that?'

He laughed, looked perplexed, and headed back inside. A minute later, he popped his head around the door, and asked if I want to go for some food with him at the cafe by the beach. I didn't question it, and instead leapt up (sort of) and skipped (sort of) to the bedroom to throw on some clothes, shove my hair in a ponytail and grab my sunglasses.

Suffice to say, a tattooed arm draped around my shoulder meant we were officially back together and I was as happy as you can be when you're at a holiday camp with a hangover and your insides on your outsides. He proclaimed the bag to be nothing but 'a big plaster'. I felt a little more confident knowing that he still fancied me. As he said, 'you're exactly the same, baby, you just been sliced up and put back together a bit wrong'. Really, you had to hand it to him - he had quite a way with words!

After that, we started off where we'd left off. Rolie booked us a holiday to Ireland. Not exactly the trip to the Seychelles that I had dreamed of, but it would give us a chance to put everything behind us and explore some countryside. I said: 'I can't be bothered to have to learn another language just to go away for a week,' to which his reply was, 'you ain't got to, you daft cow, it's Ireland,' to which I said, 'ah, don't be fooled!'

A week before our trip, as I was wondering how many pairs of socks and how many stoma bags I needed to take with me to Ireland, I felt a sudden stabbing pain in my left hip. I couldn't believe it. Not again. I stood up, gasping for breath. It hurt like hell. It was back: after all I'd gone through, here we were again.

I made an appointment with the doctor. He referred me to a rheumatologist at the hospital. Before my hospital appointment, I asked if I could have some crutches. I could barely put weight on my left leg, and my other hip wasn't feeling too good either. I also had muscle pains in my upper right side as well.

My doctor arranged for the physiotherapy department to loan me some crutches. I was determined to go on holiday - again, mental - but the pain was excruciating. I took a taxi to the hospital which almost killed me in itself as I'm so tight I'd never have paid for a cab if I wasn't in so much pain, and collected the crutches. I then had to take a taxi home as I lived too far from the bus stop to walk, even with the crutches. Plus it was up a very steep hill. It seemed like the minute my body had started to heal from the operation it decided it was OK to bring the joint pain back.

I pretty much went nowhere and did nothing for the next two days. I took strong painkillers and hobbled around the flat, heaving myself in and out of the shower, sometimes unable to get dressed. I packed my case and within a few hours, the pain began to abate, even without painkillers. I felt that perhaps God was cutting me a little slack, for once, and would let me get through this week without any trouble. At least I hoped this was his plan. He certainly hadn't done me many favours up until now, had he?

Our trip started off OK. We hired a car. We met some sheep, Rolie ate his dream dinners (cottage pie, cottage pie, cottage pie) and I felt like we were on a trip back to the 1970s. By day three we had started to argue, mainly about cottage pie. We were polar opposites when it came to food, for a start. He loved boiled potatoes and frozen burgers. I would sooner eat my own hair than eat that. Things started to wind me up, and vice versa. In between snappy moments we saw some llamas - one spat at me as Rolie took our picture - and a deer ate a slice of potato from my head (long story), so there were good times.

We also finally consummated an actual 'proper relationship' (with a leopard print vest staying very much on, to cover my stupid bag) but it was pretty testing, to say the least. We spent an afternoon horse riding. I love horses, and had had a few lessons when I first went freelance. I didn't like to tell Rolie that the pain caused by a horse trotting along a country lane was like having my hip excavated by a pneumatic drill. I just tried to stay focused on not falling off, and stroking the horse's mane. Every bounce hurt like hell.

Unsurprisingly, the next morning I awoke in agony. The pain in my left hip was so bad that I couldn't put one foot in front of the other without crying out. I'd decided at the very last minute to leave my crutches at home, because I was feeling OK before I left. What an idiot. I had to stay at the B&B, and do just what it said on the tin - bed, breakfast. I was in so much pain I could barely catch my breath. Rolie had a wander around the gardens, I told him to say hello to birds and worms from me while I sat in the conservatory, attempting to concentrate on a book. To top it off, it was raining. I've had better holidays, to be honest.

The next day, both the pain and the rain had eased up a bit and we went for a drive in the mountains. Unfortunately, I hadn't accounted for not being near a toilet. Halfway up a winding mountain road, I looked down to see that my stoma bag was about to explode under my T-shirt.

Oh dear. Thankfully there weren't any people around, but there were sheep looking at us. Rolie had to pull over, and I had the undignified and somewhat difficult task of squatting down behind a rock and emptying my breakfast of muesli and wholemeal toast into Cork's beautiful countryside. People of Ireland, I'd like to apologise for that.

On the last night, I took two tablets in succession as the pain was so horrendous. We were looking for a place to stay and had subsequently been driving around for what felt like about three years. There was some big horse race on and every hotel was booked. We finally arrived at someone's house which masqueraded as a B&B (it was literally a bedroom in their house. Eeek) and weird as it was, I didn't have time to look around. I promptly threw up in the en-suite toilet the minute we walked in. The painkillers were too strong for my stomach, and that was that. I was in such a mess. I can honestly say that outside of hospital, I had never been so glad to know I was going home the next morning.

I ended up having to ask Mum and Dad to pick me up from Gatwick upon our return, taking me to the flat to get some things (my crutches were top of the list) and going back to their house. Again. I had to have help up and down the stairs, and the worst thing was, the hip and lower back pain would just strike out of nowhere, and I'd be completely unable to move, stuck in whatever position I was at the time. If I was half way up the stairs or just about to sit on the toilet, it wasn't easy.

I was waiting for the hospital to get in touch with the date for my next operation. I wanted what was called 'reversal' surgery, where the stoma is brought back inside and various bits and bobs are pulled apart and put together so that you end up with a 'pouch' just above your bottom which holds all your food. It then comes out of your bottom, as God intended. It'd come out a lot quicker than if you had a colon, but even so, the idea of being able to get rid of the bag which was, by now, making my skin so sore that I yelped whenever I had to spray the glue on it was a nice idea. I was sick of the blisters, the sores, the bleeding. It repulsed me, too, and that's pretty hard to put up with.

After much discussion with Mum and Dad as to the risks of having more surgery ('uh, death, that kind of thing') I went in to hospital to see my surgeon so that he could give me the once over. He deemed me fit and healthy (in operational terms) to have the surgery, and scheduled me in for June, less than two months away. He said that because I still had my - wait for it - 'rectal stump', I would stand a good chance of the pain I had in my back and my hips disappearing.

'You've still got the remains of colitis, in the sense that you still have a piece of your colon near your bottom,' he explained, 'so we'll get rid of all of that, and then you'll have no colitis at all, and it's the best way of getting rid of the pain.'

I was a bit perplexed; surely pain in my hips and actual bones had nothing to do with my internal organs? It didn't sound right to me, but then I failed my biology exam so I didn't think I should argue.

A couple of weeks later I finally got a letter from the rheumatology department. My doctor had told the consultant that I had mild scoliosis (curvature of the spine), and inflammation of the sacro-iliac joints (where the base of your spine meets your hips). The rheumatologist told me that he too believed that the operation would be the best way to get rid of the pain, and that it was most definitely the colitis that was causing it.

So, two expert opinions later, I decide to go for it.

At this time I'd also put my flat on the market. I couldn't face the stairs, the lack of parking space and the mad neighbour. I needed more space and I didn't want to have to park three streets away, nor climb three flights of stairs. I'd put an offer in on a flat in Hove. It had two bedrooms and a roof terrace. I was going to get a rabbit. Rolie was going to build it an outside hutch and I planned to keep it indoors and outdoors, and scatter big cushions on the terrace in summer, with fairy lights around the edge. The bedroom had sliding doors that opened on to the terrace and I imagined sitting out there on my cushions, reading a book and nursing a glass of wine, cuddling up with my rabbit. The parking wasn't great, but the road was flat, the shops and restaurants were a couple of minutes' walk away and it was 10 minutes walk from the beach. It was absolutely ideal, and my offer on it was accepted.

Alice and Ryan were getting married on June 15th, and naturally I wanted to be at their wedding with Rolie, have a dance and a drink in case either would be my last one (I wasn't too optimistic about my odds at this stage, unsurprisingly) and I asked if I could go into hospital the week after. Now I just had to wait, all the while trying not to think of the fact that I had to go back to that place, that same ward, to the same sounds, same smells, same everything, and go through it all again. That was the first time I decided that people were right when they said I was brave. I was going to face my absolute hell all over again. How would I get through that? It wasn't any comfort that I knew what to expect - far from it. I was absolutely dreading it, yet I knew I needed to do it.

I went back to Brighton to pack the entire contents of the flat. I knew I'd be in hospital for a while, then recuperating at my parents'. I realised that they might have to organise my move for me. It was due to happen mid-July as the survey had been done and I'd got a buyer for my place. I looked at all the boxes, piled up on top of one another, and smiled. I was so looking forward to a new start – a new tummy and a new home, and a rabbit. I was feeling really positive for the first time in a long time.

Before I knew it, it was June 23rd. Time for my next fight.

CHAPTER THIRTEEN
'ALL OVER AGAIN'
JOHNNY CASH

Going in to hospital on the Saturday afternoon wasn't as simple as it should have been, as it turned out that the hospital weren't sure that there would actually be a bed for me on the Monday that I was due the operation. Mum and Dad waited patiently in Orpington while I called the hospital admissions desk every hour from 9am on the Saturday morning. At 2pm, no doubt feeling a bit anxious and restless, Mum and Dad decided to head down anyway, despite my protestations that I could go in on my own. Finally, I agreed that it would be nice to face my worst nightmares with them beside me instead of alone.

Eventually, we made our way to the hospital and sat there and waited instead of waiting at home, although I was beginning to think that this would be a good time to back out, as I was really feeling anxious being back in the same department, never mind the fear of surgery and the hell which would follow. I asked Mum if she thought it was a sign that we should just go home and forget about it. After all, it was 5pm. I'd been waiting all day and I don't think my nerves could take it anymore.

'I can't answer that, sweetheart. It's up to you, but you're here, and you hate the stoma and all the soreness, so maybe it's a good idea to just hang on for another hour or so and see what happens.'

I nodded, and paced the room. A nurse came in at 6.30pm and said, 'Juliette, it's all happening for Monday, so let's get you admitted.' Well, Mum was right, as always.

I signed some forms, told them I was allergic to penguins and jazz funk (I was bored with saying 'none' to the 'any allergies?' question) and again asked if I could go home that night and not have to stay in all weekend when I wasn't actually ill. I didn't see the point of being in a hospital bed, surrounded by sick people. I'd have done anything not to spend a minute more than I had to in that place.

'You're such trouble!' said one of the nurses, winking at me. Then she said, 'actually, you'll have to stay as we start you on a barium flush out tomorrow morning to prep you for the op.'

'Balls!' I hissed, under my breath, and followed the nurse to the bay and my bed. Just as we approached the bay – the same one as I was in before, I began to shake with nerves. The nurse smiled and gestured that we turn right... and led me to my own room. My own room! I couldn't believe it. Mum and Dad settled me in then went home. I really wish they hadn't come down as it was such a long journey and in my mind, a waste of petrol, and therefore money. I hadn't needed them there, but on the other hand, it was nice to have them around, I'll admit that. I read some of my book (couldn't concentrate as usual), flicked through magazines, wandered around the room, looked out of the window. I snuck in a Diazepam at 10pm and got into bed, thinking how strange it was that I could climb in and out of this, and go to the bathroom as easy as pie. I was told no food or drink other than water or squash, and so talked to my Orange Barley water for a bit and said goodnight to Pantouf.

I slept the whole night through. On the Sunday morning Rolie came in and we went outside for a little walk. I'd had the first of my barium things, a vile, thick orange liquid with gritty bits in. It was like drinking wet sand. After 30 minutes of sitting outside, my stoma went bananas and I had to come in and use the loo. I went back outside as it was a sunny day, with my book, and just looked at the pages while Rolie went off in to town.

He came back a few hours later with a get well card, saying, 'I know you ain't even had it yet but you can put it up there,' and placed it on the cupboard next to the bed. I kissed him and off he went, leaving me to it. I had to have the other glass of wet sand at 6pm, and felt that everything, including my stomach lining and internal organs had been flushed out of my stoma by 9pm, so I called Mum and Dad from my mobile outside, then had a bath, washed my hair, did all the things like shaving my legs and plucking my eyebrows, things I wouldn't be able do again for a while. I went to bed, and back to my old habits, lay awake until the sun came up, peeping through the blinds, shadows dancing on the wall as the breeze blew through the window.

I was shattered, and must have fallen asleep for all of ooh, 10 minutes, because at 8am, I was nudged awake by the anaesthetist.

'Eh?' I said, all sleepy, 'I didn't order breakfast in bed, did I?'

'Afraid not, sweetheart - you're on,' said someone in surgical scrubs, 'time to get you down to theatre.'

I leapt out of bed, washed my face, brushed my teeth, all the while being hurried up a bit. I'd already given my consent and signed my life away - quite literally in the case of the things which might go wrong when you're having your entire plumbing system re-built - and hopped on the bed to be wheeled down to theatre, which is when the fear set in.

Just before we went through the usual 'count backwards from 10' the anaesthetist had leaned over to put a tube in somewhere, and I'd said, 'Oh, how disappointing, I thought you were going to give me a kiss!'

He laughed, saying 'you can have one if it makes you feel better,' and I replied that it would. He duly gave me a kiss on the cheek and ruffled my hair. The surgeon found it quite amusing, I think. I figured that if I was going to die this time, the last thing I wanted was a kiss from a handsome Italian anaesthetist. I was out.

The first thing I heard when I woke up was a nurse talking about going to lunch. She said it was half past one, and I did a quick calculation. I was on a trolley, not in a bed, so I was alive and I'd had the operation. I'd been in theatre around four and a half hours. I should, in theory, be upstairs in the HDU (high dependency unit) in an hour or so. In practice, of course, things rarely go as planned. My blood pressure was so low that I was kept down in recovery for another two hours, Mum and Dad frantically wandering the corridors of the hospital, being told I was 'OK' when I quite clearly wasn't. It was a repeat of the first time and I couldn't bear to think that they were going through this again. When I was finally brought up to the ward a team of nurses swarmed around my bed, fiddling with machines and looking concerned. The situation was more serious than the first operation, and I knew it. I didn't feel that I had any of the fight I had the first time. I could feel my fight just pour out of me with every breath.

Mum and Dad stood to the side of the bed with Rolie, unable to do anything to help. Mum held my hand. I was shivering despite being wrapped in the silver blanket that's pumped with warm air, and knew that my heart might fail if my blood pressure wasn't stabilised soon. A doctor told them I'd lost a lot of blood during surgery which was why I was in such a state. Mum asked if I'd be alright, and his reply was:

'We're doing our best.'

I heard Mum gasp and tell Dad that 'her blood pressure's going through the floor!'

I couldn't believe that this was happening again, that I'd come through such a complicated and risky operation only to fail at the last hurdle. Maybe my body just couldn't take any more. It didn't make sense, but I clung on to Mum's hand as hard as I could and every now and again, I'd open my eyes and just look at her, unable to say anything, but I knew she could see how terrified I was that this was going to be it.

Several hours later my blood pressure had crept up slightly to the normal blood pressure level you'd find on, say, a tortoise on lithium. I was stable, but the doctors were still concerned. I fought to stay awake despite my eyelids feeling as though they were made of lead. The surgeon came to see me. He then delivered the shattering blow that I don't think my parents were aware of - I still had the stoma. I was in such a state during surgery that he couldn't finish the job. There was too much scar tissue from the first operation surrounding all the places he had to fiddle with, so they'd tied up the end of the pouch they'd made, and basically formed a new stoma from my small intestine that this time was lying flat against my skin rather than poking out.

'I'm sorry, Juliette,' said the surgeon, holding my hand, 'we'll finish the job soon, I promise.'

Mum was in tears, Dad too. I turned my head to one side and tried to blink away my own. I couldn't believe I'd been through all that and still had the stoma. I just wanted to be left alone. I wanted to drift away. I didn't even care anymore. I felt nothing but utter despair.

My parents finally left my side at around 8pm. They'd not eaten since lunchtime and were staying at my flat that night with Rolie, with them having my bedroom and him on the sofa. It turned out that every restaurant and take-away place was shut as it was Monday and they had to make do with egg on toast at the flat. Poor Mum still ended up cooking even after all that! I don't think they got much more sleep than I did, which, of course, was none at all. I'd been through this nightmare once already. I couldn't believe I was doing it again. The panic had set in the moment I'd regained consciousness, and it showed no signs of abating. This time, I wanted it to stop, once and for all. I couldn't do this again, I just couldn't.

I had a tube in the left side of my stomach, the thickness of a McDonald's milkshake straw. Red liquid drained into a plastic container beside me in bed. There was a tube going up my nose and down my throat, a line in my neck, and the oxygen mask holding them all in place. The tape over my earring had caught my hair and pulled like mad if I moved my head. I had the epidural in my spine and this time around, my pain was controlled by diamorphine and a local anaesthetic as opposed to pure morphine. I also had a thick, hard tube coming from inside my bottom that was stitched, on the outside, to the underside of my right bottom cheek. This curled up my back and came out by my ribs and down past the bed into a plastic container that hung on the bar of the bed. Next to that was my catheter, which of course meant another tube through my urethra. I also had a line in my left hand. I couldn't move. I was pinned down by all these tubes and needles and containers, and by my own wretched body. I felt like an animal in a laboratory. All I needed now was someone to squirt shampoo in my eyes and force-feed me cleaning products and I might end up with a new career as a lab rat.

I was monitored every hour for the first two days and nights through which again, I was awake. I wore earplugs, an eye mask and tried so hard to relax, despite the fact that I wasn't allowed to sleep on my back, and nurses had to turn me on to a different side every couple of hours. Add to this I still had the ileostomy bag on the right side of my tummy. It's no wonder that I couldn't relax enough to sleep, despite being exhausted. A slight tug on the drip in the back of my hand and the needle would press into the flesh and hurt like hell.

The lights stayed on in the ward until half past midnight, when the nurses had done all their rounds, and two old ladies either side of me snored so loudly I swear I could see their curtains shake. Somebody was brought in to the ward at around 3am and the noise was unbearable. Porters stood about shouting in the ward, nurses rushed back and forth across the floor like ants and I just lay awkwardly on my side, propped up by pillows because I couldn't support my own weight and cramps came and went in my legs all night. Morning came with the breakfast trolley at seven. It was like *Groundhog Day*.

I had plenty of visitors. Alice and Ryan came in and brought their wedding pictures, which was a welcome distraction. Alice had been an absolute angel through all this; she was always there for me and nothing was too much trouble. I don't think I'd have got through it without her, and whenever I saw her she cheered me up and gave me a big hug, afraid of hurting me but not put off by all the tubes and monitors and bags which surrounded my bed.

Looking out of the window to my left, I could see that the weather was glorious, and it made me cross because I was missing the sunshine. On the Friday after my operation it had been five days since surgery and I was finally given permission to eat something. I had half a slice of toast and a few baked beans. I sneakily took vitamins and arnica homeopathic tablets to help heal the internal bruising. I was able, by the Saturday, to shower and wash my hair on my own, although it was a real struggle. I still had the catheter and what I called the 'bum tube' in, and by now, with the epidural out and my pain being controlled by codeine and paracetamol tablets, I realised just how uncomfortable the tube up my bottom was. I couldn't sit straight; I had to lean onto my left side as the tube was made from such hard plastic that there was no give in it at all, and it was pressing on the stitches that held it in place.

On the Saturday afternoon Mum and Dad came down and brought my lunch - a ham and lettuce sandwich with salad cream, and a packet of ready salted crisps. That was my favourite packed lunch at school – clearly I was regressing, in need of comfort food to get me through it. How it hadn't occurred to them to bring me food before I'll never know. It was wonderful. I ate it outside in the sunshine with them in my wheelchair, swathed in blankets with Dad keeping an eye on the seagulls perched above my head, ready to swoop on any crumbs. The seagulls, I mean, not Dad. Helen visited and stayed the whole day, bringing me the best present ever - a soft, cuddly monkey (not a real one, one from a toy shop) whom I named Daniel. Pantouf was a bit put out, but after a couple of days they got on like a house on fire and he was so cuddly I had him on the bed all the time.

A week after my operation, the surgeon paid me a visit, and told me I could have the catheter removed. He looked at my bottom where the tube was really hurting. He told me it was no wonder it hurt so much, one of the stitches was infected. He instructed a nurse to sort it out and re-position it with tape rather than a stitch, which helped a lot.

A couple of days later I was sent to ultrasound to have the dye test which would determine whether my insides had healed, or whether there were any leaks in the tissue of the new pouch. I was frantic with worry -

if the test was anything but 100% successful, I would have to have further surgery, be opened up again and start all over. I couldn't stand the thought of it. I was wheeled down to X-ray and told to lie in this weird *Stargate* style white cylinder, my bare bottom facing the doctor. I couldn't imagine anything more unpleasant than having a bottom with recently infected stitches presenting itself to you before lunch. Ugh. I listened to him explain what he was going to do. I held the nurse's hand as he slowly pulled the tube from my back passage and swiftly attached a new tube into which he squirted the dye. It was icy cold and it shot up inside me like a bullet. I screamed out in agony. The nurse told me to squeeze her hand as hard as I liked. She let out a squeak.

'Not that hard, though,' she laughed. Tears rolled down my cheeks as the pain took over my entire body. The doctor re-inserted the drain and pulled my gown back over. I cannot tell you how undignified I felt at that moment. It was beyond anything I have ever endured, and I've been through some seriously humiliating crap in my time, including watching Tottenham lose to Port Vale in the FA Cup and wetting myself in front of the whole school assembly when I was seven.

I was taken back to the ward with the test results in an envelope. I read them in the lift as the porter negotiated the ridiculously long journey back to my bed. The test showed no leaks, no complications, and no build up of fluid. It was clear. I was overjoyed. I felt terrible, but now I could make real progress and get out of here.

A couple of hours later, the doctor came round to get the results, so I told him I'd already had a look and knew that as I was eating properly and that there were no leaks, I could go home.

He looked astounded.

'Who said you could go home yet?'

'Me. I want to go home. I don't need proper hospital care anymore, I just need to sleep in my own bed and eat vegetables. If I stay here any longer I'll go bonkers or die of malnutrition.'

'Well, I suppose the drain can come out now and we'll see how you go tonight. The usual recovery time is about three weeks, but then it's you, and I know how you like to set new recovery records, Juliette, but it has only been 10 days. Just 10!'

No more stomach drain! I was ecstatic. Stop reading and just imagine for one minute how it must feel to have a hard, plastic tube up your bottom, stitched to your infected, inflamed skin for days on end, to have tubes in your side, your neck, on your wrists, a giant needle in your spine, a hole in the middle of your stomach and a bag stuck to that, to have liquid draining from your stomach and your bottom (which, incidentally, was green and foul smelling, what the doctor called 'dead tissue'). You can't, can you? It's indescribable, the discomfort, the pain and the continuing struggle just to be able to sit in a chair or lay in a bed. It's a never-ending mess of panic, pain and despair.

I struggled out of bed after a little rest from the tube palaver and went to the nurses' station to call Mum, asking her and Dad to come and pick me in two days' time. She didn't ask if anyone had officially made that decision, and I didn't want to tell her that I was pretty much discharging myself. Despite Diazepam and sleeping pills, I still hadn't slept properly and I was going nuts. I needed to get out of there and get home. I was sick of being sick, and I couldn't stand the fact that I had no control over anything in hospital. I was at the mercy of everyone else to make decisions for me, to tell me what I could and couldn't do, I was being prodded and poked and needles were stuck into me, blood was taken, pills were going down my throat, stuff was leaking out of my bottom... it was too much. On top of that I was still the only patient under 75 and that just served to make me feel even more upset.

Over the next two days I started to imagine going home. The liquid crap was coming out now whenever I went for a wee, as if my half formed pouch was competing with my bladder. That night the old lady next to me took her laxative solution to prepare her for surgery the next day. Her commode was stationed just the other side of my curtain and I could hear - and worse - smell *everything*. It must have been awful for her but it wasn't a bunch of roses for me, either. Here I am, I've just had major surgery, almost died (again) and now my numerous open wounds were inches away from someone's faeces. That's basically what we're talking about.

It went on all night and the stench was intoxicating. I had asked for a little 'packed lunch' tea of a sandwich, some crisps (I loved my ready-salted crisps!) and an apple. I managed half of the sandwich, a few crisps, and a couple of bites of the apple before giving up. Someone's bowels exploding next to you does not make for a good appetite. To make matters worse, she'd had chili con carne for her lunch. Well done to the nurses for not monitoring that choice.

That night I felt really nauseous, and I don't think it was just the old lady's exploding bowels. I had a fever, headache, the lot. I was still being prodded and it didn't seem too much of a concern for the nurses, so I didn't say anything. I just wanted to get out. I didn't sleep at all, and threw up a couple of times, which was nice, but the following morning after keeping down some Weetabix and a cup of tea, Mum and Dad arrived with Jonathan. A quick call to the doctor confirmed that I could indeed go home if that's what I really wanted, as they were fairly satisfied that they'd done all they could from a medical point of view and were OK with Mum looking after me 24/7. I'm not sure Mum was OK, but then she knew how stubborn I was, and also how important it was to my recovery to actually leave the hospital, if that makes sense. I still hadn't told anyone that I'd been sick the night before, nor that I felt feverish and, in all honesty, not ready to go home at all.

I showered, washed my hair and got dressed in the clothes that I'd kept in the bag for going home. I felt really hot and sick, though, and Mum looked worried, so she asked a nurse to give me a quick once over. Everything was deemed safe and sound, which I was surprised by, so I stood around by the window looking at the sea while I waited for Dad and Jonathan to load the car and for Mum to take my cards down from above my bed as I could neither bend down to pick anything up nor stretch to reach things. Mum held my arm and we walked very, very slowly out of the ward, stopping to hug some nurses who wished me well, and then I was in the car, on the motorway and on the way home.

I had thrown up anything that was residing in my stomach from the night before. That afternoon, back at home, I had a Marmite drink and a slice of cheese on toast, my obligatory 'I'm home' meal. I headed to bed, helped up the stairs by my brother, stopping at the bathroom to clean my teeth. As I was brushing, I felt a rush of hot liquid under the stoma bag and down my tummy. Acidic stomach contents slid down my thighs. It transpires that nurse sent me home with the wrong kind of bag on. It was a bag for an 'out' stoma, not a flat-to-the-skin one, and there was a big difference. Mum had to get on the phone the next day to get some emergency supplies from the local hospital; meanwhile I had to clean myself up and be bandaged up in bed to try and control the leaking. My bed was covered in towels. I was freezing as I couldn't wear my pyjamas as I would just have made a mess of them. I lay there in the dark in tears, hoping Mum couldn't hear me because there was nothing she could do to make it better. The hospital just kept letting me down, time and time again. It was one nightmare after another.

I'd been home a whole 24 hours – which was mainly taken up with me trying to control the leaking by not consuming anything other than water - before Mum called the doctor out. I felt terrible now and I was in a lot of pain, particularly when I went to the toilet. It felt as though I had razor blades up my bottom. I was feverish and by now I was really afraid.

The doctor suggested I do a stool test. I had no stools, I said. She meant to test the mucus that was passing from my back passage, my new 'pouch'. Off it went to a lab - those poor people, what a horrendous job they spend their days doing after passing all those science exams - and it came back a couple of days later with the news that I had not one but three infections; bugs in my gut picked up from the hospital. No surprise there after my last night on the ward. By this time I was really, really sick. My parents were extremely concerned, and I knew I was in a bad way, but so determined was I not to go back to hospital that I tried to play it down.

'I'll be alright,' I said, shivering like mad.

'Juliette,' said Mum, covering me up with my leopard print blanket, 'you're shivering. You've got a really high temperature. You're in pain. I can't let you stay like this.'

Mum rang the hospital and spoke to the surgeon. He told her she should bring me in. She reminded him that we weren't in Brighton and that she really thought I was too ill to travel. He said I should get the doctor back to prescribe Metronizadole, a strong antibiotic, and some other weird sounding pills to kill the bugs. I thought Domestos might be cheaper but Mum gave the doctor the information. She came round with the prescription, suggested I might be better off on an antibiotic intravenous drip in hospital (you can imagine my response to that given that it was the hospital which gave me the bugs in the first place), and told me to rest. She spoke to Mum in the kitchen, thinking I couldn't hear them. I have ears like a bionic fox. Nothing escapes me.

'She needs to go back to hospital,' said the doctor, 'she needs antibiotics and a drip. She's very, very ill.'

'I can see that,' said Mum in response. I could hear the panic in her voice, 'but this is Juliette. You know her. We know her. She flatly refuses to go, and I can understand it. I'll have to just get the antibiotics and hope they work and drag her to hospital if they don't. She's just come out, she's doesn't want to go back in again. She doesn't trust them to make her better, and I'm not sure we do either.'

The doctor poked her head around the door.

'Right. You're to go to hospital if you get worse, or if they antibiotics don't start to work. I know you don't want to go, and I don't blame you, but we can't have you in this state, Juliette.'

'I can't go back,' I said, shivering and shaking my head, 'I can't.'

'There's another option,' said the doctor, sitting in the chair opposite me, 'and that's to take you to Queen Mary's. Then you're just down the road, rather than an hour away.'

That was the hospital I was born in. Imagine if I died there as well. How weird would that be? But admittedly, it sounded nicer than being sent back to Brighton. I knew that if I had to go in, I wanted to be five minutes away from home. It didn't make sense to send me to Brighton.

I knew Mum was in a real panic but I stood - or rather sat - firm.

'I'm not going to hospital, I'd rather just die on the sofa, I really would. At least nobody goes to the toilet next to me here. If I don't get better in a couple of days, I'll go to Queen Mary's. But I'm not going back to Brighton. I'm not.' I could hardly move. I almost wanted to say, 'You know what? You're right. Of course you're right. I'm going to die if these tablets don't work. Take me to hospital.'

My whole body ached as though I'd been run over by a tractor and my head was spinning, I felt like I was going to throw up whenever I lay down. It hurt to lie on my side because my hips were so bony, although I wasn't as thin as I was after the first operation, weighing in at a more respectable seven stone this time. I couldn't sit up because my stomach muscles hurt had been cut. I prayed the antibiotics would work.

After 48 hours of being constantly monitored by Mum, the fever seemed to be on the way out. She rang the doctor, and my surgeon, and then said she'd been worried sick that I might die in front of her. I realised what I'd put her through by refusing to go to hospital, and I said sorry. We had a little hug, she re-positioned my pillows and I had a nap.

A few days later, Rolie came up and brought my post from the flat. According to my parents, who had been in touch with my solicitor whilst I was in hospital, I was a week from completion on the flat. Mum and Dad were going to go to get the keys to the new place while I stayed at home, and they'd also planned to supervise the removal men with all my boxes, and then I'd move in once I was well enough. It would be a nightmare and the timing wasn't ideal, but it would be worth all the effort. Rolie said he'd help out and really, it didn't matter about unpacking. We could do that when I was better. I just wanted to be rid of my flat and have the keys to the new place.

I was chatting away to Rolie when I noticed that he was holding a letter from my solicitor. I thought it would be confirmation of the sale going through, and a moving date. Instead, it was informing me that my buyer for my flat had pulled out, that the people selling my flat had subsequently pulled out. The sale was off.

'What's the matter, darlin'?' asked Rolie, putting his arm around my shoulders.

'My flat,' I said, 'my buyer, she's pulled out. I can't believe this is happening. How can this be happening?'

Mum came in and I showed her the letter. I burst into tears and she hugged me and wiped the tears from my eyes with a tissue and shook her head. We were stunned. Rolie was staying in the flat while I was in Orpington, boxes were piled up everywhere and I should have been moving the following week. It transpired that the buyer had found a hitch with the freeholder of my flat; my seller in Hove had got fed up waiting and taken their flat off the market. The whole chain had collapsed, I was a thousand pounds lighter thanks to solicitor's and surveyor fees and I had no new flat to move into. No roof terrace, no rabbit. No spare bedroom to make into an office. No two flights of stairs instead of three. Nothing. I would have to unpack and start all over again. Not only had I still got the stoma, I still had the flat. I couldn't move on no matter how hard I tried. Every time I tried I hit a brick wall.

The next week was as dull as dull can be. I half watched a lot of television and dozed during the day. I felt as though my brain was shrivelling, but I knew I had to rest, and if you can't walk further than 10 steps without keeling over, your entertainment options are somewhat limited. Like last time, I didn't want to listen to any music, and I'm still not sure why. Each day I showered, dressed and inspected the ileostomy bag on a regular basis just to check it was all working OK.

I read magazines, too spaced out to concentrate on books despite a pile of unread novels waiting in my bedroom. When the sun shone, which wasn't too often because this was England, and it was July, Mum helped out to the garden and Dad even bought a new garden chair for me to sit on, propped up with plenty of cushions from the lounge. Mum would bring me lemonade and cheese on toast (really, those cheese cravings were insane) and I'd read the paper or talk to Pebble as she roamed the lawn looking for a nice patch of grass to munch on, before promptly throwing it all up again, usually right in front of Mum in the kitchen.

Two weeks after coming home I finally felt as though I was making progress. I could feel my body responding to the antibiotics, hurrying to get better. Mum and Dad live less than a mile from a rock and roll club called The Rosecroft, and this week's band was one of my favourites - Darrel Higham & The Enforcers. Darrel was engaged to Imelda Clabby, a stunning and very talented Dublin-born singer who would hit the big time a decade later as Imelda May.

I couldn't bear to miss it but I was still incredibly weak. I'd only taken a few steps up and down the garden and around the patio at this point, and Mum was certain I wouldn't make it. I said I'd see how I felt, but I was determined to go. Dad looked worried.

'If I feel ill, or flip out, or anything, you can bring me home in five minutes and tuck me up in bed and I promise not to try and go out again ever. But I so want to see Darrel. I think it will cheer me up. I know it will. We'll work something out.'

Friday came and I felt pretty dreadful. I had a nap in the afternoon to try and muster up some energy, but by 7pm, I had to admit defeat. I wasn't sure I could sit down long enough to see Darrel's two sets as it was still so uncomfortable to 'fold myself' as I'd explain to my parents.

I wasn't strong enough to stand, so I couldn't really see how I'd do this. At home I'd lie down, propped up by pillows. I was also thinking about the smoke - I hate cigarette smoke at the best of times but I didn't fancy exposing myself to it all, I didn't think it'd do me much good to say the least. Mum was relieved, but both her and Dad knew how upset I was at not being well enough to make it.

At 8pm, Jonathan came in from his part-time job at the local supermarket to find me in the lounge, dressed (albeit in flower-fronted flip-flops, soft denim skirt and black vest, not the most wonderful of outfits for a rockabilly) and standing by the front door. I'd put some make-up on and that was it. I was ready to go.

Dad met us at the door. People stared at me, probably wondering why on earth I was so skinny and unable to walk without being supported, and even then taking only a couple of steps at a time before stopping for a rest. It must have been a peculiar sight, but I didn't care. Mum had spoken to Donna who runs the club, and she'd told her I could sit by the open door in her chair, out of the way of the crowd and with a nice gentle breeze to help me breathe through the smoke! It also offered me a perfect view of Darrel, who was just picking up his guitar as I sat down.

Half an hour later, I was still sitting, but in a lot of pain. I was sipping a Coke (on the house, and which I could barely hold upright it felt so heavy) but it was so nice to be doing something 'normal' that I didn't care. I was so tired I could hardly hold my head up. Afterwards, I had a chat with Darrel and a very gentle hug.

'There's nothing of you,' he remarked. I squeaked, 'I know'. I actually couldn't wait to get home. I was in so much pain it was unbelievable. I stumbled through the front door and said, 'please don't let me tell you I'm OK ever again, I'm mostly lying and I'm an idiot' and fell asleep as soon as I got into bed.

A few days later it was my 30th birthday. I asked Mum for a paddling pool and she laughed. I said I was as serious as mustard, whatever that means.

'No chance! Your Dad would be emptying the bloody thing every night; we had enough of that when you were little!' I was resigned to cooling my feet in a washing up bowl of cold water when it was baking hot. I was in the garden each day from morning to afternoon, slathered in sun tan lotion, and to my delight, picking up a great tan. The forecast for my birthday was hot - around 88f - perfect barbecue weather, and I'd invited a few friends down from London and a few up from Brighton to mark my turning a whopping 30-years-old. I think they all knew it was more than a birthday celebration - it was a 'look guys, I'm still alive!' celebration.

Barbecue jobs were allocated that morning: Dad would borrow next door's gazebo and clean the barbecue, Mum and Dad's friends Maureen and Alan would arrive at midday and while Alan lit the barbecue, Maureen would help Mum with the salad. I was busy peeling the skins of roasted red peppers, placing them on chunks of goat's cheese and making a sort of tower thing with pieces of French bread. There was so much to do and so little time to do it, but we finished just as Alice and Ryan turned up, chilled drinks in hand and birthday presents galore. I was so touched I cried a bit then sent them to the garden.

I hadn't invited Rolie. I felt really mean but it wasn't his thing and besides, I'd not seen some of my friends for months - them being in London, me in Brighton, me in hospital - and wanted to talk to them all day, was afraid that if Rolie came it'd just be awkward. He never liked being in a crowd he didn't know and was only really himself when at his clubs in Eastbourne. I knew he'd hate it as he'd often told me he was out of his depth with my friends. I found it really weird, but then his friends weren't really my cup of tea either. We were worlds apart and I knew it'd just make for an uncomfortable day.

I did invite Ross, with whom I'd stayed friends since our last break-up, and he showed up dead on time from London with good gifts and a big smile, and despite only knowing one person aside from me and my family, got on a treat with everyone. I had a great day. It was gloriously hot, the food was fabulous, of course, and the garden looked beautiful. Dad had worked all day on Saturday mowing the lawn, trimming the edges, watering the rose bushes, tidying every blade of grass there was. In the morning I gave him a pile of my monkeys (not real ones, sadly) to hang from the cherry and apple trees by their Velcro hands. There were balloons and flowers everywhere. Champagne flowed but I only had the tiniest sip as I couldn't bear the taste of alcohol since the operation and also knew I'd be on my back within three seconds had I swallowed a whole mouthful.

I thanked everyone for coming and Mum and Dad for making it so special, high on helium from one of my balloons. I was ecstatic, if not a little worn out. My brother provided a free taxi service to the station for everyone, and Mum and Dad began to clear everything away. It was so warm we were still out there at midnight, which is when I realised Ross hadn't left.

'You div! You've missed the last lift back to the station. Are you staying?' I asked, between tiny sips of juice.

'If that's OK,' he smiled, 'I didn't realise it was so late. Is it OK?'

Of course it was OK. Mum went up to make up the put-you-up bed in my room and he gave my hand a gentle squeeze, asking again if I was sure I wanted him there.

'It's fine,' I said, 'you'll just have to be up really early for work.'

'Don't worry about work,' he laughed, 'I'll skive. It's your birthday. I'll take you out for lunch instead.'

I couldn't argue with that.

Later that night we were in my bedroom, me in my bed, him struggling to get comfortable in the put-you-up bed, his six-foot frame squashed into a space a good twelve inches shorter. We held hands between the beds, the glare of the moon darting through the curtains so that we could just about see each other. I felt pretty weird - guilty about him staying because of Rolie, happy that he had stayed, confused about who I actually loved - either, neither or both of them, and eventually I fell asleep, still wondering.

The next day Ross phoned in sick then took me to lunch as planned and I polished off mussels in garlic and white wine and French fries like there was no tomorrow, because these days I can never be sure that there is. It probably wasn't the best thing to order; mussels are pretty hard to digest if you've not got a colon and before we even arrived home I could feel them pushing their way out of my side and into the bag. Ugh. We fed the ducks at the pond, which I'd always loved doing and which he'd always indulged me in doing when we were together, then went home.

On the way home, he pulled over and told me to close my eyes while he disappeared into a shop. Two minutes later he appeared with a big grin on his face, three ice lollies - 'one for me, one for you and one for your little mum' - and a paddling pool! I laughed so hard I'm surprised I didn't literally split my sides.

Once home, he blew up the paddling pool and a couple of hours later Dad came home from work to find the two of us, our feet in the pool, holding hands and giggling like a couple of kids. He smiled a great big smile and fed the fish in the pond their dinner. I hadn't seen him look that happy in a long time.

'I like Ross,' he said, 'he's a good bloke. You look really tired, baby. Are you OK?'

'I'm alright,' I sighed, 'really worn out but I don't care because I've got a paddling pool to be worn out in.'

I felt a sense of rejuvenation after that. I had more energy, more motivation to get better. Alice sent a little card to my parents to thank them for a lovely day. Mum and Dad remarked on what a great bunch of friends I had, and I agreed. All I wanted to do now was sort out the mess I was in with Rolie as I knew my feelings for Ross were going to get in the way eventually. I just didn't know if I was still in love with him or simply just loved him as a friend. Talk about confusing.

I called Rolie that week told him that I couldn't imagine us being together forever, or getting married. That I wanted a smoke-free house with lots of light and I didn't want to live in Eastbourne.

'You can sell your flat and buy somewhere and I'd give you money or we could go on the council list,' was his answer.

'How can that be your life's ambition - to go on a council house waiting list? Are you joking?' I spluttered.

'I want to settle down. All my mates are settled down. I want kids. You don't want kids. So what's the point?' He almost spat the words out.

A week later he rang to announce that he was 'seeing someone else and thought you should know before someone told you'. I was stunned. I went back to Brighton that weekend with Dad to get some more things from the flat. The place reeked of economy burgers. My grill pan was swimming in congealed fat. 'What a lovely parting gift,' I thought. If you're wondering if he ever did get married and have kids, the answer is no.

CHAPTER FOURTEEN
'TICK TICK BOOM'
THE HIVES

I returned to Brighton at the beginning of September. Ross and I were officially back together, and I was glad to have his support. It was comforting, though, more than exciting, but I thought that was normal after everything I'd been through. He loved me before all this happened, he loved me after. I wasn't embarrassed about anything, and felt completely at ease with him. On my first day back in Brighton I drove along the seafront, the window wound down, and breathed in the salty air. It smelled like home. Builders were working on the house next door, so I didn't sleep well but it was quieter than Ross's flat, which was on a four-lane ring road in Swiss Cottage in London, and about as peaceful as a tour of Afghanistan.

I caught up with friends, struggled around the supermarket and up all my stairs, looked out of the window towards the sea a lot and called my Mum every five minutes, or so it seemed.

It was now the end of October and I'd heard nothing about my next operation, which was supposed to have been scheduled for September. Whilst I wasn't exactly looking forward to another trip to hospital, I really wanted to get rid of the stoma. I felt as though it completely controlled me, which is the opposite effect that it was meant to have. I suppose because I never had a problem with constantly needing the loo, unlike the majority of colitis sufferers - this was the tell-tale symptom, after all - I didn't feel I had gained any benefit other than not being dead. That was it. The surgery had simply saved my life, not improved it. It was made worse by the fact that my skin was so sensitive to the glues and sprays. I just couldn't bear it any longer. I didn't seem to be suffering with the joint pain, though. I reasoned that the consultants must have been right, that it was the colitis all along.

I needed 2003 to be a New Year in more ways than one. I wanted the old me back - at least as much of it as I still had - and I dreamt of holidaying somewhere hot, lying on the beach in a bikini, scars on show and explaining to intrigued strangers who wouldn't be able to help stare that I'd been mauled by a bear in the woods. A whopping 13-inch scar and a covered-up hole beside it would no doubt convince them, not least coupled with my acting skills and ability to embellish a story with gusto.

Ross and I talked about marriage. He told me that I wouldn't have to worry about anything, that he'd look after me.

'I'll even come home at lunchtimes and make us a nice lunch,' he said. I mean, honestly, I couldn't have asked for more. I would have emotional and financial security and although I wanted to work, it meant I wasn't in any hurry to rush into anything. It all seemed to make perfect sense. The ties I had with Brighton, aside from my friends, were not good ones. Brighton, to me, had become associated with hospital, with relationship break-ups, with mentally ill, threatening neighbours and all the bad things that had happened in the last three years.

I wrote to my surgeon, and asked if he could do anything to whizz me along a bit. I stressed how hard I found this second stoma, told him how sore my skin was and how I wanted to put it all behind me and get on with my life. I couldn't move on until I had the next operation.

Ross took me to France for a little break; we went on the Eurostar and stayed in Le Touquet. We had just enough time for me to go on a carousel (I love carousels!), walk along the beach, have a fabulous dinner and a nice breakfast, and come home again. The only thing wrong with the dinner was me thinking I should give oysters a go for the first time in my life - when I have a stoma. I had learned nothing from my experience with mussels. I swallowed two of them before I decided they were disgusting and subsequently spent the entire night awake while my small intestine attempted to push them through out of the ileostomy. Whole. Suffice to say, I wouldn't recommend oysters *unless* you have a colon and also enjoy eating what I call 'dinosaur snot'.

A week later I was packing to go to London for the weekend when I got a letter from admissions saying I was to come in for my operation on November 2nd, a mere five days later. I couldn't believe it. I rang the surgeon's secretary again to thank him via her, rang Mum, rang Ross and felt really weird. I was excited, but terrified. It was so unexpected having resigned myself to waiting another four or five months. It would be exactly a year to the day that I was first admitted, at death's door. I would again hear the fireworks that rained down on the seafront, unable to go to the window to see them. I would imagine them shooting towards the sky, exploding in a mass of vibrant colour and dropping into the ocean to be washed away under the darkness of the night. And to pollute the sea and scare off the last of the cod, but I tried not to think about that.

I had to check into hospital on the Saturday afternoon, even though my operation wasn't booked in until Monday. I hated that rule. Again, I was determined not to spend a single minute more than I had to in hospital, so I asked if I could stick my toothbrush and pyjamas on my bed so it looked occupied, and then go home again.

After a quick consultation with someone on the phone, the nurse said that I could go home if I promised to come back on Sunday evening. I punched the air, said 'whoohoo!' and off I went before she changed her mind. I think they knew by now that even if I was quite naughty, they could trust me to do as I was told. Either that or the idea of me being on the ward for two whole days and nights before I needed to be was more than they could bear.

I drove home like the clappers, stopping on the way pick up a lovely stone baked pizza from my local pub. If I wasn't going to be able to eat for the next few days, I wanted to have something indulgent while I could. I watched the football and rang Ross, and had an early night. I was actually excited about going in, as I knew it was a relatively minor operation compared with the horror of the last two, and I was physically well and feeling pretty strong.

On Sunday Mum and Dad came down for the day, so of course, it poured with rain. They ate scones and crumpets in a teashop in Rottingdean; I looked on wistfully while my stomach growled like an angry dog. By the evening, I was feeling nauseous I was so hungry.

Mum and Dad were staying the night, and I'd cleaned and tidied the flat and got some milk and a few bits in for them. We took my things down to the car and Mum and Dad drove the two miles to the hospital and dropped me off.

'Make sure you go in,' said Mum, 'you'd better not arrive back home in five minutes!'

I announced to the nurse on reception that I'd duly done as I was told and turned up. She said she had no idea I'd been allowed to go home last night. Apparently they'd been looking for me until one of the patients said, 'she went home!' I thought it was pretty funny.

I sat on my allocated bed, read my book, walked around a bit, thought about food a lot, thought about it some more, sat down again, and finally saw the anaesthetist at 8pm who told me I was now last on the list and wouldn't be going down to theatre until gone 3pm tomorrow.

'I'll have died of malnutrition by then,' I said, 'are you sure it's not a conspiracy by the NHS to cut costs?' He ignored me, of course. I then asked if I needed to stay tonight, now that I'd seen him. He was somewhat taken aback.

'Why? What's wrong with being here? Is it really that bad?' he said, rubbing his brow, to which I nodded heartily.

'I never sleep in here,' I said, 'and am already a bit scared about it all. I just want my own bed while I can. I promise I'll come back in the morning. Pleeeeeeeease?' I was on my knees on the bed in front of him, hands clasped to my chest. Yes, I was begging. No, I'm not proud.

He sighed, shrugged his shoulders then relented with a smile.

'You won't get to sign a consent form until tomorrow so you could spend the night at home I suppose. Make sure you're back in by 8am, though, or I'll be in trouble.'

I gathered up my things (again), put a tiger mask Ross had bought me at the zoo on the pillow, put my pyjamas underneath that, and rang Dad to come and pick me up, saying goodbye to the other patients who must have wondered what on earth I was playing at. Dad said, 'are you sure you're allowed out? I know you!' and I said, 'I am, but even if I wasn't, you know I'd still sneak out, so just come and get me please!'

I slept on the sofa - or rather stayed awake on the sofa - Mum and Dad had my bed, and at 7am I got up, showered, made myself a cup of tea which I then remembered I couldn't drink, and shakily drove back to the hospital. I was so faint having had nothing to eat since Saturday night that I probably shouldn't have been in control of a car. Pffft!

I'd left a note at home saying that I'd driven, and where I was planning to park, and then Mum could get my keys from me and drive my car back to the flat with Dad following in their car. It didn't actually occur to me to get a cab. What?

I saw my surgeon's charming registrar who explained the procedure - nip and tuck, essentially - and the risks that went with it, including permanent incontinence, peritonitis, loss of sexual feeling, you know, nothing major - and I duly signed the form. After I'd seen another doctor, I decided I was bored already. It was 8.45am. I asked a nurse if I could go for a wander and said I'd have my mobile with me if they needed me.

'Have you seen the doctor and the anaesthetist?' she asked, writing down my phone number.

'Yes,' I nodded, 'and my lawyer in case it goes wrong,' I said, completely straight-faced.

It took her a minute. 'Juliette,' she laughed, 'you're a nightmare you are. Go for a wander if you must. But your operation's at three. Be back here by 1pm at the latest. Don't disappear on us and be ready to come in at a moment's notice if someone's operation is cancelled. In other words, it's probably best not to leave the hospital grounds.'

As if! The hospital didn't have 'grounds', it had a car park. Had it been built with a nice garden area attached to it, I might have been happy to stay there. As it is, I knew where I was going. I got in the car and drove home. It took five minutes. I pressed the buzzer and Mum looked out of the window and shouted, 'Christ! Not again!' while I cackled on the doorstep.

It was a bright day, and a very mild one for November. After I'd had a bath and washed my hair - despite my earlier shower I already felt tainted by hospital germs - we went for a stroll around Queen's Park. We fed the squirrels monkey nuts, wished we could feed monkeys squirrel nuts, watched a robin hop about by the duck pond and saw a cat chase a squirrel up a tree. We were all fairly quiet, I suppose, thinking about the operation, but enjoying the sunshine and the fresh air. Mum couldn't believe I'd run away from the hospital again and in her usual fashion, was worrying that they might be searching for me.

'Honest to God, they know I'm not there. It's OK. Well, I'm not meant to be at home or in the park, but it's not like they need me, is it?'

'What do you mean, you're not meant to be here?' questioned Mum, stopping in her tracks, 'you said you were allowed out!'

'Yeah, I am. Out of the ward. Not really out of the hospital per se. It's alright, if they get a cancellation we can be there in 15 minutes!'

Ross was on the train on his way down from London, and I said we'd go back to the hospital for good once we'd picked him up. I directed Dad to the station as I felt far too faint to drive. I knew full well what the time was, but here I was, in the sunshine, with the people I loved and nice little animals everywhere, and I can't say as I really wanted to swap that for a hospital ward full of old people with prolapsed bowels.

When we walked into the ward, lunch was being served. I never thought I'd say it, but even the hospital food made my stomach grumble. I was starving, and so thirsty I could have drunk from a puddle. I also felt as though I might faint at any moment. I suppose that's why you're supposed to sit in bed and do nothing when you're nil by mouth. D'oh.

The nurse came to see me.

'Thank God you're back,' she said, writing something on my chart, 'we were worried you'd left the hospital.'

'I had,' I said, cheekily, 'I've been in the park all morning playing with the squirrels.' Mum glared at me and Ross and Dad laughed. The nurse then explained that an emergency had come up and I was now not going down to theatre until much later. My heart sank. I wanted to cry, but instead I said, 'that's rubbish, I'm getting well bored,' and suggested that we go to the canteen so that everyone but me could have some lunch.

After I had the pleasure of watching everyone else eat, we sat in the waiting room just to escape the ward, and put the television on. It was 4.45pm. I was so hungry it was untrue. I was trying to decide whether or not I'd stay in hospital until the operation could be done, or bail out not, go home and go back on the list when, halfway through *Ready Steady Cook* (not the best TV show to be watching when you haven't eaten for two days) a nurse popped her head around the day room door and said, 'Right, Juliette! The surgeon is calling, he's ready, get your gown on!'

'I hope he's washed his hands after the last one!' I squealed, hurrying back to my bed while Mum drew the curtains. I clambered out of my jeans and pulled on the gown. Backwards. I did it again the right way round, jumped into bed and simultaneously had a thermometer shoved in my mouth, my blood pressure taken and my heart rate recorded as the porters - already waiting by the bed - wheeled me down to the operating theatre. Mum, Dad and Ross followed, jogging along beside the bed, and then I pulled the tiger mask from under the covers and popped it on my head. Ross shook his head and called me a 'silly idiot'. As the doors to theatre opened, the team of surgeons and anaesthetists burst into laughter. As they wheeled me into my allotted position, I shouted, 'see, the side effects of these steroids are horrendous!' What it must have looked like I don't know, but it certainly made everyone laugh. If one moment could sum me up I guess it would be that - trying to avert my fears, and my family's, by making a joke of surgery. Because it's so funny! Not. I was terrified, but I wouldn't let them see that. I waved goodbye to my parents, held Ross's hand for a second and then got down to answering the serious questions, such as:

'Do you have any metal on your body?'

'Yeah, I've taped up my weird earring because it doesn't come out. And there might be a pair of scissors and a spanner in my tummy from last time, but you'll soon have them out.'

The line went in the back of my hand, and I didn't even bother to count. I was asleep. The next thing I knew I was coming round from the operation, pain free. I coughed ever so slightly, and realised that I didn't have a tube down my throat. This was a breeze!

'Has it gone?' I asked the nurse who was putting a blanket around me, 'has it gone?'

'The stoma's gone, Juliette, everything went well. It was very quick, and it's all gone fine. I've told your Mum and Dad you're OK and we'll get you back up to the ward in a little while. Are you in any pain?' she asked, leaning over and stroking my hair.

'Not really,' I said, 'but for some reason my stomach hurts.'

She laughed, and said she'd up my diamorphine a bit. I asked how many tubes I had in me.

'Only one this time,' she said brightly, 'how good is that?'

I smiled the biggest smile I could, and closed my eyes.

Back on the ward I was full of it.

'It's gone!' I said to Mum and Dad, 'it's really, really gone. My insides aren't outsides anymore. I can't believe it. Well, at least that's what they're telling me. I'm too scared to look. Can you peek for me?'

Mum pulled back the covers, lifted up my hospital gown and pointed to my stomach where a dressing lay flat against the skin. There was no bag. No lump. I thought it looked beautiful, this clean, white dressing, my stomach all swollen from surgery but my insides where they should be - on the bloody inside. I wanted a photo. I couldn't believe I had my tummy back. Mum, Dad and Ross all gave me a gentle hug and a kiss, then after collecting coats and bags and making sure I was OK, they went home.

I couldn't get over the fact that I only had one tube in my entire body, and that was thoughtfully placed in the wrist of my left hand, rather than my right - makes things easier when you're right handed and the cupboard with your water and lip balm and tissues is on your right hand side after all. I put my earplugs in and went to sleep. Yep, sleep. How mental is that? I honestly didn't feel panicky or frightened at all. I was so relieved that it had gone well I wasn't really bothered by the fact that exactly a year ago to the day I was dying in the very same room. Halfway through the night I woke up in agony, and put in a request for some more diamorphine. I got myself a nice 'clicker' which meant that I could control the amount that I had pumped into my blood, and boy did I click it! I felt as though I was being jumped up and down upon by a dog in concrete boots.

I managed to vomit out my general anaesthetic as soon as I sat up the next morning. It went on forever, a sea of yellow liquid spewing forth from my stomach. It was quite impressive. The surgeon came to check on his handiwork about three minutes after the nurses had finished clearing it all up. He was relieved to see how cheerful I was. I told him about the vomit. I was quite proud of it.

'You're doing very well, sweetheart,' he said, patting my knee, 'we'll have you home in no time.'

'You should look pleased with yourself,' I said, pointing to the floor, 'because if you'd turned up any earlier,' I said, wiping specks of sick from my knees with a paper towel, 'I'd have made a right mess of your shoes!'

I left hospital on the Friday morning, having been told I'd be in a week.

'No chance', I'd said at the time, 'I'm not spending the weekend in here.' One skill I do have, other than the projectile vomiting, is to make my body compete successfully with my mind. My brain said, 'hey, let's get out of here by Friday even though you only had the operation on Monday night,' and my body said, 'Yeah, let's do it, dude.' And so it all comes together, and despite much discomfort, a lack of sleep and the pain, I managed to get myself out of there way ahead of schedule. Mum couldn't believe I was ready to be picked up so soon. I'm sure she was worried that it was too early, like last time.

'I'm fine,' I said, 'I've eaten a tuna sandwich and everything seems to be working. Well, it came out of where it's meant to rather than out of my ears so I reckon my plumbing is fine.' She spoke to Dad and he came to the phone to tell me that he'd be delighted to come and pick me up in the morning. I was ecstatic. The Health Secretary should come and thank me personally for freeing up hospital beds.

At home, things were so much different than before. I could walk around, get dressed in jeans after 10 days and felt on top of the world. The internal pouch took some real getting used to - I read in a leaflet given to me as I left the hospital that I had to 'train' it. It was literally a pain in the backside. I kept thinking I needed the toilet and when I'd get there, I didn't. I'm sure I heard my pouch mocking me. It was driving me mental as I'd be up every 10 minutes to go to the loo for nothing.

The registrar had asked me before I left hospital what it felt like now I had the pouch. I said, 'it's like a little mouse tugging at my bottom with his little hands to tell me I need to go to the toilet'. She shook her head, laughing, but wrote that on the form anyway. That's how it felt - a little tugging sensation right at the end of my, uh, bottom. It twitched, it sort of pulsated, and while it was very strange, it was exciting to think that my food would be processed in yet another way. Christ, within a year I'd had three different digestive systems. My poor body.

With the pouch, I had to really learn the different feelings, and not rush to the loo all the time. I suspect it was a bit like having a puppy – I had to train it, hope there weren't any accidents and watch what I ate. My food still passed through me at an alarming rate, and that what came out was even more liquid than when I had the stoma, which I couldn't understand. It was like pond water. There's this feeling, officially known as 'phantom rectum', which sounds like a death metal band, but is in fact a recognised medical condition, rather similar to amputees thinking their missing leg itches. I could feel things that weren't there – strange internal tickling, wobbling feelings, and the desperate urge to go to the loo when in fact, my pouch was tricking me into thinking I needed to go.

I was told to avoid anything too fibrous for the first month, and lived on jacket potatoes, mashed potato, chicken, fish, rice and pasta. I rubbed Vitamin E cream into my new scar which was as neat as a pin.

I went back to Brighton after two weeks. It was odd, being able to sit on the toilet again, and odder still that what came out wasn't anything like pooh, it was more like runny porridge. I discovered how to get the pouch working - by contracting my pelvic muscles - and how to make my food exit a bit easier (by putting my feet up on a box). It was all very strange. The scar from the stoma was healing well and I felt pretty good, albeit kind of tight and a bit constricting. I certainly couldn't bend much, but then my back hurt too much for that anyway. Yep, the pain had started up again, albeit fairly mildly.

The control I had over the pouch was fantastic. It was perfectly normal after reversal surgery to have a few accidents and I'd been warned not to expect too much too soon. There is also a big risk that it wouldn't work at all – that the muscles of the rectum (bleuch) would be too weak after the surgery, and then the pouch itself wouldn't hold the waste and it'd just come straight out, but I felt I had to take a chance and hope for the best. The list of 'maybes' on the pre-op form didn't make for great reading. I didn't fancy being incontinent for the rest of my life, but I couldn't also envisage putting up with the problems I had with the stoma, not least the severity of the soreness of the skin surrounding it. In time I found that there were some foods that I couldn't tolerate too well at all. Obviously, they were all the good ones. Chilies, funnily enough. Eggs. Fish - my god, the stink! - and even salad was tricky as that seemed to come out almost whole. As did bits of mushroom. Beer led to pure gas. That I could live with, though. To have my tummy back was great, even if it was covered in big, ugly scars.

Ross came to stay, but something wasn't right. This time, it wasn't my body, it was my head. I knew that I didn't want to marry him. It hit me as suddenly as that, one night, lying in bed, when he fell asleep, I just knew. I didn't really want to move to London either. In fact, I didn't know what I wanted, other than to go out dancing. That was all I was clear on, and I wasn't going to get that with Ross. I couldn't compromise on something that had become such an important part of my life. It was so much more than a hobby to me, and I knew I'd never be happy with someone who mocked the music I loved. I knew that most people in my situation - with more scars than a trainee stuntman - might have been glad of anyone who loved them, but I felt different. I've never felt the need to 'make do'. OK, Ross wasn't what you'd call a 'make do', far from it, because he was great, and I really did love him (and his mum - I was on course to have the best mother-in-law on earth) but I just loved him in a different way to how I had years before.

I told him exactly that one night as we lay side by side in the dark. He simply said, 'well, hurry up and make up your mind.'

That morning I awoke at 5am in agony. The muscle pain that had burned through before my flesh was back with a vengeance.

'It can't be coming back. It's not meant to hurt anymore. I can't bear it,' I cried, unable to even turn over. At 8am, I slowly and agonisingly got out of bed. I gasped out in pain as I sat up. I went into the lounge, put the kettle on, made myself a cup of tea and pulled my dressing gown around me. I was freezing. I just sat there waiting for the pain to subside. An hour later, it was almost bearable.

Later that morning Ross got up, and began packing his bag. He said he was going home. I burst into tears; a mixture of pain, frustration, sadness and disbelief hit me all at the same time. A few minutes later he said he'd decided to stay. At that point, I didn't know whether I wanted him to stay or go. He was angry with me - humiliated, no doubt - but he didn't want to leave me in agony. I had a hot bath and took some more painkillers. The painkillers made me nauseous.

Ross stayed, in the end.

'It's like I'm unraveling,' I said to him that night, 'like an old cardigan.' I woke up in the same state the next morning and took painkillers and a Diazepam, so I was too drowsy to drive. Ross drove my car back as far as Orpington on the Sunday morning, stopping at the station on the way and taking a train back to London. I drove the last bit of the journey to Mum and Dad's. Things were tense, to say the least, but we had a big hug and I promised I'd try and sort out what was going on in my head. I needed a few days rest. I also had some work on a new magazine booked in for the week. It was a new launch, so it'd be frantically busy. How I was going to manage a train and tube journey, twice, as well as a full day's work was beyond me, but I had to.

CHAPTER FIFTEEN
'VIVA LAS VEGAS'
ELVIS PRESLEY

I'd arranged to meet Ross at a coffee shop across the road from the office. He'd brought the bag of things I'd left at his flat - including my stoma kit and various creams that I suddenly felt embarrassed at him seeing - and I cried. He was quiet. We walked to the tube station, and at Baker Street we said goodbye. He told me he didn't want to hear from me again, that it would kill him to just be my friend. I didn't know what to say, so I put my arms around him. He kissed me on the forehead, then he went one way, and I walked into the tube station with tears streaming down my face. I didn't know whether I was doing the right thing or not any more. I loved him so much but that spark had gone and I didn't feel that it was fair on him to pretend otherwise. I cried all the way home, wondering if I'd made the biggest mistake of my life. I would wonder that for the next few years, and regret my decision quite often. I think I was just unable to cope with a relationship at that point. I needed to come to terms with everything that had happened to me, to work out where to go from there. I had to get my career back on track, I wasn't sure where I wanted to live, and all the big stuff was unclear and undecided. I should just have said I needed a little time, and we'd probably have worked things out. As it was, I just took the usual 'all or nothing' route. I also felt as though I was punishing myself yet again, that perhaps I felt I didn't deserve him. All in all, it was a mess, and it was all my own doing. A few years later Ross married a delicate-looking blonde girl from good Yorkshire stock who liked snowboarding and mountain-biking with whom he now has three very blonde children. I am not from good stock, do not like extreme sports (and couldn't do them even if I wanted to) and could not have children. I think he had a lucky escape. I still have his grandmother's cat-sized ceramic leopard that she gave me one Christmas back in the day; he has stood proudly in every living room I've had, and will do for the rest of his or my life.

All that after my first day back at work was enough to wipe me out completely. I kind of staggered home on the tube and train and Dad picked me up from the station. I had four more days to go. I managed it, and produced some of my best work in years.

It was two weeks before Christmas when I went back to Brighton. I missed Ross like hell, but we weren't talking. I couldn't blame him for feeling like that. I'd managed to lose Rolie and Ross, both of whom I loved, both of whom who loved me. I didn't really know what I was feeling, other than the need to push people away.

I put what little energy I had into work. I had a meeting in Canary Wharf about a big project that might take off in the spring. I was also writing a column for a new football magazine, along with a cover story about David Beckham. It would later turn out that the magazine would go bankrupt and I would be owed enough money to have funded a fortnight in New York. I saw Alice for lunch, wrapped my Christmas presents, had a few early nights and listened to a lot of Gene Vincent, though certain songs made me think of Rolie, which wasn't ideal.

Three days before Christmas I went to see my doctor. The pain was now making itself apparent every morning. My whole back felt as though it had been trampled by a horse. It was a constant, white-hot ache which stretched from my hips (and on this occasion, my ankles) to my shoulder blades. I felt as though the pain was pouring out from the top of my spine, all around my body. It actually hurt to breathe, which really frightened me.

'The trouble is,' said the doctor, taking off her glasses, 'we can't treat you with anti-inflammatories, as you know.'

'I know,' I said, my head in my hands, 'but I'm not taking steroids again. Apart from the fact that they're destroying my bones, they obviously don't work. I'm seeing the rheumatologist soon. Shall we do some blood tests now so that he knows what's up before he sees me?'

She instructed the results to go to the rheumatologist at the hospital and wished me a happy Christmas. She couldn't have been more helpful. If only she'd been a consultant I might never have been in this mess in the first place. I thanked her and went back to my car. I could feel the pain in my joints working its way down my left hip, through my thigh, to my ankle. I sat in the car and realised that I might have gone through all these operations, this last horrendous year, for nothing. I was in the same pain as before. I couldn't see a way out. The answer a year ago was to remove my colon. It's gone, and yet the pain hadn't.

I was scared. I was right back where I'd started, but I'd lost a lot of work, a year of my life, my colon, my dignity, my independence and pretty much lost my mind. I wanted a cuddle from my Mum but she was 57.3 miles away. Instead I went to the supermarket and bought some Oreo biscuits for a treat.

Christmas Day, 2002: Mum goes mad buying tubes of my favourite sweets, socks with monkeys on them, make-up and fancy little bits and bobs. I also received three enormous books that I could only just lift. I decide to go back to Brighton for New Year's Eve even though I knew I'd probably spend it alone. As it turns out, I went into town and bought myself a new pair of shoes on New Year's Eve morning and was beside myself with excitement. They were red patent, with white piping, shinier than anything I'd ever seen. On the inside, they were lined in pink. They had v-shaped tiny heels, and a heart shape cut into the front where, on the left shoe, was a colour picture of two white kittens, and on the right shoe, a picture of a dog. How brilliant is that? If only they hadn't been as uncomfortable on as cheese graters, they'd have been a great buy. I still haven't been able to actually wear them!

I went to meet Alice and Ryan by the West Pier in Hove. During a particularly nasty storm a couple of days after Christmas, half of it had collapsed into the sea. I cried when I saw it.

The dilapidated ballroom perched precariously upon the pier, half in the water, half out. It looked as though a bomb had hit it. We took photos. It was an incredible sight, and in a strange way, I thought, utterly beautiful. It was a bitterly cold day and none of us were wrapped up warm enough because we forget how cold it gets by the sea, even though we've lived here for three years.

I said to Alice that I thought it was somehow apt that this historic part of Brighton should give up on itself, after years and years of battling against the elements. It had become home to thousands of birds that would circle the crumbling ballroom in one single, flowing movement, each bird flying in exactly the same direction, like some kind of black and white spotted balloon. It was a sight to behold, but as they swooped over and under the rotting walkway, I felt sad for them. It looked like some semblance of panic had set in, their formation ever so slightly out of shape. I wondered what would become of them if the whole thing crashed into the sea.

'The birds can have my flat,' I said to Alice, wiping a tear from my eye and watching the waves crashing against the rusty girders. At that moment, I felt such an overwhelming sadness that I identified with the crumbling bodywork which was beyond repair, waiting and waiting for somebody to help restore it, to put it back together, to give it a reason for existing.

Ryan came over with hot chocolate; they were going home to throw a little party but I didn't feel up to making small talk with people I didn't know, and anyway, I had a date with Orlando Bloom.

I took myself to the cinema to see *The Lord of the Rings: The Two Towers*, even though I still have no idea what was going on in the first film. I had brought along a tube of my Christmas sweets, and I fell asleep for ten minutes and woke to find Fruit Pastilles strewn all over my lap, and the battle of Helm's Deep about to kick off. I am officially excited and in love with a blond elf. Armour is my new fetish. I have magic but painful shoes. It's 2003 and already it's an improvement on 2002.

I decide to drive to Mum and Dad's again for a few days as I feel a bit restless and can't sleep. On New Year's night I take the train to my friend Kate's house in Brixton. She surprises me with a very belated birthday tea - fancy little things from M&S, cocktails, roast chestnuts, posh bread with bits in and a chocolate caterpillar cake. I mean one in the shape of a caterpillar, not a cake made of caterpillars. There are seven presents for me. I'm so touched I burst into tears.

'I can't believe this,' I said, completely overwhelmed, 'it's the loveliest thing anyone's ever done for me. Thank you.'

The chocolate caterpillar, *The Lord of the Rings* and my new shoes pulled me back from the brink. I was happy to be alive.

A few days later I see the rheumatologist again. He looks bored, as if he can't wait for my appointment to be over so he can get on with something more fun, like sticking pins in his eyes. I feel like an unwelcome intrusion, and I sense that he doesn't quite know what to do with me. I sit down, awkwardly, wincing as my hip feels as though it's got a screwdriver wedged in it.

'How do you feel?' he asks.

I tell him that the pain is back. Again. That it's been as bad as ever, despite having the reversal. That I don't even have a stoma anymore and yet it's still here. He sort of shrugs, and says, 'we can't treat you with anti-inflammatories. Your blood test shows high levels of inflammation.'

'I bet it does. So what do I do?'

He mentions steroids again and I shake my head.

'Well,' he said, 'I don't know what else to suggest. I might have to refer you to the Pain Clinic, see if they can help you manage your pain. They'll talk to you about it, and we'll try and find something else to try, but it's going to be difficult.'

He shuffled my file, a good sign that my time was up.

That was it. OK, it was a relief not to have the stoma, but I know full well that if someone had said that I'd still have the same pain after going through such a living hell to have the reversal, I wouldn't have bothered. It really wasn't worth the risk, pain, the near-death blood loss, none of it.

I go back to the doctors, get more industrial strength painkillers and get on with it, as I always have. What else can I do?

A week later I am on out with Aaron when I meet his friend Chris who is very drunk and dances with me (I am back on my vodka/painkillers combo to be able to have a dance) to Elvis then falls over. His behaviour is strangely appealing. He asks for my phone number and a week later he picks me up in his 1952 Chrysler Windsor for a date at the Ace Café in North London.

The car is like nothing I've ever seen before - 20ft long, matt black with a purple roof and leopard print fur inside. It has teeth (the grille does actually look like a shark's mouth) and is slung so low that it scrapes every bump in the road and there'd be no hope of a hedgehog crawling underneath, even if there was a 'Crawl Under The Car' competition in hedgehog land with a £1,000 prize. It also attracts perplexed stares from the general public and, naturally, the police. It makes the sound of a jet engine but I like it and my leopard print coat matches the interior rather nicely. I tell him about my tummy and he doesn't bat an eyelid and drives me home with his arm around my shoulders all the way, which is kind of nice and old fashioned. I know he's not going to be the love of my life or anything, but I liked his car and he seemed nice enough.

Two weeks later Chris asks if I fancy coming to Las Vegas with him and a group of friends at Easter for the Viva Las Vegas Rockabilly Weekender. I think about it for all of three seconds and say yes, even though I don't really want to be someone's girlfriend, particularly his (again, like chalk and cheese other than our love of rockabilly) but my flight's booked the next day and when I tell Mum she says I'm mad.

'It'll only be five months since your operation!' she wailed.

'Yeah, and I feel OK and life's too short and all that so I'm going. They have hospitals there and if I can't get to one then they can lay me on the roulette table and operate with cocktail sticks.'

We would be in LA for five days before a week in Vegas then back to LA for another week of gigs after that. I didn't explode on the plane and arrived in one piece. On the Saturday night in Vegas I wore my cerise pink vintage pink playboy bunny outfit (it was almost Easter Sunday) and was invited up on stage by Swedish punk/rockabilly band The Go-Getters, to play skull maracas. Chris was filming the gig with the camcorder and 20 minutes later when I toppled off the stage, job done, I squealed, 'I just played Vegas!' My hip pain was horrendous, but I just doubled my intake of rum and painkillers until I couldn't feel it anymore. For five days and nights we drank, danced (a bit) until 7am and slept until lunchtime. We did get out sometimes, and I even went on two roller coasters despite all the health warnings - I ticked just about all of them other than the being pregnant one but I just said, 'bothered!' and reasoned that it'd be a really cool way to die, on the New York New York roller coaster in Vegas. And it would have been, right?

We even went all the way up the Stratosphere Tower because I love heights, in the way that I love being *scared* of heights. We could see all of Vegas down below; the neon signs, the swimming pools on top of hotels, the cars the size of ants snaking down the Strip. We went on the roller coaster that goes around the top of the tower despite howling winds and being so high up we saw helicopters flying *below* us. I thought it was a pretty good two fingers up to all my operations, riding at the front of the roller coaster, the wind almost taking my head off, at midnight in Vegas. It was pretty surreal. I felt great, if not a bit tired, and was the happiest I'd been for a long time. My painkillers were working in conjunction with all the rum I was drinking and I didn't care if it would make me feel worse at the end of it all, I just wanted to go mad and worry about it later, and so I did.

Emma (one of Chris's friends whom I'd become close to on the trip) and I bought matching skull and crossbones bikinis, and yes, I showed my scars. Standing around the pool with a tummy you notice for all the wrong reasons was kind of liberating. All the other girls were dressed up to the nines in their vintage outfits with parasols and Carmen Miranda-style fruit hair accessories, in full make-up and looking the epitome of glamour. Whilst I admired their efforts, I couldn't understand why anyone would bother taking hours and hours to get ready for anything. It was beyond me. People did sneak looks at my tummy but I just smiled back. One girl started a bit too long and I walked towards her saying, 'I got mauled by a bear, wanna take a closer look?' I couldn't have cared less.

Although there were a few really bad days with pain in my hips - including the one where everyone left me behind at the motel to go to a theme park, which made me cry - I think the endorphins radiating from my body kept most of it at bay.

One night in Vegas I met Phil and Cherry, a couple who lived in Brighton. I'd seen Phil at a gig or two but never really spoken to them, and said to them, 'I haven't got any friends with good taste in music in Brighton, so now we've said hello you're never going to escape me!' and it would turn out that I was true to my word.

On the Friday night in the ballroom at the Gold Coast hotel, a handsome chap took my breath away, he really did. I just caught his eye as I was looking for Emma and that was it. Bam! We didn't speak, and I didn't see him again after that but I told Emma because I felt quite strange about it - 'kind of queasy-nuts-lightning-bolt stuff' I told her.

A few nights later, when we were in LA, I literally bumped into this handsome chap again at a great little club called The Doll Hut. I was walking in the door, looking behind me at Emma, and he was walking out, for a cigarette. We bumped. He was in a black suit, white shirt, two-tone shoes, bootlace tie, looking like Johnny Cash. I almost passed out. He was tall. I had bumped into his chest. He said, 'excuse me, ma'am' as he went to walk past me, then looked down, stopped dead and said, 'Well, hello again, how are you?' in a deep, husky Southern drawl. I was hooked, but then I remembered that I was with Chris. Bah! It turned out that this guy was in a band – Cash O'Riley & The Downright Daddies - and they were playing that night. It was an obscure place to end up at, and I thought, 'this is well more than coincidence,' but had to behave. Well, I had to behave a bit. I was in the loo writing my email address on a piece of toilet paper in red lip liner. I couldn't let this go, but I couldn't do much about it with Chris there.

I opened the door and there he was, cigarette dangling between his lips, whisky in the other hand. I felt my knees buckle. He patted the red plush seat next to him. I looked around. I could see Chris on the other side of the bar with our friends. I sat down for about 20 seconds. He asked my name, I asked his - 'Cash' - and he said, 'Oh, man, I love your English accent,' and a two-way infatuation was born. I went a bit mad and suddenly kissed him hard on the lips, just for a second, which was really naughty.

Emma raised both her eyebrows, so I knew she'd seen it all. I also knew she wouldn't say anything, so we had another beer and I tried to not spend the rest of the night staring at Cash as he played. After the show he then sat at the bar with his back to me, and I pretty much stared at the back of his head. I'd never felt anything like it. If I'd been on my last night in LA, I'd have just told Chris, 'Sorry, bye!' and sorted myself out to go home. As it was, we had another week left. Gah!

Cash stole a few glances my way when he got the chance. He came over when he was leaving, handed me a copy of the band's CD, and said, 'I'll be seeing you, Juliette, take care.' But he didn't turn to leave, he just stood there. The electricity was so mental that I'm surprised my hair wasn't standing on end like it does when you rub a balloon on your head. Cash told me he had a girlfriend when I asked (I like to know these things before I bother having crushes) and although I was really disappointed with that snippet of information, at least he was honest and at least I had asked. The sparks flew until he went out of the door and carried on his tour of the West Coast. I thought of nothing else but him for the rest of the week.

Once I'd got back I rested at Mum and Dad's for a few days before going back to Brighton. I needed to - I could barely walk at this point and was in terrible pain. Of course, I'd completely overdone it, and now I was paying for it. I hadn't heard from Cash, so I did a little internet research, listened to the CD and emailed the band. I got a reply the same night, explaining that he'd lost my note in Nebraska (how cool does that sound?) when the wind blew everything off the dashboard of his van one night, and was hoping I'd get in touch. My note had fallen in the snow. Poor note! That started a long line of emails, some a little cheeky, often just nice, friendly 'I did this at the weekend' type ones, and I really began to fall in love with him, in a 'I met you for 20 seconds' way.

Just over a week later was the May Hemsby Rock 'n' Roll Weekender in Great Yarmouth which Chris and I had booked a few months previously. I was so besotted with Cash that I really didn't want to go, and should have just backed out. A trip in the Beastmobile turned out to be a disaster as the engine blew up a bit on the way from Chris' house to pick me up at Mum's in Orpington. It was smoking on the driveway, basically. It then exploded in Ipswich and we had to get an AA lorry to tow the car back to Dover to pick up Chris's old Cavalier. By the time we got to Hemsby it was 2am and we'd been travelling for almost 12 hours. As I got out of the car outside reception, I felt my hip go and that was that. Chris then managed to lock the keys in the car, which meant that we spent two more hours waiting for the AA. By this time I was ready to join the other AA, I needed a drink so bad.

Subsequently, I spent the entire weekend aside from an hour or so on the Sunday night in the chalet on the sofa, unable to move, knocked out on painkillers and bored out of my mind. At one point Chris had to help me up to get to the toilet and to bed. We had to call a doctor out for stronger painkillers and I was absolutely distraught. Not only was it £100 down the drain but I had never had this pain in my hip so bad. At one point it took half an hour to get to the bathroom, all of ten feet away from the sofa, and then I couldn't sit on the toilet anyway because I had just seized up completely and couldn't move. It was terrible. I sent Chris out to the hall to see the bands and try and find someone to have a dance with but he was very upset by the whole thing and it was a waste of time and money for both of us. I felt completely hemmed in by my stupid, useless body. I'd had enough. Poor Chris had probably had enough too.

Vegas had clearly been too much. I'd done it again, completely ruined things by denying how fragile I was, not taking care of myself, pushing my body to the limit - beyond the limit, in actual fact. He had to drive me home with me lying across the back seat, wrapped up in blankets, trying not to puke (that car sickness again). It wasn't much fun. After three days at my parents' place I was just about able to drive myself back to Brighton, but I didn't feel much better, with the pain staying with me for weeks. I had an MRI scan a few weeks later that confirmed I had severe inflammation in both hips and scoliosis of the spine. I knew there was something wrong, but I couldn't understand why it had taken so long to investigate it.

When I came down with a fever and excruciating pain whenever my pouch did its stuff in July, I went back to see my surgeon. He reasoned that I might have a couple of staples lose in my back passage (nice) and tried to examine me. The pain was so excruciating that I'm embarrassed to say that I shouted, 'f*cking HELL'S BELLS!' as he prodded me. My symptoms were pretty unpleasant. After going to the loo I'd curl up on the bed, shaking with the pain and trying hard not to cry. I had a raging temperature and felt sick and dizzy. I told Mum I felt like I was passing shards of glass. I'd gone back to their place again when I started feeling unwell as I was worried I might black out with the pain, hit my head and be left to rot if I was on my own. I'd got pouchitis, which is inflammation or an infection in the pouch, on this occasion due to the wayward staples, which meant I hadn't been able to sit down properly for almost five weeks. Anyone with a brain would have put their flat on the market at this point and moved back in with their parents for good. Well, maybe not for good but for a while. I didn't. I'm an idiot, and I'll regret not making that decision for the rest of my sorry life.

Work was impossible as I couldn't sit at the computer and I spent most of the time lying on my side on the settee, standing up and walking about or sitting in the garden, just like the previous summer, although at least this time I had emails from a guitar-slinging hillbilly to keep my spirits up.

Back in Brighton I got sent for a CT scan as I'd also developed weird lumps on my legs that hurt like hell. The MRI radiologist pointed out changes in my lymph nodes that apparently meant I might have lymphoma, so that was nice and cheery. I went for the scan at 7am on my 31st birthday - happy birthday to me, right? Three weeks later I was still waiting for the results. I still felt weak from the infection, and pretty scared by then that I'd have even more bad news. I felt as though I was falling apart. I headed back to Orpington again. Mum cheered me up with a bottle of Pimm's that replaced the painkillers for the most part and generally made a fuss of me, which she excels at. After three weeks of sitting in the garden (not permanently, I mean just when it was sunny) I was ready to go home again, though I really didn't know what to call home any more. I had still not received the all-clear, or the not all-clear, from the hospital.

I was so desperate to move. My flat had been up for sale yet again since February and wasn't shifting, so I decided to drop the price to rock bottom and look for a two-bedroom place in Hove, just like I had the summer before. I found a purpose-built place on a tree-lined avenue with a parking space and a lift and put an offer in, which was accepted. I remember being in the bath at the time, bluffing at crossing my fingers under the water, then getting the answer that I wanted at the price I wanted to pay. Hoorah! I finally got a buyer for my place - good riddance to that - and we were all systems go.

I then got an appointment with my rheumatologist, who said that the CT scan just showed scar tissue and some sort of fleshy mess (I'm paraphrasing here) rather than anything sinister. I was somewhat relieved.

I was given physiotherapy sessions at the hospital that I felt were helping in two ways - physically and mentally. I described the pain and the physiotherapist agreed that it couldn't be colitis if I no longer had a colon, something I'd been telling the consultants for a year. There wasn't any particular explanation for it other than the steroids causing the thinning of the bones and probably the inflammation, but at least someone was now doing something to try and help me. Someone was listening, and understood that living every day in constant pain is not something most people are able to endure.

To continue my lucky streak, I then developed bronchitis upon the anniversary of Elvis Presley's death in August, and so I had that to deal with and again, was back at Mum's being fed antibiotics, throat sweets, Bonjela and cough syrup. I felt like a sick child in a Dickens novel, begging for help and coughing at everyone like poor kids did in the olden days. Only difference was I got brought honey and lemon drinks, had a cat on the bed that loved me and I wasn't dressed in rags. Mind you, I think Dad might have had me going up the chimney and giving it a clean to earn my keep if Mum had let him.

To top it all, I then developed an allergic reaction to the antibiotics, coming out in red, itchy lumps from head to toe. If I wasn't scratching, I was coughing. We spent almost an entire day in A&E with me saying, 'Uh, my throat's closing up and my eyes are the size of golf balls, I reckon I'm allergic to something. Any chance of a shot of antihistamine?' until four hours later, someone with a stethoscope said, 'you're allergic to something. We'll have to give you a shot of antihistamine.' Genius.

I had to go on television two days later. Talk about lousy timing. It was for an ITV documentary about David and Victoria Beckham, explaining how I'd set them up. I don't mean set them up as in done them over, I mean as in romantically. As a journalist I sometimes got asked to do odd things on TV and radio and duly said yes. Fortunately my itchy blobs began to fade and by the day of filming, they had gone completely. I was told I'd have my make-up done professionally, for the lights, so I barely wore any. When I got there, there was no make-up and no make-up artist, so that didn't exactly go to plan. I still had trouble saying a whole sentence without waving my hands around half way through to indicate that I was about to cough my lungs up. I got through it in the end, despite not having any idea what I was going on about.

I had another check-up with my surgeon in August during which I asked him if he would be able to sort my out with a pair of elf ears (I was a bit obsessed with *Lord of the Rings*). He thought I was kidding, but I wasn't. I thought it'd be great. I asked how much it'd cost and but he wouldn't even give me a quote. I told him I'd ask my dad to do it with a Stanley knife and some Sellotape if he wouldn't do it with a proper scalpel. I worked out that if I cut a triangle bit out of the top of each ear and sewed that bit together, it'd heal into a point. Obviously after they'd got septic and I'd contracted blood poisoning.

He shook his head, again, and dismissed me.

'I seriously want it done!' I shouted down the corridor, 'I'll go to Harley Street, so I will!'

September 2003

The pain that hit me in the early hours of the morning was still hanging around. Some days were excruciatingly painful, and for a couple of days a month maybe I'd just ache a little and that, compared with most days, felt like heaven. My new flat had a bedroom and a spare room (an office at last, even if I didn't have any actual work!) and a lift so I could carry my shopping upstairs. I had a parking space all to myself and in the meantime, I'd also sold my 'normal' car and bought myself a 1965 Triumph Herald on a whim.

I figured I'd be staying for five years at least, so I wanted to decorate this place properly. In the bathroom I went for black gloss tiles all around, a black bath panel, black and white floor tiles and a bubblegum pink wall. It was as far removed from a hospital bathroom as possible, and that's just what I wanted. The living room went from baby pink and mint green to cream, to a kind of grey/stone colour. I just couldn't decide on anything. The bedroom was blue, but I have no idea why as I hate the kind of blue I chose. Three weeks later, I repainted it white with a sage green wall behind the bed. Much better. The kitchen, of course, ended up being candy pink. It wasn't my dream home but it was spacious and I felt safe there. Mum and Dad were so relieved that I'd bought somewhere 'sensible', as in two floors up (less chance of being broken into) with parking (no driving around for 10 minutes and having to park three streets away) and a with a lift (I wouldn't have to climb any stairs).

I finally mustered up the courage to break up with Chris in October, and just felt relieved the minute I told him. He's a nice bloke, but I didn't love him, never set out to and I knew it wouldn't go anywhere. I would have been better off just being friends with him from the start as I never fancied him either, he was just fun to be around. I wanted to be on my own for a while. Turns out Chris had cheated on me before we went to Vegas so in the end, I didn't feel too bad about writing that lipstick note and actually wished I'd given Cash two kisses rather than one!

I had an overwhelming desire to jump on a plane and go and see Cash, honestly believing that fate had brought us together and that I was destined to live in America with a man whose only possessions were his car and his guitar. He could spell, he wrote beautiful songs and he looked great in a cowboy hat, though. It was just a matter of him having a girlfriend. And a daughter. And living 4,000 miles away. You know, little obstacles. I really felt we were meant to be together. I just couldn't figure out how.

Two weeks before Christmas I went to a gig in London with Phil. He and Cherry had become firm friends since Vegas and we only lived 10 minutes' walk from each other's flats. Cherry was stuck at work, so Phil and I got the train up together. I felt a bit awkward about borrowing my friend's husband-to-be, but we had a great afternoon and at the end of it, I spotted a very handsome young man on the dance floor, drenched in sweat and screaming with passion at the last record. I'd never seen anything like it - someone who felt like I did when they heard the music, and someone ridiculously good-looking too, which is a rarity on the scene (other than Cash, of course!).

I decided to ask him for a Christmas kiss as it seemed like a good excuse, and he duly obliged. Just a little peck on the lips, and then I backed away. He leaned in as I leaned further out and said, 'I only wanted a little one, thank you,' and he said, 'OK, but give me your phone number'.

I thought that was a bit odd, as he was clearly very young and I was clearly not, plus I was also drenched in sweat from dancing, so not the best I've ever looked.

'Give me your phone number,' he said insistently, 'please.'

'Hang on, how old are you?' I asked him, thinking he was about 18.

'Twenty,' he said, 'How old are you?'

'Bloody 32,' I said

He looked somewhat surprised.

'You're not 32. I thought you were about 24!'

'I wish I was. But I clearly remember seeing my birth certificate once and it said 1972 on it, so it must be right.'

'Well, I don't care,' he said, 'I'll ring you anyway.' I handed him my card with my mobile number on it and he stuck it in his pocket. He asked me my name, I asked for his, and I said goodbye. Phil and I got the train back to Brighton and I'd already decided that he wouldn't call and that he was too young anyway.

'I reckon he'll call,' said Phil, texting Cherry to let her know we were on our way home, 'he looked like he meant it.'

Phil was right. I got the call the next night, and somehow John invited himself down to Brighton for the weekend. I had no reason to say no, other than for sensible reasons such as I didn't know him, he could kill me and eat me, that kind of thing. He came down four days later on the train from the Midlands, and when I met him at the station I could have sworn he was 16-years-old. He looked very, very young. Cripes. Fortunately, despite being 32 I didn't look it, so the transport police didn't arrest me. We got back to the flat, I made him a roast chicken sandwich and after three and a half hours, we had a kiss. That weekend we visited my sponsor dog at the Dogs Trust - where he copied the dog and rolled around on the grass with his feet in the air, which I found hilarious - and listened to a lot of rockabilly.

'So,' I said, four days into his stay, 'when are you going home? It's nearly Christmas.'

'I'll go home tomorrow,' he said, 'I promise. And then I'll come back in a couple of weeks to see you again.' I thought for a moment, and before I knew what I was saying, this came out:

'Why don't you just move in? It'd save a lot of bother.'

Yes, I actually said that. I know. Really.

He looked very happy. Despite seeing how much pain I was in every day, and knowing that it was unlikely to get better - if anything, it would get worse - he wasn't fazed. I was worried that he would be too young to cope with it, and that it would be unfair of me to pursue a relationship with him on this basis. He insisted that he could handle it, and I couldn't really argue. Here was someone so handsome I almost fell over when I looked at him, who had my warped sense of humour down to a tee, who loved the same music as me, and who talked to Pantouf as if he was my real son (which he is, sort of). I decided I had nothing to lose, which is unfortunate, because it would turn out that I was quite wrong about that.

On the Monday night we went out to a rock 'n' roll club and I'd asked him if he could dance. 'A bit,' he said. We danced to *Santa Bring My Baby Back to Me* by Elvis, a great Christmas song and I'd never had a dance like it. OK, so I grimaced the entire way through due to the pain, but it was still exhilarating. He was absolutely amazing. I'm sure I had a smug face all night, but I couldn't help myself.

My joy was interrupted the next morning with a bang. As I stood by the kitchen while he made me a cup of tea, I said, 'I feel well sick,' and the next thing I knew I was sliding down the wall and my head smashed onto the floor. I came round to him leaning over me, gently slapping me on the face and calling my name. He helped me up, and got me to the settee. After a few seconds, the pain in my head set in, and I started to cry. Before I could get the tears out, I had to leap up because I knew I was going to be sick. I stumbled to the bathroom, still reeling from the shock and the pain.

I was duly violently sick, and to top it all, lost all control at the other end of my body at the same time. Nice. And all this in front of someone I've known for only four days. Not the best start. He held my hair back while I was sick, stroked my back, helped me take my pyjamas off which were soaked through with last night's dinner, and didn't bat an eyelid. He put me in the bath, and I insisted I was OK now I'd been sick and motioned for him to wait outside. I was crying now, with embarrassment more than anything. I sat under the shower and cleaned myself up, then put my dirty pyjamas in the bath along with the bathmat, and turned the shower on them. He came in, dried me off, and brought in my tracksuit bottoms and my comfy warm cardigan (how did he know where to find them? Most men would have brought in flippers and a cocktail dress, something completely inappropriate) and got me into my clothes, telling me all the while that it didn't matter.

He put the dirty things in the washing machine, rang my doctor for some advice ('tummy bug') then I called Mum. I asked her to ask Jonathan to pick me up that afternoon. I was meant to be driving to their house the next morning - Christmas Eve, nice timing - but I knew I couldn't drive in this state. Jonathan jumped on the phone and said no problem, and once I'd got the duvet, pillow and Pantouf next to me, John got his stuff together and called a taxi.

'I hate leaving you,' he said, 'I want to know you're OK.'

'I am now,' I said. I still couldn't believe that he'd witnessed that. Not the most romantic start to a relationship, is it?

His taxi arrived. I was fine by the next day. Unfortunately, Mum and then Jonathan got it 24 hours later. I felt terrible that I'd inflicted it upon them, but hey, that's what families are for. Happy Christmas.

CHAPTER SIXTEEN
'THRU DREAMIN''
BIG SANDY & THE FLY-RITE TRIO

The next few months were difficult. John had moved down right after Christmas, and it was then that he decided to be honest with me about his job. Oh, and his age - he was 19, but had been too scared to say so because he thought I'd say he was too young. He was right! Even though 20 isn't exactly ancient, not having a 'teen' on the end of the number didn't seem quite so bad. He'd told me he was training to be an accountant, and I'd had visions of him doing some temping in Brighton until he found a job. He'd told me he'd handed his notice in and his boss had wished him well. I found it a bit weird that he was allowed to leave his job at a moment's notice, but didn't think too long about it.

The truth was somewhat different. He'd drifted in and out of a few menial jobs and was, when he met me, working as a cleaner for the company where his mum worked. I found out the truth when I took him to the Job Centre and he had a form to fill in. He looked panicked, stood up and walked out, and wouldn't tell me what was wrong. In the end he mumbled something about not having GCSE's and completely withdrew, wouldn't talk to me. This should have served as a big enough warning sign, but it didn't. He said he was renting a flat back in his hometown, but he actually lived with his mum. Oh, he'd also told me he could drive, and guess what? That was a lie too. How mental is that? I had too many problems myself with work, or rather the lack of it, to worry about supporting someone else. I'd been completely duped and felt like a fool, but instead of asking him to leave, I let him stay, and it would be a decision I'd come to regret.

He spent the first month glued to his PlayStation, bereft of any desire to explore Brighton, get a job or do anything. I didn't know what to do with him. I didn't want to admit I'd made a huge mistake, but I felt completely duped. Several times I told him to leave. I couldn't look after him, couldn't deal with trying to get him on his feet and me back on mine. I didn't have the energy. Half the time I felt like his mum, not his girlfriend, but that was my fault for thinking that living with a teenager was a good idea.

At the end of February I finally gave him an ultimatum - get a job, or go home. He did do the odd weekend here and there helping Phil on private plastering jobs, and on Valentine's Day came home with a pair of beautiful Marc Jacobs stilettos (I hasten to add that they were for me). He'd spent his entire day's wages on them (yes, they were in the sale, I'd have gone spare if they hadn't have been) and although I was cross with him for blowing his hard-earned cash on something so frivolous, it was the sweetest thing anyone had ever done for me. He was trying to make amends, and if shoes can't make amends, I don't know what can.

That weekend I asked him what he'd like to do if a job with Phil didn't come up, and he said building work. With a little (oh alright, a big) nudge, the aid of the Yellow Pages and some help from me with what to say on the phone, he got himself a job with a fencing company.

The money was reasonable, the hours were good, and he was happy. For three months he worked every day that he was asked (although that turned out not to be every day, and sometimes his boss just didn't pick him up at all, with no explanation). We had a little money, John had some direction in his life and things were looking up. He'd give me 75% of his wages to help with the bills and the mortgage, and I'd sit on the sofa with him plucking splinters from his fingers with my tweezers after dinner. I hoped that things would continue to get better; I really did love him and I knew he could make me happy if *he* was happy.

The good times were really good: we spent weekends on the beach with Pantouf, having picnics and swimming. We went dancing when I could, and even when I couldn't - I'd dance in agony reasoning that it was better than doing nothing in agony. I paid for it the next day, and would barely be able to move, but just one dance made me feel so alive, as corny as that sounds.

We were still short on money, even though we never spent any. I needed a job; my writing work was really thin on the ground.

I applied for 15 part-time jobs, and had one interview and only three replies. They were all reception or administration jobs, mostly in estate agencies, an area I was interested in, yet my experience as a journalist counted against me. I rang several of the companies to ask why I'd not been selected for interview, and was given the classic 'you're over-qualified, we just want a secretary, not a journalist,' line, and when I did get an interview with one letting agent, I still didn't get the job. I was asked if I had any medical conditions, which is the norm these days, even on an application form. I felt I should explain that very occasionally I might be in too much pain to come to work, but that I was such a hard and fast worker that I'd do more in a day than most people would in three. I was told that this was fine, and we shook on a job offer. I was to start the following week, three days a week, 9am to 3pm. The hours were perfect.

I felt as though I could manage that, even if I had to rest when I got home. I could get through it, I was sure.

Two days before I was due to start, I received a letter from the company stating that they felt I was not right for the position, and the offer was being retracted. I felt as though I had no control over any aspect of my life. This black cloud that hung over me every day wouldn't shift, and no matter what I did to try to get a job, nothing went my way. I couldn't believe I was being turned down for a role that I could do with my eyes shut. I saw no way out of the mess I was in.

'I think I'm properly fed up, like medically fed up,' I told Mum, 'I just feel like whatever I do, and no matter how hard I work or try to work, everything's against me. I don't know how I'm supposed to survive, let alone pay the mortgage.'

'I'm not surprised you feel like that, dear,' she said, sighing, 'you've been through so much, and you're still going through so much. It's alright to feel fed up.'

'Not for me it isn't, but I am. Part of me wants to stay in the flat all day watching TV and eating crisps and reading magazines. I want to give up, really. I wish I'd been renting; I'd have had so much financial support I wouldn't need to worry. It's too hard.'

Council tax, half the mortgage (I had switched to interest-only as I couldn't repay in full), food, petrol, water, gas and electricity set me back around £1,000 per month. Had I been renting, I'd have had housing benefit (no rent to pay), income support, incapacity benefit, council tax benefit and a whole host of other add-ons, like free prescriptions. Because I owned my own home, the Department of Work and Pensions' suggestion was that I 'rent out a spare room for extra income'. When I explained that I didn't have a spare room, and besides, I was very ill and wouldn't want to share my living space with a stranger (as much as they wouldn't want to share a bathroom with someone with colitis), the bloke just shrugged and said, 'well, you just need to get a job, then.' Next to me in the Job Centre was a mother with five kids running around who was demanding more money for 'taxis and that'. Yep, she took her kids to school in a taxi each day, paid for by taxpayers. She would have been pulling in more in child benefit alone than I was living on each week. Meanwhile, I struggled on.

John and I began arguing. A lot. He had lost his job with the fencing contractor (through no fault of his own, it turns out that his boss was nuts) and because of that, he was angry, but angry with me. He refused to apply for Job Seeker's Allowance as he was 'too proud'. I could to keep our heads above water. The rows quickly became nasty and I soon saw a side to him I was afraid of. His behaviour became more erratic, more controlling and more manipulative by the day. He ordered me to throw out all my old photographs of other boyfriends. It made him angry to know I had them; he couldn't accept that I had a life before him. He would ask my how many men I'd slept with, saying 'if it's more than five, you're a slag'. Honestly. When he was nice to me, I couldn't imagine life without him. When he was angry, I couldn't stand to be in the same room as him.

His lies became more frequent, more elaborate. He told me how he'd played youth team football with West Bromwich Albion, and was let go when he was 17 due to a knee injury. I thought it was questionable, to say the least. He went on to embellish it to such an extent that he told my parents the same story, even making up entire tales about games he had never played against players he had only seen on TV. I knew he was lying. My parents knew he was lying. He'd say he played against players who were twice his age, for a start. Dad said at the time, 'how come you got to play against David Ginola when he was in the first team at Aston Villa and you were in the Youth Team at West Brom?' and obviously he didn't have an answer for that, because there wasn't one. His lies were embarrassing me, but they didn't seem to embarrass him. He told me he had videos and photos of him playing; when I said, 'ask your mum to send them down,' his reply was, 'they're in the loft, and the loft door is stuck so she can't get them.' Right.

Another time I heard him telling our neighbour that he'd won £3,000 after a bet on a snooker tournament. He hadn't, but he had started gambling. He was completely out of control and I just got swept along with it, too afraid to admit I'd made a terrible mistake.

He would play mind games with me all the time, and I didn't have the energy to fight it. He'd start an argument half an hour before we were due to leave the house, for example, and once he'd reduced me to tears, and to a point that I didn't want to go, he'd go on his own, deliberately goading me by putting on whatever vintage shirt or jacket he knew I liked best on him, taking ages to quiff his hair, all the while smirking, knowing that he was hurting me. He'd walk out of the door shouting, 'have a good night on your own, Juliette,' and actually took real pleasure in upsetting me. It was awful. I was too ashamed to tell anyone what was going on, humiliated that I had let things get this far.

We went on holiday to Spain, for a rock 'n' roll festival. I was doing my make-up in the bathroom, fully dressed after my shower, and had just dried my hair. As I opened the bathroom door to ask John what time he wanted to head to the venue, a bottle of water fell on me, soaking me from head to toe and hurting me in the process. He had put it up there while I was in the shower.

'You can't go out like that, can you?' he said, smirking. As I stood there shaking, he said, 'you're a joke, Juliette. Look at the state of you.' He was lying on the bed, one arm behind his head, mocking me. I was furious, and couldn't understand why he'd do that to me. I went straight over to him and hit him; I couldn't help myself. Of course, that's what he'd wanted. He then had the excuse to 'restrain me', as he called it, by grabbing me by the hair and throwing me to the floor, all the while with this vile smirk on his face.

As I lay on the floor wondering what I'd done to deserve that, he calmly picked up his wallet, opened the hotel room door and went out without me. I followed him outside, barefoot, wet, make-up sliding down my face, but so angry I didn't care what I looked like. He walked on ahead, then suddenly turned and ran back towards me, and grabbed me around the middle, my arms blocked against my chest. He was still laughing. He dragged me back to the hotel room and pushed me onto the bed.

'Don't you follow me, Juliette. I'll drag you back again, and you know it.' I had no idea where the venue was, it was late, it was dark and it was a long walk anyway. He knew I wouldn't go there alone. I took my make-up off and went to bed in tears. He stumbled in 5.00am, got into bed and went straight to sleep beside me, no doubt having spent the night chatting up and dancing with other girls.

I could go weeks without an incident and then he'd just blow up out of nowhere. Most often he would accuse me of flirting with someone (I had no need to flirt with anyone, I was in love with him, besides I was a hopeless flirt anyway). After one particularly bad row at home, in which he'd been so vile to me verbally that I'd slapped him, and he'd restrained me a little too forcefully by throwing me up against the wall in the hallway by my throat, I took his Stanley knife from the cupboard and fled to the bathroom, locking the door behind me.

I cut my left arm, but nothing happened. The blade was blunt. I screamed in frustration and threw the knife to the floor. I was leaning over the sink, hands on the black tiles behind it, my head hung, tears streaming down my face. I turned around and picked up the knife again, this time I cut as hard as I could. It grazed the skin, and drew a little blood. Typically, I couldn't even get that right. It sort of gouged a line instead, as if I'd caught it in a door. I think that hurt as much as if I'd slit my wrist. The frustration I felt was nothing compared to the guilt and the anger welling up inside me. I thought of how John would have to call Mum if he got me to hospital. I couldn't bear to put them through any more pain, but at the same time I realised that I couldn't deal with my own pain anymore, at least not alone.

John banged hard on the door after a couple of minutes and told me to let him in. I did. He saw the knife in my hand, glanced at my wrist, and grabbed the knife.

'It's blunt,' I laughed, 'I can't even kill myself.'

'You want to kill yourself?' he said, 'then I'll sort you out.' He left the bathroom and after a few minutes' rummaging in the cupboard, came in with the brand new Stanley knife that I hadn't been able to find.

'You can have this,' he said, putting the knife in my hand, 'or do you want to take some pills?'

'Not pills,' I said, now crying so hard I could hardly breathe, 'it takes too long and gives you liver failure instead of killing you. Then you just die in hospital. I need to get in the bath, a hot bath, and cut myself.'

He pushed me out of the bathroom.

'OK, I'll run you a bath,' he said, turning on the hot tap. He poured in some coconut bubble bath, still holding the knife in his left hand.

'I don't want bubbles,' I sobbed, 'it'll sting.'

'Too late, so do you want a drink to help dull the pain?'

I was in such a state that I didn't even question the idea that he was helping me to end my life. I nodded, confused, distraught and desperate.

'Will you just shut the door and let me lock it and go out,' I pleaded. 'Give it a couple of hours then come back and you can call an ambulance or whatever, it'll be too late anyway. All my bank things and stuff for the flat are in the office, in the cupboard on the left. All the bills are paid up. My mortgage details and all of that stuff, Dad will need it, it's in the same place. You can sort it out with them.'

I'd just distanced myself from everything and everyone. Panic gave way to a surreal sense of calm. I knew what I was going to do. It would be OK. I'd tried everything else. I felt totally in control of my own destiny, of being able to tell my body, my diseases that actually, I'll decide when I've had enough, not you. I didn't want to call my parents, because obviously they'd be in hysterics so I just thought I'll go quietly and then it's done. It'll be more peaceful that way.

The bath was ready.

John came back in with half a tumbler of neat gin and I drank it straight down. As I put the glass back down on the tiles, I knew then that I couldn't back out. I had to do it, for everyone's sake. I felt terrible for my parents, but I didn't give John much thought. After all, he was often the root of the problem and the cause of so much of my misery. He brought as my happiness to my life as he did pain, but at this point the pain - both mental and physical - had taken over my life. I had nothing else.

I climbed into the bath. He turned out the lights and lit two candles. I didn't even question the absurdity of it all. John brought Pantouf in and placed him on top of the vintage pink linen basket next to the bath. I couldn't stand to look at him.

'Say goodbye to Pantouf, then,' said John, 'give him a kiss.'

That really set me off. I was crying like I used to cry when I was three or four-years-old at the end of a temper tantrum - big, uncontrollable sobs. I didn't want to leave Pantouf - or his brothers Warm Bear and Daniel (the monkey, remember?) - without their mum.

'But I don't want to leave him,' I sobbed. I couldn't stand this. I looked at him and felt total despair. I didn't know what I was thinking, never mind doing. I wanted out, but I didn't want to hurt my family. What was I supposed to do?

I put my head under the water and lay down. The water was so hot that I knew it would help with the pain. My wrist stung from where I'd tried to cut it. I didn't think I'd be able to go over the same spot. I decided to do my other arm first. I was even contemplating cutting my throat, when I think all I really wanted was a cuddle.

John was watching me as I sat up in the bath. He held up the knife in front of my face. I went to take it off him. He pulled away.

'You're ready to leave Pantouf, are you?' he hissed, 'you're going to leave him without his mum?'

I nodded, tears streaming down my face.

'Do you think I'd let you cut yourself?' he shouted, 'do you think I'd let you do that to yourself?'

He was screaming the words at me. He opened the bathroom door and flung the knife out into the hall.

I didn't know whether I was relieved or not. Probably half and half, but by now I was so hot and drunk I wasn't sure what was going on inside my head. This was a build-up of years of unhappiness that had been festering away like the diseases that had taken hold of my life and smashed it into million pieces.

I looked at John. He was crying, kneeling beside the bath, his hands over the edge, fingertips dangling in the water.

'I would have done it,' I said, 'I would have done it.'

'That's what makes me so upset. I thought you were kidding. When you drank that gin, I knew you meant it. You hate neat gin.'

'I did mean it. I still mean it. I think. I don't know. I can't go on like this, I just can't. The pain is so bad, I can't do it anymore. There's no point. What will I be like in five years' time, let alone 20? I don't want to fight anymore. I'm tired. I'm so, so tired.'

He motioned for me to sit forward, and began to soap my back. I was crying still, but quietly.

'Can I get out, can I get a cuddle?' I said, shivering again.

'Course you can, stand up.'

He wrapped me in the big, white towel, dried me off, got me into my pyjamas and held me to his chest for a while. Somehow I was *still* crying - I could have been in the Guinness Book of Records by now - as he led me into the lounge, holding my hand and telling me it'd be OK.

I lay on the settee, wrapped in the leopard print throw, just as I had the day I'd blacked out and been sick.

'Don't tell Mum,' I said, 'please don't tell her.'

'I won't', he said, 'but don't ever do that again.'

He lay behind me on the sofa, holding me tight. From zero to hero, every time. I didn't know what to make of any of it. I hated and loved him in equal measures.

As it turned out, I did tell Mum, and I also told Alice. In doing so, a huge weight lifted from my shoulders. I wasn't embarrassed about what I'd done - or tried to do - I was more embarrassed that I hadn't been honest with the people I loved, who I know would have tried to help, or at least offered me a hug and a biscuit. Alice cried, Mum was alarmed, and I was still surprised that I had come so close. Had that knife been sharp and John not been in the flat I have no doubt in my mind that I'd have attempted suicide. Whether or not I'd have succeeded I don't know, but I'd have given it a good go.

I'd been to see a doctor at the Pain Clinic a week prior to my 'episode'. The Pain Clinic takes referrals from consultants who basically don't know what to do with patients who aren't responding to conventional treatment. I'd been through all the painkillers, but couldn't take half of them because of my colitis history. Anything which served as an anti-inflammatory, even Nurofen, could inflame the lining of my stomach or gut, and I didn't really need that. Because I also had an ileo-anal pouch, my digestive system was extra sensitive, and very strong painkillers made me nauseous. I'd tried everything, to no avail. I preferred to be in pain than feel as though I was on the verge of throwing up all day and night.

The consultant decided to try me out with a painkilling patch, which released a morphine-based substance into my bloodstream rather than via my stomach, which the consultant told me would be easier for me. I was advised to cut the patch into quarters and build up to a whole one if my stomach could tolerate it.

I cut the patch into quarters and stuck one of them on my right shoulder. Within half an hour I began to feel a bit sick, but shrugged it off. I got in the car and drove to the supermarket, and by the time I had picked up a basket and decided to get broccoli instead of green beans, I thought I was going to pass out. Waves of nausea washed over me, and I wondered which would be the best aisle to throw up in. I put my basket down and left the shop. I got in the car and sat with the window open for a few minutes, hoping it would pass, but instead, it got steadily worse. I decided I had to drive back now or I'd throw up in the street, so with my head swimming and my stomach turning, I drove home.

Those five minutes felt like forever, my vision starting to blur as I pulled into the car park behind my flat. I opened the front door, lurched towards the bathroom and positioned myself over the toilet. Within 30 seconds I was throwing up so hard I thought I'd lose my feet through my throat. It was horrendous. That was what a quarter of it did – thank God I hadn't gone with a whole patch. I sat back, exhausted. Another treatment had failed. I had been told that this was my last hope; the despair hit me like a truck.

John had started work earlier that week at the local supermarket. It was far from his dream job, but he had to do something and I kept hoping that he would get a building job – a proper, regular one – and that it might sort him out. Now he was back to long hours and minimum wage. I had a little freelance writing for Brighton creative agencies, but it didn't amount to much. One day, after another argument, John pretended to take an overdose of my painkillers, just to get my attention. He was sobbing, telling me he didn't want to break up with me, that he was sorry. That was not the kind of stunt I needed. His histrionics were getting more and more ridiculous. He was starting to scare me; I wouldn't know from one minute to the next whether he'd kiss me or threaten me. I calmly handed him the phone and told him to call an ambulance. Needless to say he didn't make the call because he was lying. Again.

In the same week, Ross - my ex-boyfriend - came down to Brighton to take me out to lunch. I hadn't seen him since we broke up but we'd started talking (via email) occasionally about a year after. That morning, before he left for work, John asked me what time Ross would arrive. I told him around midday. John went off to work at 9am and I pottered around and got ready. At 11.15am I heard a key in the front door. It was John.

'I don't feel well, I'm taking the rest of the day off,' he told me, looking sheepish and ducking into the bedroom.

'You were fine two hours ago,' I said, 'what's wrong?'

'Don't question me, Juliette,' he spat, the all-too-familiar sly look coming over his face, 'when's your ex-boyfriend turning up?'

So that was it. He was so jealous that he couldn't bear me to have lunch with my friend. That he had to be here when he arrived, to show him I was in a relationship? He'd changed out of his work clothes and was sitting on the sofa when the buzzer went. He sneered at me as I walked towards the front door.

Ross walked in and looked suitably surprised to see John sitting on the sofa. I introduced them, glared at John and left the flat with Ross. As we crossed the road, Ross put his hand on the small of my back (he was holding an umbrella over us with his other hand). We got into the car, and drove off.

When I got back, John answered the door before I had a chance to put my key in the lock.

'Why did he put his arm around you, Juliette? Why did he do that?' He followed me into the kitchen, asking me over and over again. He insisted Ross and I had gone to a hotel together - really, can you believe that? I ignored him. He was following me from room to room, jabbing me in the back and repeating it over and over again like a stuck record.

'I know you did it, Juliette,' he kept saying, 'don't you lie to me.'

I couldn't stand another day of this. I then thought about taking every painkiller I had and just going to bed. I didn't know what to do. The reality was that I didn't want to do anything anymore. If someone had offered to shoot me, I'd have said, 'sure, go right ahead.' As it was, I grabbed my keys from my bag, opened the front door and let myself out, then locked the door behind me so he couldn't come after me. I just sat outside the front door with my head in my hands, sobbing my heart out, wishing someone would take me away from all this.

October 2004

'There is a treatment which is being considered for sufferers of ankylosing spondylitis,' said my consultant, leaning to one side in his chair and clicking his pen in and out, 'however, it's very expensive. You probably won't get funding for it,' he continued, waiting for a response.

'Why not? I can hardly walk, I can't sleep, and I'm so much pain all the time. I can't work, I can't even move around until lunchtime. I've tried everything else. That's all I've done for four years - try, hope, try again. There's nothing left to try. I can't go on like this. I won't go on like this. I really won't. I can't do it.'

'The Primary Care Trust would have to approve it for you. And you are not in a wheelchair. So you are not that bad.' He shrugged, as if to say, 'that's it, end of discussion.'

I couldn't hold back the tears at this point. I was absolutely desperate, yet I was still being told to get on with it. How? And, just as importantly, why? Why would I want to carry on if my life was going to be like this?

'I'm not in a wheelchair because the pain isn't in my legs, it's in my upper body, so how can I push myself around in a wheelchair when I can't even lean on my elbows to sit up in bed? How? Can you at least tell me what it is?' I begged.

He sat forward in his chair.

'It's called Etanercept. It's an injection which you have to do yourself, twice a week, into your tummy,' he explained, pointing at, you've guessed it, his tummy.

'My tummy?' I squeaked. Of all places!

'Or your thigh, but mainly in the tummy area. It's for people with rheumatoid arthritis who haven't responded to other treatment, and who have a very severe form of the disease.'

'I'm so tired,' I sighed, 'and in so much pain, with nothing to look forward to but more pain and losing my home that I've worked so hard for. I don't get income support because I have my own place. I have to pay for my prescriptions, and there are a lot of them. I can't get a job, but I can't get funding to train in something I could do from home, again because I don't get income support. I wish I'd never bought my flat. I'd have been better off if I was renting. I get less financial help than my friend receives in child benefit. And that's just the basics. I can't go on like this. I've already discussed it with my parents, and they completely understand how I feel, and what I am prepared to do to not put up with this any longer.' I continued, the tears giving way to anger again.

I drew breath, finally.

'You said it works for ankylosing spondylitis. Is that what I've got?'

'Well, yes,' he replied, nodding. 'I would say so. Inflammation of the spine, the sacro-iliac joints… it's possible the drug could work well.'

He was quiet. I wanted to shake him.

'I'll write to them,' he said, 'I will try for you. That's all I can do.'

'Please. That's all I ask.'

As nobody seemed bothered whether I knew anything about this disease of mine, I decided to look into it myself. A couple of years previously I'd read a book based on symptoms of disease and asked my doctor at the time if I could be given the blood test for AS, as I thought that's what I had. He'd said: 'the tests are really difficult. It's probably just your colon.'

Yeah? Probably bloody well not. At last I had a diagnosis. I felt as though it should have been accompanied by a fanfare of trumpets rather than practically dragged out of my rheumatologist.

The thought of injecting myself in the tummy, full of lumps, bumps and scar tissue didn't get me too excited. However, four years of agony meant I was willing to try anything bar supporting Arsenal or eating a cat. I logged on to the internet.

'The tendency for developing AS is believed to be genetically inherited, and the majority (nearly 90%) of patients with AS are born with the HLA-B27 gene.' Makes sense, Dad has arthritis, a slipped disc and his Dad stood around like a bendy straw, always with his hand in the small of his back, as I'm now doing. I read on.

'The initial inflammation may be a result of an activation of body's immune system by a bacterial infection. Once activated, the body's immune system becomes unable to turn itself off, even though the initial bacterial infection may have long subsided. Chronic tissue inflammation resulting from the continued activation of the body's own immune system in the absence of active infection is the hallmark of an auto-immune disease.

'The symptoms of AS are related to inflammation of the spine, joints, and other organs. Inflammation of the spine causes pain and stiffness in the low back, upper buttock area, neck, and the remainder of the spine. The onset of pain and stiffness is usually gradual and progressively worsens over months. Occasionally, the onset is rapid and intense. The symptoms of pain and stiffness are often worse in the morning, or after prolonged periods of inactivity. Patients who have chronic, severe inflammation of the spine can develop a complete bony fusion of the spine (ankylosis). Once fused, the pain in the spine disappears, but the patient has a complete loss of spine mobility. These fused spines are particularly brittle and vulnerable to breakage (fracture) when involved in trauma, such as motor vehicle accidents. A sudden onset of pain and mobility in the spinal area of these patients can indicate bone fracture. The cervical spine is the most common area for such fractures.

Chronic spondylitis and ankylosis cause forward curvature of the upper torso (thoracic spine), limiting breathing capacity. Spondylitis can also affect areas where ribs attach to the upper spine, further limiting lung capacity. Ankylosing spondylitis can cause inflammation and scarring of the lungs, causing coughing and shortness of breath, especially with exercise and infections.

Patients may notice pain, stiffness, heat, swelling, warmth, and/or redness in joints such as the hips, knees, and ankles. Occasionally, the small joints of the toes can become inflamed, or 'sausage' shaped. Inflammation can occur in the cartilage around the breast bone (costochondritis) as well as in the tendons where the muscles attach to the bone (tendinitis) and ligament attachments to bone. Some patients with this disease develop Achilles tendinitis, causing pain and stiffness in the back of the heel, especially when pushing off with the foot while walking up stairs.

'Advanced spondylitis can lead to deposits of protein material called amyloid into the kidneys and result in kidney failure.

'The treatment of ankylosing spondylitis involves the use of medications to reduce inflammation or suppress immunity, physical therapy, and exercise. Medications decrease inflammation in the spine, and other joints and organs. Physical therapy and exercise help improve posture, spine mobility and lung capacity.

And then we got to the most interesting bit.

'Newer, effective medications for spine disease attack a messenger protein of inflammation (called TNF).

'These TNF-blocking medications have been shown to be extremely effective for treating AS by stopping disease activity, decreasing inflammation, and improving spinal mobility. Etanercept is an injectable drug that blocks tumour necrosis factor alpha (TNF alpha). TNF alpha is a protein that the body produces during the inflammatory response, the body's reaction to injury. TNF alpha promotes the inflammation and its associated fever and signs - pain, tenderness, and swelling. Etanercept is a synthetic (man-made) protein that binds to TNF alpha. It thereby acts like a sponge to remove most of the TNF alpha molecules from the joints and blood. This prevents TNF alpha from promoting inflammation. Since Etanercept is a relatively new drug, there is limited information on long-term risks.'

Other than that, it sounded great. Later on, having done some more research on my lovely diseases on the internet, I would find that about 1 in 800 people in the UK develop AS, and many more go undiagnosed. Then I remembered the pooh tests the nutritionist had arranged had flagged AS when I was first told I had colitis. I was stunned.

It is estimated that around 1 in 200 people suffer with the disease without diagnosis. Hugely relevant to me and providing an answer as to why I had AS and UC, was this little known fact: the highest incidence of UC is in people descended from Ashkenazi Jews, who originated in Russia and Eastern Europe. Given that my dad's father was Jewish, and from Russia, I had my answer. My granddad had also been diagnosed with AS. My poor Dad was forced out of the army at 21 years of age with a duodenal ulcer. So, ulcers, slipped disc, arthritis = ulcerative colitis and AS in daughter. That's not lucky, is it? I'd managed to get the lot, while my brother and two cousins avoided both. I thought that was a bit unfair. I didn't wish either disease on any of them, obviously, but it would have been nicer for me if they'd been shared out a little, right?

A month later I was given the go-ahead to begin treatment. I thanked the consultant and called Mum to tell her the news. She was excited, as was I, but I was pretty nervous too. I'd thought long and hard about all the possible side effects, and talked through things with my parents about whether or not I should chance it, but the pain was so unbearable I had no choice.

'I'd sooner have 10 pain free years on this drug than 30 terrible ones without it,' I reasoned. It's not much fun, deciding things like that, but I felt I had to take one day at a time, something I wasn't used to doing, and see how I got on with it. If an ear started growing out of my back, my hair turned green or my palms sprouted eyes, I'd stop the drug, sell my flat, and go to Rio with all my tablets, sit on the beach, drink cocktails and walk into the sea late at night in a sapphire blue, sequined 1950s mermaid dress (look it up, it's worth it).

The drug arrived a couple of weeks later. The next day the nurse came round to show me how to prepare the drug and inject it. I wasn't very good at this bit and got into quite a pickle. It seemed so complicated - lids off this, twisty caps off that, pulling down one thing and pushing up another, then pinching the skin on my tummy into a big fat lump, injecting it in one quick swoop - ouch - and pushing down on the vial. All in all, there were about 245 steps to the instructions.

Three days later when I did it myself, it took me half an hour to complete the process as I'd forgotten everything I'd done before and had to read the leaflet. Nowadays it takes no time at all. Caps off, twisty bits off, join two bits together, wait for it to dissolve, pinch my skin, jab it in, pull it out. It reminded me of the stoma in the sense that I couldn't cope at all with that the first few times I had to go through all the palaver of setting everything out and remembering which order to do it all in. I soon got the hang of that and whilst this wasn't as bad - I didn't have blisters or old lunch to deal with nor did I have to strip off to do it - it wasn't much fun.

After the second injection, later on that week, I went to bed at midnight. The next thing I knew the alarm was going off and it was 8am.

I looked at the clock again to make sure, and then I realised that by the simple fact that I could look at the clock, I wasn't in pain. I turned over. That's right, turned over. I haven't been able to do that for years.

I woke John up.

'Hey, I can breathe, I'm not hurting, I can move, I can turn over!'

He woke up to find me leaning over him, waving Pantouf in his face.

'What's going on?' he said, rubbing his eyes, 'are you alright?'

'I'm fine. I don't know if this is some kind of trick but I really don't hurt. It's mental. I've slept right through.'

It was mental. And from that day on, I had actual good days. Pain-free days. Not every day, by any means, but I'd gone from seven terrible days to four. My pouch and my tummy still gave me twinges and some pain, and I was exhausted from having to get up in the middle of the night to go to the loo (at least twice); my bottom still hurt most days either from the pouch being a little bit inflamed, or because what comes out is so acidic and burns the skin (nice).

But I could get out of bed, kicking off the covers along the way, stand up straight, just normal things. The next step, now that I felt up to it, was to try again with getting a job. Admittedly, I'd have liked to have just enjoyed my life for a while, but I couldn't afford to.

Things with John actually got worse as my health improved. I thought that my feeling better would make him happy, but actually, when I felt up to going out for a drink one night with a friend (without him), he kicked off about something before I left, made me cry, then kept calling me while I was out, demanding to know when I'd be home. I had to turn my phone off. He did everything he could to keep me to himself; one night he went as far as telling me he was sick so I would stay home and look after him. I didn't, but when I got home, he was blind drunk and waiting for a fight. I needed my own money so I could pay the mortgage and the bills and get him the hell out of my life.

When I first moved to Brighton, I'd had regular work on a magazine called *Business Edge*. I wrote a lot of their cover stories - interviews with local business people but not dull ones, people who were doing something a bit different, or were well known nationally, like hairdresser Trevor Sorbie. The place that published it also doubled up as an advertising and marketing agency, and they were looking for a receptionist, 9am-3pm, five days a week. I knew I would find that physically hard-going, but I was determined to give it my best shot. If I had any writing work I could do that in the evening, I reasoned (which was madness; I was still ill, just in less pain than I had been).

I had a very informal interview with the MD that lasted all of thirty seconds and went like this:

'You're a journalist, what do you want to do this for, Willsy?'

'I need the money, I already know you, your tea and coffee making facilities are excellent and I can park right outside.'

'We'll see,' he said.

A couple of days later they rang to say sorry, that they'd found someone else. They knew I 'didn't really want to do reception work'. I tried not to feel set back, but I did. I had no idea what to do. I as more exhausted than ever; since starting the drug, I felt even more tired than before, but I think that's because I was pushing myself to do more, to get out of the house, rush around the supermarket, dump papers and bottles at the recycling plant, visit sick cats at the Cats Protection League, cook chicken for the sick cats, cook and clean like crazy and apply for at least 20 jobs a week, both part-time in Brighton and on magazines in London. I was finally catching up with my sleep, and it felt as though my body wanted this time to relax, to sleep 10 hours a night because it could. I had completely useless days where I could barely move, and then I'd have two days where I could. I'd then push myself to do all the things I couldn't do the day before on the day I felt OK. Naturally, I'd feel worse the day after, but what could I do? In the end, the reception job came up again. I did three days a week from 9am to 3pm for three months, then the company suddenly announced that they were declaring bankruptcy. Oh well. I was a lousy receptionist anyway.

CHAPTER SEVENTEEN
'TAINTED LOVE'
DAVE PHILLIPS
& THE HOT ROD GANG

One night I invited Phil and Cherry over for dinner. I made a joke, I can't even remember what it was, and John didn't think it was funny. I had no idea that anything was wrong until they left. I asked him to help me clear up after dinner and he pushed past me, saying, 'you wanted them to come over, you wanted to cook, you can clear up your own mess.' He sat down on the sofa and turned the TV up to full blast. I went back to the kitchen and washed up, wondering what I'd done to deserve that. He told me I'd humiliated him on purpose. I had no idea what he was talking about, but he'd been charming until the moment they had left, then as soon as he'd shut the door behind them, off he went.

In April he went into hospital for an operation on his right knee. I'd pushed him to have it done. I couldn't understand why his mother hadn't sorted it out when he was at home. He'd had terrible problems with his ligaments for years, and would often dislocate a knee just walking down the street. They told him he'd be on crutches for six weeks, and just as he would begin walking unaided, he'd have the left knee operated on. In all, it meant 12 weeks at home, then a further six weeks after that before he could go back to work. I still can't believe I went through with it. That would have been a great time to tell him to move back to his mum's.

I said I'd support him throughout his recuperation and we'd spoken to Phil about him working as his labourer once he was fit enough. It seemed like it would be a good new start - new knees, new job, good prospects, the lot. I was still hoping it would also put him in a better mood, that his anger might abate and that our relationship would be better. I kept hoping, kept trying, kept thinking that if he could work with Phil, he'd be happy, and everything would be OK.

When I picked John up from hospital, it sunk in that I'd be caring for him. I wasn't really sure how I'd manage that, and I'm still not entirely sure how I did. I had to do everything for him. He couldn't even wash the dishes because he needed both crutches, although he gave it a good go one night, with me saying 'Nooooooo! Sit down!' as he wobbled about at the sink. I'd got a big project to work on and I needed some peace and quiet to be able to work. I asked John to call his mum and see if she could take him back to her house for a week so I could focus. On the Friday, I went back to Mum and Dad's to write. On the Saturday, John called me, saying his brother had come down with his mum and his nephew. They'd been to the pier and had a nice day out, and they were all staying over before taking him back to Birmingham. I found that a bit weird as we only had a sofa bed and sofa, so unless they'd brought their own beds I couldn't see where they would sleep. I didn't think too much about it. On the Sunday, when John was supposed to be on his way back home to his mum's, he called from the flat.

'Why are you still there?" I asked, my heart sinking.

'Because I miss you, I didn't want to go,' he said.

I was furious. I took a deep breath.

'I really needed a break,' I said, 'surely your mum can see that.'

'Well, I didn't want to go,' he answered.

I told him I wasn't coming home until Tuesday and that he'd have to manage without me. He told me his mum had been to the supermarket so he'd be fine. When I got home, I found a bin full of empty crisp packets and chocolate bar wrappers and an empty box of Rice Krispies. Looking back, I don't think his family came down at all; I think he took a cab to the local shop to buy crisps and chocolate and cereal and had just eaten that for three days. It was like living with a child.

In the end, I worked from Cherry and Phil's flat for a few hours a day, just to get some peace. John had taken to antagonising me as I tried to work, by turning the TV up to full volume, playing music or constantly interrupting me, even yelling 'hey, Juliette, blah blah blah blah blah,' and laughing at me, just so I lost my train of thought. I couldn't understand his behaviour. Why would he not want me to work?

I asked him that exact question. He just laughed, turned the TV up to full volume and said 'it's not my fault you can't concentrate, Juliette. Maybe you just don't know how to write anymore.'

I overheard him lying to friends about all kinds of things; from what he did for a living (at one point he told someone he was a graphic designer!) to telling people we were going on holiday when we weren't, or that we were looking at buying a bigger flat - together - and even that he was learning to drive. Can you imagine what it's like to love someone like that? He would go from being loving, kind and funny to a narcissistic monster that enjoyed nothing more than making me afraid of him. Outside of the flat, he was the most charming, funny person you could meet. He'd be telling Cherry how nice she looked one minute and whispering, 'you need to be nice to me, Juliette, or I'll go and find someone else,' a second later. He was also demanding I put him on my mortgage. I thought that was pretty hilarious. He hadn't a hope in hell of that ever happening, but he kept on about it, even getting his mum to call me and tell me I should do it. Can you believe it? I felt trapped, backed into a corner like an injured animal. The walls were closing in on me. I couldn't make things better. I just wanted him gone.

January 2006

John had been at his mum's for Christmas and New Year. I had managed to convince him that I needed looking after at my parents', and that he should spend some time with his family. Whilst he was away I had borrowed a book from a friend. The book was called *Power & Control* and was about being in a relationship with elements of abuse. I'd never read a 'self-help' book before, but I read it cover to cover in one sitting during an afternoon and identified with so many of the case studies that I knew John had serious problems which weren't going to go away. He was narcissistic, manipulative, violent, controlling and a compulsive liar. Worse still, he was so young I thought he had plenty of time to get even more extreme, whereas I had first thought he was young enough that I could 'make him better.' Pretty much everything he had told me was a lie. He lied to me, to my parents, to my friends, to complete strangers. He'd embellish every single story he told. He told so many lies that he couldn't keep up with whom he'd told them to, giving one story to one person and another to someone else. I made up my mind there and then that it was over.

He arrived back at the flat four hours later than he said he'd arrive, stinking, hangover and looking like he'd slept exactly where he had - on the floor at someone's party. He was more threatening and abusive with each row over the next few weeks, and his threats were becoming more menacing. In between these rows he'd shower me with compliments, help me around the house, take me out dancing - when I could - make me laugh my head off and tell people how lucky he was to have met me. He was utterly charming to everyone with one friend saying 'you can see how much he loves you by the way he looks at you, Juliette. He's always looking at you.' I almost said, 'no, he's just watching me to see if I flirt with your husband.'

Everyone thought he was completely besotted with me. I honestly had no idea what he felt.

He accused me of sleeping with every man I ever spoke to. He had 'banned' me from seeing my friend, Mark, because he felt threatened by him, refusing to meet him when he offered to come to Brighton to take John and me for lunch. I just met him for dinner when I visited my parents instead.

He was so jealous when we went to rockabilly clubs he'd pretend to go to the bar, then actually stand across the other side of the room, watching me, presumably to see if I spoke to another man. He thought I didn't know that he did this, but I did. I laughed it off with my friends at the time (they all knew he did it), but it made my skin crawl; it scared me, and it must have rattled them, too. I was embarrassed by his behaviour, trying to find a way to justify the things he did, but the walls were closing in and people around us were starting to see him for who he really was.

I told him to move out the weekend before Valentine's Day. I think we'd started arguing in the living room. He'd then got in the bath. He was shouting at me from the bathroom.

'You're so *old*, Juliette. You look like shit. Your hair is so grey you have to dye it black, like an old woman. You can't even dance. You limp when you walk. You're boring. You're disgusting. Who'd want you?' He was really yelling now. It wasn't the first time he'd launched a tirade of abuse.

I walked into the bathroom and he kept saying the same thing over and over again whilst smirking at me.

'Nobody else would want you, Juliette. You're damaged goods. You're useless. You haven't even got a job. I have to help you clean the flat. You can't even do that on your own. Your shoes have been on the floor for three days now. You can't even put your shoes in the wardrobe. It's pathetic, don't you think?'

I was so angry that when he lay down in the water and closed his eyes, I pushed his face under the water. It was a heat of the moment thing. He reacted immediately, grabbing my arm and my hair and pulling me half into the bath, smacking my head hard against the tiles. I screamed, prised his fingers from my hair and ran to the bedroom where I sat on the bed, wet, shocked and shaking. He got out of the bath, got dressed in a flash and then came into the bedroom, still taunting me. I got up to leave the room, and he pushed me down on to the bed. He held me there, leaning over me, laughing at me. He spat in my face. I had reached the lowest point in my life. I moved to get up a third time, and he said, 'go on then, I'll let you walk out, but if you do, I'm not letting you back in again. Do you hear me, Juliette? You go out, you stay out.'

'It's *my* flat!' I screamed. I grabbed my Converse, my phone and my keys and reached for the door handle. Just as I opened it he pounced, pushing me back against the wall with one arm and slamming the door with the other. He had his left wrist across my throat, and his body was blocking mine. He was still smirking, and then he let me go. He just stood there, laughing at me as I slumped to the floor, trying to catch my breath. I stood up slowly, and said, 'I'm going now. If you lock me out, I'm calling the police.'

I drove straight over to Phil and Cherry's and although I didn't tell them exactly what had happened, I explained that I could do with a cup of tea because John had had one of his 'moments' again. Cherry gave me a hug, and Phil asked why I let him stay there. 'I can't afford not to. I can't pay the mortgage, can't pay the bills. Without him carrying things, I can't even go shopping. I can't do anything. I don't know what else to do. And besides, he won't leave.' I'm pretty certain that if Phil had offered to round up a few mates and remove him for me I'd have been delighted. I honestly didn't know how to get rid of him.

I came back to the flat after an hour. He'd calmed down. I avoided looking at him, and went in the bathroom to run myself a bath. I locked the door and stayed in there for an hour. I came out, and went to bed. He came into the bedroom, and climbed into bed beside me.

'Come on, give me a kiss. You know you love me. Say it. Say you love me, Juliette.' He was stroking my hair and leaning over me.

'Just leave me alone,' I said. He made me feel sick.

'Seriously. Leave me alone.'

'Are you crying?' he asked, sitting up, a big grin on his face.

'Are you? What are you crying for? Are you sorry, Juliette?'

I couldn't believe what was happening. He was asking me if I was sorry. Christ. It was like reading the book all over again. He was ticking every box and more. I was really afraid of what he might do to me. I ignored him and tried to go to sleep. After 10 minutes, I got up and went into the living room where I lay on the sofa under my leopard print blanket. He was already sound asleep beside me, clearly without a care in the world.

Fortunately the next day was Friday, and John had to be up at 6.30am for some plastering work with Phil. Phil picked him up. I got up, took a shower and packed my bag. I rang Mum and said I was coming to see her. I left a note and told him not to call me. He got home early, and naturally, he did the opposite. On the seventh call, I switched my phone off. He called the house phone, and Dad said I didn't want to talk to him.

I was drying my hair on the Saturday morning, getting ready to go and meet Charlie for lunch in London, when Mum popped her head around the bedroom door. She saw the cluster of bruises - his finger and thumb prints - on my upper arm as I lifted the hairdryer.

'I take it that's John's work,' she said, and I cringed. At that point it occurred to me how much it must upset them, all the arguing and the constant battles. They'd still be nice to him when he came to their house with me, and it must have been so difficult.

'I'll sort it out,' I said, 'I promise.'

I still didn't understand how I could leave my own home. When you read advice for domestic abuse situations, they always say to pack a bag and go when the coast is clear. If we were renting, or I was living in his place, or even if we owned the flat together, OK. But walking out and leaving him when he threatens to smash my things up? That wasn't an option. I wouldn't let him drive me out of my own home.

Two days later I came home. It was Valentine's Day. I hadn't even remembered, and besides, I'd never been bothered about it. On the table was a bottle of Chanel No.5, a box of fancy Belgian chocolates and a beautiful bunch of pink and yellow tulips. John had obviously arranged it all before he went to work. If we'd had a normal relationship, I'd have found it absolutely wonderful. Instead, I actually found it a bit disturbing. I thought I was going to throw up, and had to steady myself. He was clearly in denial and hoping that this would persuade me to change my mind. I knew I really had my work cut out. He came home that evening and kissed me as if nothing was wrong. It was so weird, and it scared me.

'You need to leave. I can't live with you anymore.'

'That's the thanks I get for buying you presents, is it? I'm not leaving, Juliette,' he said, slowly and again, with that nasty smirk: 'I'm not leaving because you owe me money,' he said, jabbing a finger in my face.

Once again, in less time than it takes to boil a kettle, it escalated into a violent row, and once again it went on for a good couple of hours and ended with me in tears and him hysterical. It wasn't pretty. He'd gone to grab me as I'd turned to leave the room. I dodged him, and ran into the bedroom. I had taken to keeping a spare set of keys - car and door - and £20 in one of my boots in the wardrobe. My phone was in the bedroom, so I put that in my back pocket. I could hear him taking my keys off the hook in the hall. I laughed, because he thought he was so clever.

'I've got your keys,' he said calmly, through the bedroom door.

'I've got your keys, and I've got your shoes. You're going nowhere, OK? You can't even stand up straight, how are you going to run away from me?'

I wasn't crying anymore. I thought it was hilarious that he'd said he had my shoes. 'I've got 78 pairs of shoes,' I said in response, half crying, half laughing, 'what are you going to do about that?'

I pulled on another pair of Converse and slid my keys into the side. I put the £20 in the other and opened the bedroom door. He was standing against the door.

'You're not leaving,' he said, 'I just told you. Don't you listen? I've got your keys.' He was holding them in front of my face.

'You'll have to get them off me if you want them.' He laughed, and walked towards the living room, expecting me to follow him.

As soon as he was a good few feet away from me, I flung open the front door. I wasn't quick enough. He was on me in a second, slamming the door shut and pulling me in. His fist was in my face.

'You think you're going to go, just like that, do you?' he spat, 'I swear to God, you push me so much, Juliette, one day, maybe today even, I'll break your f*cking face.' His knuckles were white. He pushed his fist into my cheek, gently.

'I swear to God, I'll break it. Just here,' he said. He pulled back his fist, and mimicked a punch, shouting 'bam!' as his fist came down, stopping a when his fist touched my cheekbone. The tears were rolling down my face. He suddenly let go of me.

'Do what you like,' he said, 'you won't get very far. And while you're gone, I'll smash up your flat, cut up your beautiful vintage clothes, break your records, all the records your dad gave you, smash it all, the lot. How do you like that?'

I opened the door, walked calmly down the stairs and straight to the car. I'd parked out the front, directly below our living room window. I heard the window open as I approached the car.

'You can't go anywhere, Juliette,' he yelled, leaning out of the window, a big grin on his face, 'you left your key behind. Come and get it.' I totally ignored him, and quickly unlocked the car, got in, turned on the engine and did the quickest three-point turn in history.

I pulled up outside Hove police station two minutes later. I sat in a room with the police officer and told him, in short, that I wanted my boyfriend out of my home but he refused to leave. That he had threatened me on several occasions, but that he didn't actually hit or beat me. That I was sure the next time we argued, he would. I even told him I'd lashed out at him several times, but only because the things John would say to me were designed to make me react like that. I told him that he'd once taken my dinner plate from the table into the kitchen, and put it on the floor, telling me that I was so disgusting I should eat off the floor like a dog. Sometimes, if we were eating when he kicked off, I calmly picked up my plate and took it outside, and finished my dinner in the corridor. He enjoyed seeing me angry, laughed at me when I cried, and threatened me if I stood up to him. He knew he could really hurt me and he thrived on it. It was all about control, and the reason he behaved so horribly was because he knew he *wasn't* able to control me. I was frightened of him when he lost his temper, but I never believed the nasty things he said to me, and never blamed myself for how he treated me. I think was the problem - my reluctance to become a 'victim' and his inability to control me just caused him to be even angrier. I was afraid he'd kill me, or in a fit of anger, that I might kill him.

The police officer suggested I change the locks while he was at work. I said that John would kick the door in. I didn't want a scene - I was in a flat, not a house, and I thought our neighbours had heard enough as it was. In the end, he picked up the phone and called him. No answer. He said he'd try again and would tell him he had 24 hours to get out. He asked if there was anyone in Brighton he could stay with, and I said, 'no, he doesn't have his own friends here. He needs to just pack a bag and get on a train and go.'

I left the station with the assurance that the officer would keep trying until he got through to him. I sat in the car and rang Mum and Dad. I told them what was going on.

'But you say this all the time, dear,' sighed Mum, 'then you change your mind.'

'I know, and I hate myself for it. This time it's final - he just threatened to break my face and smash up the flat. I think that's kind of enough. I'm at the police station now.'

When I told them that, I think they knew I meant business. Dad offered to come down to Brighton with my brother and physically remove him from my flat. I said I wanted to leave it to the police; the last thing I needed either of them getting punched in the face. This was my problem, not theirs. When I got home, and unlocked the door, wondering what was waiting for me, John was on the phone to his mum in hysterics. I felt so strange. On one hand there was this huge relief that I had finally come to a decision and executed it in the best way - by involving the police, there was no going back. I was handing the problem to someone who could sort it out in no uncertain terms. I just made a cup of tea while he screamed down the phone at his mum, and ignored it all. The wave of relief was indescribable. He came into the kitchen. I couldn't look at him.

'What have you done, Juliette?' he screamed, 'what have you done, ringing the police, telling them I hit you, why do you keep lying?'

'I didn't even say you hit me. I just told them everything else. Don't speak to me. Seriously. Pack a bag, and get out. I'm not doing this anymore. I don't care where you go, just go.'

I stirred my tea. I felt completely numb.

'I'm packing everything I've ever paid for,' he said, opening the retro pink bread bin he'd bought a couple of months before, taking the food out and hauling it into the living room.

I just wanted him to disappear. I can't even remember what happened that night, but I do know that he climbed into bed next to me and put his arms around me, crying and begging me to let him stay. I was too scared to move for fear of setting him off.

He went to work the next day, which I thought was really weird, telling me that his mum and brother were coming down to get him and all his stuff that night. It was a Friday. He collected his wages, and came home. I can't explain how I felt when he was packing his things, haphazardly throwing clothes into bin bags, picking out CDs, unplugging his PlayStation.

That night we started talking, even got a takeaway. We held hands on the sofa, and talked and talked. We were both in tears, but I was telling him that if he just went away for a few months, had some anger management therapy or something to calm him down, and maybe got his own place and grew up a bit, that I'd have him back. Looking back, I was completely insane to still be offering him another chance. I didn't want this to be the end, despite all the horror that had unfolded during the past two days.

I wanted the John I loved, the funny, daft John who made me laugh, who made me so happy so much of the time. When we weren't at each other's throats, we were great together. He was the funniest person I'd ever met. We were either crying laughing, or just crying. It was one extreme emotion after the other, and utterly exhausting.

His mum and brother arrived, completely ignoring me other than to glare in my direction as I sat in the living room with a glass of wine. I even offered them a cup of tea, but they shook their heads. They loaded up a van full of his things. I'd given him cutlery and plates and all sorts of things 'for your own place, so you've got some things already'. While he'd been busy the night before collecting everything he'd bought, and anything else he decided he would imagine he had bought, I'd been busy hiding what money I had in a shoe in the cupboard. I hid the bottle of Chanel No.5 he'd bought me two weeks before in the washing machine so he couldn't take that and the lovely Marc Jacobs shoes in the boot of my car. I then put my painkillers and Diazepam in my sock drawer so that he couldn't take a handful of them as an attention-seeking tactic. It was surreal. He demanded the Chanel 'for his mum' and I laughed. She'd stood by and watched him abuse me at her house on several occasions, and always took his side. She was in complete denial about how monstrous her son was. To her, he couldn't do any wrong, it was always my fault. She'd say, 'well, you must have done something to set him off,' as if she was addressing a child who'd upset a dog.

'I earned that,' I told them both, calmly.

I watched the van pull out of the car park and pulled the blinds. I poured another glass of wine and sat on the sofa, staring blankly at the wall. The quiet that had descended unnerved me. I let out a sob, and cried until my eyes ached. I called Mum to say that he had gone, and she simply said, 'thank god.' It was over. I felt angry, sad, relieved, terrified, lonely and empty but I also felt an amazing sense of calm.

He called me almost every day, until I asked him not to. I was trying to be supportive, and knew how hard it must have been for him to leave, but I had to be quite hard about it. He'd not told Phil he was leaving, so I had to do it the morning after he'd left. Phil was understandably furious, having got work booked for the following week.

'I'd labour for you if I could lift the plaster bucket,' I said, only half joking.

Whenever I was really down from then on, I'd email Cash. I had this fantasy that I'd head off to America and spend a week with him, eating steaks, smoking long white Menthol cigarettes (me, not him, he was a Camels man through and through) and being made a fuss of by a *real* man. I knew it was all just fantasy, but it made me happy in a little corner of my brain and heart. This time I dropped Cash an email and told him that it was finally over with John. He asked how I was doing, and if I felt happier. I said I did, although it was weird being without John. Then he gave me his number and asked me to call him.

Somehow he'd always had this hold over me, though, and clearly I had the same. I couldn't ignore it any longer. I called late one night about a week later after a couple of glasses of wine.

'Cash, it's your fantasy wife calling from England,' I stammered, nervous as hell. There was that awkward transatlantic pause on the line.

'Well, praise the good Lord!' he yelled, 'if it ain't my favourite girl in all the world!'

He was driving to a show, so he pulled over, telling me it was snowing and 'cold as hell'. I loved his accent. He had a really deep, gravelly voice. It was melting my heart there and then. We chatted for a few minutes, then I said, 'let me know if you're ever single and I'll come and see you.' He laughed, then said, 'baby, I'll write you in a coupla days. I'll have to have a think about that.' When we said goodbye, I almost said 'I love you.' It took everything not to say it, which was ridiculous. Two days later I got an email saying, 'when we hung up I wanted to say something... I don't know. More than just goodbye. I don't know what you did to me since that night I first saw you, darlin', but you've always been in my heart, and I can't stop thinkin' about you.'

'Blimey,' I thought, 'he doesn't mince his words.' He went on to say that he was single too - he'd broken up with his 'girl' a couple of months earlier but didn't tell me because he knew I was with someone. Turns out he'd actually been married, not to the one who was the mother of his child, nor the girlfriend he'd had when I first met him. 'I don't go in for tryin' to wreck someone else's relationship,' he said.

I squealed down the phone to Mum, 'how mental is that?'

'Very,' said Mum, 'but it's just a fantasy, dear. You can't actually go.'

'Why not?' I laughed, my heart going nine to the dozen.

With that I emailed him back and said if he really meant it, I'd come. I thought it was the maddest thing ever, but I didn't care. Later that week I went up to see my parents for a couple of days. I told Dad that I wanted to go and see Cash. Weirdly, I seemed to be in remission, pain-wise, and put that down to the relief of having kicked John out of my life. I decided to make the most of it.

'You're mad. You might not even like him,' he said, shaking his head and eating his roast chicken.

'No, Dad, you're mad,' I said, shaking my head, 'as if I won't! He sounds like Johnny Cash, his name actually is 'Cash', he has it tattooed on his knuckles, and he makes me laugh. He's a *musician*. He's the perfect pick-me-up,' I laughed, prodding him in the arm with my fork.

'Anyway,' I continued, 'you brought me up on rockabilly and country music, encouraged me to fall in love with Eddie Cochran and Johnny Cash and now you're trying to tell me it's no good. You can't have it both ways!'

Sadly Cash didn't live in Kentucky which is where he spent a lot of time as a kid. His grandfather grew tobacco and brewed moonshine. His mum lived in Florida. I like Florida (even if I don't like the mosquito bites). I was looking at flights to Florida online and then I remembered him talking about Detroit a couple of times. Michigan. Oh well, you can't have everything. I asked Dad if he'd lend me the flight money. Incredibly, he said yes. I think he just wanted me to get over John as quickly as possible.

How cool is my dad? Honestly, he's just as nuts as I am!

CHAPTER EIGHTEEN
'HAVE LOVE, WILL TRAVEL'
HOT BOOGIE CHILLUN

Emotionally I was all over the place, but a week later I'd got my flight to Detroit booked, and while I was exciting and nervous as hell about going out to see Cash, I spent more time wishing he lived in Miami or New York instead of the murder capital of the USA than I did anything else. My pain seemed to have lifted, despite all the stress and emotional upheaval. I knew the pain would come back, but at that moment, I felt like a new person.

Whoever invented aeroplanes should have made them faster. I know they're bulky and have lots of stuff on board, but it felt like I was on that plane for a week. I was a bundle of nerves, both excited and terrified. Three hours into the flight I started to wonder what I was doing. I'd spoken to Cash in person for 30 seconds. We'd had one quick kiss. We'd spoken on the phone twice, and here I was spending £348.00 of Dad's hard earned money to go and kiss him again. Dad had a point, it was a bit nuts. But then he gave me the money, so what can you do?

Having been on a plane for eight hours I was a bit hungry and tired when I landed. He was late. My phone didn't work in America despite me ringing up the mobile company to ask them to switch it to international the week before I'd left. A nice man who I'd sat next to on the plane bought me a coffee and a bar of chocolate. If I'd been half my age I'd have been worried; as it was, I thought it a very kind gesture. I also borrowed his phone to call Cash. He was stuck in traffic.

'Have you changed your mind?' I squeaked, terrified that I would be spending the week with the stranger who had just bought me sweets.

'No, baby, I'm just a little late is all' (there he went with that Southern drawl again. It got me every time).

'I'll see you real soon,' he said, and hung up. I went back inside the airport, which was tiny and didn't even have a place to sit down, and brushed my hair, cleaned my teeth again, put my lipstick on again, wondered whether to have hair down, plaits or a ponytail while I waited for him to arrive.

Finally, an hour late, he pulled into the kerb, leapt out of the car, engine running, scooped me up, swung me around, and gave me a huge smacker on the lips. 'I've waited three years and an hour for this!' I squealed. He had a grin the size of Oklahoma on his face. He also looked completely different to how I'd remembered him, so I stood transfixed, confused and excited all at the same time. Plus, I'd forgotten how tall he was and I do love tall even though I'm only 5ft 2in.

The week flew by, despite the fact that we did the same things almost every day. It was nothing like I had expected. For one, he didn't own cutlery. That was weird. He lived on fast food and egg mayonnaise sandwiches (there were eggs in the fridge. And mayonnaise. But that was it). What I was expecting was a trip to Lake Michigan and the zoo, for starters. Instead, to see the great outdoors I had to take a chair outside and sit in the front yard. Not garden, nor porch, but yard. The neighbours opposite were insanely obese and shouted at their dog all day. The dog was obese too. It kind of went like this for seven days:

Obese mother: 'Dammit, will you kids get in here and eat your goddamn corn meal before I whip your fat asses!'

Kids: 'We ain't comin' in 'til daddy tells us to come in, so stick your corn meal up *your* fat ass!'

Daddy: 'Your momma said git, you dirty little f*ckers, so git!'

There were good times, though. What I thought would be great was great. No need to elaborate, I'm sure, but suffice to say it was worth the £348 based on a daily rate of £49. And there were some romantic touches. He told me he loved me out of the blue during a break at one of his shows, dedicated a song to me and told everyone in the bar how far I'd come to see him (3,478 miles) and how long he'd waited for me to be there, to a round of applause. He wrote a song about me, and put it on his album. He held my hand everywhere we went and once he realised that I actually ate food, like most humans did, he managed to cook me some eggs, some more eggs, and then some eggs again. I must be the only person who goes to America for a week and loses weight rather than gains it. We drank whisky, he played his guitar, and he even bought some cutlery from the dollar store 'because I got a classy English girl now, I gotta have knives and forks, right?'

He constantly told me that I was beautiful. He looked at me in a way I don't recall anyone *ever* looking at me. He made me feel like a gazillion dollars, never mind a million dollars, despite the scars which ravage my stomach and my chest. I was pretty shocked at how he lives, and knew that if he came to stay with me (fat chance of that, he didn't have a passport) he'd probably think I was a millionaire just because there's food in my fridge, but it didn't really put me off. Living hand-to-mouth had never appealed to me, but in this instance, I think I could have lived on love and cigarettes alone.

I met his 10-year-old daughter and despite my lack of maternal instinct towards anything other than an animal, we got on great. I felt like more than a passing phase in his life, with him asking me to spend time with her. By the end of the week, he was talking about moving down to Florida where his mum lived so that I could come and live with him (Michigan is way too cold). I'd spoken to his mum on the phone (her name is Wanda Sue, how brilliant is that?) and she said she'd heard all about me for many years and would love to meet me.

'It's too damn cold in Michigan,' he said, 'we could set up in Florida. I could teach you to shoot 'gators and move the band down there.' I was astonished. Not just at the idea of setting up home (quite possibly in a trailer seeing as he had zero funds) in Florida, but at the idea that alligators needed to be shot. If they need to be shot, I reasoned, it's because they come too close to your trailer. That was something I never thought I'd need to consider when choosing a property.

Me: 'How are the neighbours?'

Real estate agent: 'Oh, you don't have neighbours.'

Me: 'How come?'

Estate agent: 'The 'gators got 'em!'

Hmm. Oh well, it seemed like a good idea at the time.

As it was, I came home, all messed up but totally into the idea of moving to Florida and becoming a step-mum. Actually, I wasn't embracing the second bit. Cash called every night for two weeks, and then I called him more than he called me. We talked about getting married and I looked into health insurance for my drug, how to obtain a visa, blah blah. This went on for a month or so, and then his calls became less frequent. I suspected that he was getting cold feet. I'd mentioned that the idea of being a full-time step-mum to a teenager whilst adjusting to living 4,000 miles away from home with a disabling condition and a man who views cutlery as a luxury item a bit daunting. I didn't say I was giving up, but after three months, his emails were more distant, hurried and casual. I was beginning to panic about what I'd do for a living, too, given that I couldn't find a job in my own country. I also hated driving in America so much that I imagined being stuck in a shack 24/7 eating eggs with my fingers. Hmm.

The week after I'd flown home from Michigan I'd bumped into Bo, a delightfully impatient, sarcastic and impossibly tiny Irish girl whom I'd met at a hair show that we had both been asked to model at earlier in the year (she had long red hair, mine was blue-black Bettie Page style). We'd hit it off straight away, and we'd said we'd meet up for a coffee sometime. Here I was, on my way to take my photos to be developed, when we saw each crossing the street in Hove. We were going in opposite directions, but neither of us was in a hurry to get anywhere, so we went for that coffee.

'What have you been up to?' she asked. I told her. She thought it was hilarious, but was also a bit afraid that I was, and I quote, 'a bit unstable in the head, there, to be honest'. After that afternoon, where neither of us could get a word in because we both talked incessantly, we saw each other all the time. We kept each other company all summer, partaking in picnics on the beach with Pantouf, me picking her up in Teddy, my lovely 1965 Triumph Herald, and going for days out. We were pretty much inseparable. We were there for each other, night and day. I'd not had friendship like this before in my adult life - it was magical.

One day, on our way back from the beach, we were talking about me disappearing to America, with me telling Bo that I might have to move to Detroit first if Cash didn't sort out going to Florida anytime soon.

'I don't fancy that,' I told her, wrinkling my nose, 'what would I do for a job in Detroit? Sell anti-freeze? Make bonfires in bins like tramps always seem to be doing in films set in Detroit?'

'You could get a job as a rapper or a murderer,' she replied, helpfully, 'or a rapist?'

We were laughing so much I thought I was going to burst. Eventually, the whole thing with Cash just stopped. I got tired of making all the effort and feeling like he didn't want me to call. Because of the time difference I had to stay up half the night to call him at 2am my time, so his phone would accept my call for free (after 7pm his time). He'd then complain because I hadn't called. It was falling apart. I wanted him to visit me; he said he couldn't come ask my dad if he could take me back to Florida to be his wife without having any money. D'oh.

What he did have he seemed to spend on cigarettes and uh, stronger cigarettes. He had no money for gas, let alone a flight. By September, things were strained, and I told him I wasn't coming out to see him. I'm glad I did. I had my fantasy, then the reality, and finally the realisation that sometimes, fantasies are much more entertaining. I still loved him - I genuinely did - but I wasn't prepared to live on Mountain Dew (it's a green soda which looks like plutonium but is probably even worse for your digestive system) and eggs for the rest of my life.

Just as well, really, because a month later I met another musician.

I was on instant messenger, chatting to my Portuguese pal Ana, a delightful little country/rockabilly singer whom I'd met at the Rockabilly Rave. We were both small and hot tempered and we got on like a house on fire. I'd tell her about my woes with Cash, she talked about her crazy cats and her long-distance relationship with another rockabilly singer from Denver who was making a big name for himself on the scene.

Ana was typing away in her apartment in Limoges, France, her two cats beside her on the sofa. Whilst moaning respectively about the trials and tribulations of being involved in extremely long-distance relationships with easy-on-the-eye musicians with no money but great clothes and bags of talent, she came up with a suggestion.

'Why don't you date my guitarist?' she said, matter-of-factly.

'Eh?' I said, 'where's that come from? We're just talking about how hard it is to have a relationship with a musician, and now you're trying to get me into trouble with another one who *still* doesn't live in the same country as me!'

'Yeah, well, Gautier's different,, he's really nice. And handsome, too.

And clever. You should date him. I did. Seriously. Get yourself away from that hillbilly fool.'

'I love the hillbilly fool, Ana. I even love his non-existent cutlery, which for argument's sake I can't love, because it doesn't exist. I'm not interested in anyone else. You'll see Cash when you do your show in New York, and then you can pick up my CD from him and post it to me. It's got songs about me on it. I think that's well cool. And anyway, there must be something wrong with Gautier if you used to date him but don't anymore. I'm not sure I want your cast-offs...'

'Gautier's great,' she said, 'He's a good guy. He'd treat you right, that's for sure. But yeah, when I see this Cash in New York I'll tell him you said hi, or maybe punch him in the face, depends how much whisky I've had and how he's treating you.'

In the meantime, Ana was to play a gig in London in two weeks' time, and kept trying to distract me from Cash with tales of how nice Gautier was. I looked at his profile on MySpace, and indeed, he looked quite handsome. But I wasn't ready to move on just yet. I'd always overlapped boyfriends and needed to get Cash well out of my system before embarking on anything more than a cup of tea with another man. And who's to say he'd give me a second - or even first - glance anyway?

October came around pretty quickly. At the gig, Ana introduced us with a big smile on her face. Gautier looked tremendously underwhelmed, and I said hello but was embarrassed because I knew she must have told him I was great just as she had told me he was. And I wasn't. I kind of nodded hello and slunk off to the bar to get myself a drink while Ana got ready to go on stage. I'd seen her play with other musicians, but suddenly my ears perked up at Gautier's guitar solos and I thought, 'he's a bit good!' That was as far as it went. The next night, they were playing in London again.

We were at the Bloomsbury Bowling Lanes, but I'd never bowled in my life. A few minutes later I had the ingenious idea of bowling myself - yes, you read that correctly - rather than bowling a ball, and I thought I would slide along the maple if my friend Bill, another singer, who was even more stupid than me, kind of slung me along the floor. He pulled me up by my jeans loops, and then did just that. Turns out I just crashed to the floor, really hurt my knee, smacked my chin on the wood and cried. According to Gautier, as I lay helpless, face down in the middle of the bowling lane, being lambasted by security for whatever I was doing (I said I wasn't really sure but it seemed like a good idea at the time), he decided, 'that's the woman for me!'

Bill then bowled himself, which consisted of him running half way down the bowling lane and launching himself, face first, at the pins. He almost had his head chopped off by the thing that comes down and swipes the pins away. The security guys were a bit annoyed by this point. I tried to rescue Bill by limping down the bowling lane and pulling him out of the head chopping thing by his ankles. Unfortunately, I didn't get much of a grip and instead, just pulled his bowling shoes off. I stood there, shoes aloft, laughing my head off whilst crying with the pain.

Gautier came over and rubbed my knee, and put his arm around me. I thought it was a bit weird, in all honesty. There I was, in jeans and a T-shirt, red-faced, with a thumping knee and pounding jaw, holding said knee with one hand and my chin in the other, tears rolling down my face while everyone tutted and ignored me for spoiling their game. I managed to move my jaw enough to talk to Gautier this time, god knows what about, but when I said I had to go (I was staying at Mum and Dad's and my friend Suzy was waving car keys in my face, a general hint that it's time to leave) he kissed me.

'You can't kiss me, you've only just met me!' I exclaimed, 'I'm all sweaty and broken and stupid, what would you want to kiss me for?' I asked, putting my coat on.

'I don't know, but you are stupid, and quite a bit mental, and you are funny,' replied Gautier, before waving me off.

I'd promised Ana I'd go to Camden the next day to meet her and Gautier, but in the end, I cried off. I couldn't walk properly, which was hardly surprising, and I wanted to curl up on the sofa and rest in front of the football and a roast dinner. Ana and Gautier flew back to France on the Monday morning, and a few days later I sent Gautier a message on MySpace *(this was before Facebook, if you can even remember such a time, reader)*, probably a load of old nonsense but he did write back. He professed a keenness for 'the girl who bowl herself like an idiot' and said if I came to Limoges to visit Ana and her cats, I'd have to let him cook me dinner one night. Ana's friend Carole, who is equally as bonkers as the rest of them, emailed me too, even though we'd never met, telling me she made her own rum out of potato peelings and toothpaste and fruit or something, and was making a new bottle in readiness for my arrival. I promised Ana I'd visit her, the cats and her two best friends very soon.

Cash had a new CD out, and I emailed him and asked him to take one to New York to pass on to Ana if they crossed paths. They did, at a bar one night, where they were both playing. Ana introduced herself and he handed her the CD. Upon her return, she posted it to me. The songs were great, and he'd hidden my favourite one - *Honky Tonk Man* - at the end, minutes after the last song, as a surprise. It made me cry. I had to get him out of my mind, which was proving impossible now that I had a DVD, three CDs, fond memories and my own songs. I didn't feel like I'd ever be able to keep away from him, even if it was just the odd late-night phone call or email. I was fighting a three and a half year addiction to a man I was convinced that in another world - one where I would count a cigarette and a coffee as a two-course meal - I would live happily ever after with, and it was harder to wean myself off him than it was dairy products.

By now Gautier and I were emailing a couple of times a week now, and I was becoming quite fond of him. Note I didn't say 'falling head over heels in love with him'. I finally felt different after the whole Cash thing had twisted me this way and that, and thought, 'I'm not falling for anyone as easy as that ever again.' Gautier had his work cut out - I really wasn't that interested, but not because I didn't like him. I still had strong feelings for Cash and was sad at how it had turned out and to be honest, I thought I could do with some time on my own after all that had happened with John.

I also had to contend with the fact that Bo had moved up to London. I missed her so much it was untrue. We spoke on the phone a lot but it wasn't the same as being around the corner from each other. It's such a shame we didn't meet years earlier; it turns out she had lived in the road behind mine when I first moved to Brighton. What are the odds of that? And how annoying is it that we'd just met and then she'd moved away? Just my bloody luck. I told her all about Gautier and she was amazed at how, well, calm I was being about it all after the Cash debacle.

I was also amazed at how grown up I was being - the old me would have jumped on a plane within five minutes of being asked and rushed headlong into something which probably would have burnt itself out within a couple of months. At Christmas, I had an email from Gautier, signed 'with millions of kisses,' and I just thought it was really sweet. He wasn't over keen, he was hugely intelligent, he didn't seem like he'd be the type to play games, and he wore his heart on his (vintage gabardine) sleeve. I liked him more and more, but it was a slow-burning effect, like a candle, rather than like my usual firework-like relationships. And I don't mean a succession of quick, noisy bangs, I mean the sparks and the pace I normally go at, before an expectant crowd (friends and family) watch it fizzle out and hit the ground with a resounding thud.

I kept promising Gautier I'd go and visit Ana and let him cook me some kind of French dish which I imagined would involve a big part of a cow, some cheese and probably quite a lot of nice wine. The fact that he could cook and speak another language (by that I mean French, not English, who cares if he can speak English? There's nothing sexy about that, but French... eek!) Plus, France was a lot nearer than Michigan, too.

In January, three months after Gautier and I had first met, I decided to give him a chance, because my heart said, 'he's genuine,' and my purse said, 'he's closest'.

But I was tired of doing all the running, and my AS was giving me terrible pain again as it was so cold, so I sat tight and told him I'd come to France soon to see Ana, and that I'd very much like to accept his offer of dinner at his place. A trip to see my friend, meet a new one (Carole with her homemade rum) and have a date? How exciting!

As it turned out, Ana went to Denver to tour in January, so I told Gautier I'd see him in February instead, when he was coming back over to England with Ana for a show. I couldn't have flown over anyway - I wasn't well enough, and could hardly walk most days with the pain. I couldn't sleep, either, and I was utterly exhausted, not only by my diseases, but due to the emotional fall out from being with John. He said he was very disappointed not to see me in January, but he understood. At this point, of course, I'd not told him I wasn't well. I think, to be honest, he was getting a bit bored. He was doing all the - albeit gentle - chasing and I was giving him nothing. Mind you, that meant I was a challenge, which can only be a good thing, right?

On the night of the gig, I'd forgotten to bring my make-up with me. Yes, really. I could picture my make-up bag on the bed where I'd put it whilst packing. I didn't even have time to pop into town and at least buy some new stuff. Suffice to say Mum doesn't wear black eyeliner or red lipstick, so I was stuffed.

In the end, Suzy, who was picking me up, brought her 12-year-old daughter's clumpy old 'dressing up' eyeliner over for me. It went on like tar. Fortunately my hair was shiny and I was wearing killer leopard print (medium height) heels. I wasn't looking my best but thought, 'Oh well, it's better if I don't, then he'll just not be interested, and then I don't have to worry about whether he likes me or not, because he won't.' Like I said, I'm well stupid.

Ana walked through the door, followed by Gautier, and my heart didn't skip one beat, it skipped about four. Gautier looked so handsome I almost choked on my drink. My stomach was in knots, and I knew I'd gone red. He barely looked in my direction, then as he approached, said hello to Suzy first, and gave me a quick 'hi' before going to the stage to sort out amps and light a cigarette and leave it dangling between his lips.

'I think I'm in love,' I said to Suzy, wringing my hands in excitement, 'look at him! He's French! He's brooding and dark and handsome and has a cigarette hanging out of his mouth while he tunes his guitar. He is also ignoring me. That's cool! I can't let that get away!' and went to the loo to splash some water on my wrists, ankles and head to calm down.

Mum and Dad walked in.

'Where's this French bloke, then?' said Dad, and I pointed at Gautier who was seeking refuge at the bar.

I went to the bar. Gautier appeared beside me. I bought him a drink and he said, 'so, do you think it would be OK if I kissed you?' and I almost had a heart attack. While the barmaid waited for me to tell her what I wanted, I pursed my lips and closed my eyes. Gautier kissed me. He squeezed my hand, gave me a big smile, grabbed his whisky and went on stage. Ana played a storming set and Gautier, I think, showed off, just a bit. I was absolutely besotted. Outside we had another kiss, then at the end, another one. Dad had to drag me to the car, but he found it amusing all the same, and had been blown away by Gautier's talent, and boy does Dad know his stuff when it comes to music. He saw Gene Vincent *and* Eddie Cochran on the same night; there's nothing you can teach him about guitar players!

Gautier took my mobile number and I said I'd meet him and Ana in London the next day as they were in London all weekend. I had to go to the passport office in Victoria as I'd realised mine was about to run out.

The next day, after a swift passport renewal, I waited for Gautier to call at Victoria station, half wanting to head home but also thinking, 'if I get on that train, he'll ring, and I'll have to come back again.' He had rung while my phone was off, but I didn't know, as he didn't leave a message. I waited an hour at Victoria station and in the process missed two trains, almost cried, got the third train back to Petts Wood, drove home and just as I walked in the front door, he rang again. D'oh!

Despite the fact that I was absolutely shattered, that my back had been pretty bad that morning, that my hip pain was growing stronger by the minute, that my tummy was still in knots, I wolfed down a sandwich and a cup of tea and went back to the station, parked the car and headed back to London. Mum said 'you must be mad! You'll make yourself ill!' and I said, 'I am mad, and I am already ill, so I don't care!'

I was more concerned about the fact that I only had one more T-shirt with me as I'd been planning on going home on Saturday afternoon. This was not the weekend to have packed a sandwich bag's worth of clothes and no make-up. Gah!

We met in a dirty old pub called The Elephant's Head in Camden. Gautier was sitting with Ana and some friends of theirs of varying nationalities. He looked really, really pleased to see me (I had bought an eyeliner and lipstick at Victoria station and applied both in the public toilets). Ana gave me a wink and said, 'ha ha, I knew you'd come!' and I squeezed on to the bench beside Gautier. My back was hurting so much by now, but I didn't want Gautier or Ana to see how much pain I was in.

I'd driven to the station and had to drive home again, so I had a one gin and tonic and a couple of soda waters with them and must admit that I was very glad I'd bothered to come, despite both Ana and Gautier telling me how I should be 'drinking properly'. Gautier was charming, handsome and everything Ana had promised. I just felt really comfortable with him, if you can be comfortable with AS on a wooden chair for three hours (in short, no).

I left at 11.00pm to get the train back. Gautier walked me to the tube station. Then to the platform. Then almost on to the tube itself. We kissed goodbye and he asked me to come to London again the next day to see him. I hadn't planned to see him other than at the gig on the Friday night, so not only was I unprepared with clothes and make-up, I wasn't prepared for the energy this was sucking out of me, too. I was feeling pretty rough by now - I'd been on my painkillers since Friday evening and I was so exhausted with driving to Mum's, the gig on Friday, then London twice already that day, and couldn't face another trip to London tomorrow, even if I was smitten with Gautier. I just wanted to go home after Mum's roast beef dinner. Tottenham were playing in the FA Cup that afternoon and it was on Sky, and I'd planned a long lie-in, a hot bath and to sit in front of the football before mustering up the energy to drive home.

I said I'd think about it. He said, 'if you don't come tomorrow, I will be really disappointed and I will think you don't really care.'

The train doors shut, and I shouted, 'What are you, *a girl?*'

I missed Bo like hell, so I'd invited her to come to dinner at Mum and Dad's that Sunday - I had really wanted them to meet her - and I'd warned her that I'd be watching the football, so she either had to go home before it, at half-time, or when it had finished. Bo told me she thought I should go up to London again if I felt up to it.

'It sounds like you really like Gautier,' she said, 'and you can rest all you like tomorrow. Why don't you go, just for a while?' Mum was shaking her head, but Bo was right. I was all for seizing the moment, even if I did feel terrible.

I texted Ana, telling her I'd meet her and Gautier at the same pub as last night, at 7pm. I drove Bo to the station at half-time, quicker than I've ever driven anywhere in my life. I came home, watched the second half, and then drove back to the station the second the final whistle went. I caught the train to Victoria then the tube to Camden. I was almost in tears at the pain, but I just took more painkillers and decided to deal with it tomorrow. Gautier and I talked for three hours about how weird this was but that we really wanted to see each other again. At one point he was crouching on the floor in front of me, holding me around the hips, telling me he wished I didn't have to go home, and asking if I could come to France next week to see him. I couldn't afford to go to France. The flight would only have been about £45 but the train fare to Stansted from Brighton was £30, and I couldn't turn up with no money and expect cheese and wine and steak for free. I was also conscious of trying to take things slowly for once, not to rush in headfirst again.

I was still thinking about Cash, still dealing with the break-up with John; emotionally I really wasn't entirely sure I was ready for another relationship. Then again, I think I knew that this one was going to be different - a lot different. I told Gautier I would think about it. His response was: 'OK, I'll come back to England and see you. I waited too long already, so I'm not going to let you escape now.'

A few days later Gautier announced that he'd booked himself a flight and would be over two weeks later. I was glad I had a time to prepare for that; I was in so much pain after rushing around that weekend that I thought I'd never feel better. I'd pushed myself way too far and now my body was making sure I knew what an idiot I'd been.

On the day he arrived I was so nervous when I went to meet him at Blackfriars station that I thought I might faint. I was in my '50s leopard print coat, had put on a bit more make-up than usual and had just dyed my hair a fresh blue-black. I was as ready as I'd ever be. My heart was pounding as I looked for him. He came through the ticket barriers, took a cigarette out of the packet, a lighter out of the pocket of his leather jacket, put it between his lips and looked around for me. I waved at him, jumping up and down on the spot. He dutifully removed the unlit cigarette from his mouth and gave me a kiss. He was so handsome I did a little dance and made a 'yowzers!' face at the bemused ticket inspector when Gautier had his back turned.

We got the train back to Brighton, and pretty much fell in love immediately. We went to a rockabilly club in North London on the Saturday night - I really made sure I showed him off even though I couldn't dance, couldn't sit without wincing and generally felt terrible - and walked along the seafront and had coffee in the park during the day. As we lay in bed on the second morning, I told him I had something to tell him. He looked a bit worried.

'Don't panic,' I said, 'I haven't got a husband in the SAS who's on his way home. I need to tell you something important. Now. Before anything else happens.'

I then explained how I couldn't have children. Not only because my AS caused me such pain on a daily basis, but because I couldn't lift anything (like, you know, an actual baby), barely slept as it was, and that I wasn't to get pregnant whilst on Enbrel, but that I couldn't manage without it. Oh yeah, and that I'd had so much surgery to my insides that the idea of growing a human in there was too much to bear for my brain, let alone my body. I told him a little bit about how my AS affected me and didn't allow me to do the things I wanted to do. I needed to know before I fell completely head over heels that this wouldn't be a deal breaker. He gave me a hug and smiled.

'I really don't mind,' he said, 'I don't like kids much. They are too noisy. As for your back, I will look after you.' I'm not quite sure he had any idea what I was talking about, but at the same time, I didn't really want to say, 'I'm a bit disabled' and him run a mile.

He flew home on the Tuesday and I cried at the station. It was the beginning of March, and two weeks later was his 30th birthday.

'Check your inbox,' he wrote in an email a week later, 'I bought myself a present.' There was a ticket to Limoges in my name. Mental!

I arrived in France to cobbled streets and wobbly, ancient buildings, met up with Ana and Carole, had my slices of cow and hunks of cheese (delicious) and Carole's homemade mint rum (questionable) and met the cats at Ana's (delightful). I got quite drunk and convinced myself that I was speaking French all night. Ana described it as 'obviously just bullshit', but gave me full marks for trying. Trust my luck to get a man whose ex-girlfriend is not only slimmer and prettier than me, but can speak about 3948 languages and sing like a lark. Oh well, I can do piranhas-eating-people-in-a-river impressions; we all have our talents.

I absolutely, unquestionably knew that he was 'the one' as we walked down the cobbled street, huddled together under an umbrella. It was snowing, despite it being 80 degrees when I had arrived a few days before. I just glanced at him in his leather jacket, cigarette between his lips, and thought, 'blimey, he's lovely' and that was that. He's a quietly determined chap and doesn't talk much (that's putting it mildly) but I blame the Russian blood from his father's side. With my dad's dad being Ukranian - and Jewish - and passing on those stern, silent and brooding genes, I was used to the Eastern European side of things. My brother and my dad are both very much like that, whereas I'm more like my mum's dad, outspoken and emotional, stubborn as hell and with a quick temper. The French are brusque and brooding by nature, the Russians cold hearted and somewhat emotionally stunted. Gautier's a quiet little fish, living in his own world (Pisces) and I'm a roaring lion (Leo) who whilst generous, thoughtful and creative (true!) am also loud, bossy and opinionated. Except that Gautier was on the cusp of Aries, too, so that made him strong and stubborn as well. I knew he'd keep me on my toes.

I was so impressed by his ability to knock up perfect, buttery fried eggs that he convinced me to stay a few more days. He also took Pantouf to the patisserie one morning (snuggled inside his leather jacket) and came back with just about every pastry known to man 'so you can choose what you want, and Pantouf can choose what he wants'. If that's not endearing, I don't know what is.

I re-booked a return ticket, and joined him and Ana on a trip to Paris for two shows they had booked that weekend. I quickly washed my clothes as once again I'd only brought the bare minimum as hand luggage, so it was hard enough as it was for four days when you're trying to impress the love of your life. I borrowed a jumper, some socks, pyjamas and a jacket from Ana, and off we went.

It wasn't quite what I had in mind when I thought of a trip to Paris. The gig was not underneath the Eiffel Tower but in an illegal bar underneath a multi-storey car park. We drank neat whisky (I was too embarrassed to ask for Coke) to warm ourselves up, and by the time Ana got on stage she had forgotten most of the words to her songs. I mouthed them for her, Gautier hit her on the head with his guitar neck, and all in all, it was pretty entertaining.

At around 4am Gautier flopped down on a sofa next to me, with Ana passed out on the other side under a pile of people's coats, her '50s Western boots poking out from someone's jacket like the wicked witch's ruby slippers under Dorothy's house.

'I really fink I will marry you,' said Gautier, slurring slightly whilst lugging on a Lucky Strike and blowing smoke in the air, 'and I think not in too long,' he said, looking at me. Probably looking at three of me given the amount of whisky we'd been putting away.

He stared at me for a moment, then sort of slid off the sofa and got down on one knee, put two straw boaters on his head (we'd found them in the kitchen earlier and decided to wear one each for the rest of the night, so he borrowed mine), threw his hands in the air and said, 'Juliette, blah blah blah ma femme? (at least that's what I thought I heard).

There was a pause as I looked confused.

'Eh?' I said, not sure I'd heard him correctly.

'Do you want to be my wife?!' he shouted over the music, holding on to his hats with one hand and my right knee with the other. He toppled backwards, composed himself, took another drag on his cigarette and looked half expectantly at me and half drunkenly somewhere else. I said, 'I can do that!' and with that we were taken off into the night on a three hour car journey with a woman who had spent the entire gig in the corner of the bar chewing on the ends of her hair.

She lived in a trailer in the middle of nowhere. Her husband, apparently, was in a high security jail down the road.

'Oh good!' I exclaimed.

She insisted on us having her bed (I said I'd really rather not) as she would be visiting her husband for the next few hours anyway, and didn't need to sleep. We stood in the bedroom in the trailer and Gautier pulled me to him.

'See? You can have a very glamorous life with me,' he laughed. There were huge dog biscuits in the bed and scary porn DVDs in amongst Disney classics. I was wearing his ex-girlfriend's pyjamas. This was, I can safely say, the weirdest night of my life. We huddled together, dog biscuits between our toes and I thought, 'blimey, I've finally met someone as weird as me.'

CHAPTER NINETEEN
'GOT THE FEELING'
RUBY ANN

I told Mum over the phone when I came home from France that we were getting married. I think she thought, 'here we go again,' my having said 'I'm getting married!' exactly 12 months before. At the same time, I think she also knew that this was different to my usual mental ideas, and that at least France wasn't as far away as America. I think the fact that Gautier could cook, get out of a chair, had paid for my flight ticket and also owned cutlery helped her collect her thoughts. She was delighted - I think - and we decided not to tell Dad at that moment. Instead we arranged that they'd come down for lunch in Brighton a few days later. I was going to go in for some elaborate prank but in the end just said, 'Dad, guess what? I'm only going to get married, how funny is that?' to which he said, 'blimey!' after a 10-second silent shock reaction and gave me a hug, spilling a little wine in the process.

He hesitated, looked at Mum, then back at me and said, 'hang on a minute, to Gautier? Because I never know with you, you change your mind so quickly it could be Cash or someone else we've never even heard about!'

'Dad!' I yelled, 'of course it's to Gautier. How mental is that?' I laughed, clinking glasses. He looked really, really happy.

'We'd better meet him properly then, rather than just stand looking at him playing guitar.'

Gautier came back to Brighton three weeks later. I drove us up to Mum and Dad's on the Friday evening. Gautier was pretty nervous, but probably not as nervous as I was. I'd brought home every single boyfriend I'd ever had over the years - some good, some terrible - but this was the one that mattered. I was going to marry this one. In fact, he'd never even been my boyfriend. He pretty much went straight into being my fiancé. How mad is that?

So it was with some surprise that we arrived to find the house infested with wasps. A nest had been disturbed in the roof and they'd got through the wall in my bedroom and were buzzing around the entire house. Dad had called pest control ('for me?' I quipped) and Mum was busy putting the kettle on whilst saying, 'can you believe we're infested with wasps when we're meeting your fiancé for the first time!'

Gautier thought it was hilarious. Pest control managed to smoke the wasps out, and save for one or two buzzing around our heads that night, we were unfazed. Dad took us to dinner at a local gastro pub and we all had steak. I knew Gautier would be happy with that. That night he mumbled something to Dad about permission to marry me and Dad threw out his arms and said, 'at last, please, take her!'

Gautier's mum was very keen to meet me; subsequently I was hideously nervous because I couldn't speak French. I flew to Limoges to stay with Gautier and on the Saturday morning we took the train to a little town two hours north east of Limoges. It was early May, and the weather was glorious. His mum and her partner, Christophe, met us at the station. I think I said 'hello!' instead of 'bonjour', purely out of nerves and felt like a right idiot.

His mum was tiny and you could tell she was French by the way she was dressed. French women just look effortlessly chic. She had a warm smile and was clearly very happy to see Gautier. My nerves soon disappeared. And then came back the moment I saw their house - it was more like a castle. We sat in the impressive garden eating our way through sourdough bread, cheese, strawberries and little fancy pastries (and a few painkillers for me) all washed all down with pots of coffee and Evian, under the shade of a weeping willow. I was in some pain, but it wasn't too bad. Gautier smiled at me, took my hand under the table, and gave it a little squeeze, which all at once said everything to me - 'you're doing OK. I love you. They like you'.

At that moment I felt utterly at peace for the first time in years. I wanted to remember that moment forever. Little old me, in France, eating pastries with my soon-to-be-husband. A French husband. Seriously, how did that happen? I couldn't help but feel that after the two years I went through with John, I'd earned it. What a contrast.

I didn't have much idea of what was going on but Christophe spoke very good English and with Gautier being pretty much fluent, we got by with various bits of conversations being translated either for me or for Monique. She was a superb host and made me feel very welcome. I wanted her to adore me. I was taking her son away to another country, and I couldn't imagine how she must have felt. It wasn't as though he has brothers or sisters; he's an only child and I knew she doted on him.

After lunch I promptly fell asleep on the sofa in the living room while everyone else was clearing up. I may have even dribbled on a cushion. We went for a nice meal that evening, and I even wore ballet pumps instead of Converse with my jeans (how French!) but I got blisters within two minutes of leaving the house (how English!). Gautier and I watched Indiana Jones movies in their cinema room (I kid you not) on the top floor of their house and we awoke on Sunday morning to the smell of chocolate cake that Christophe had just baked. I ate my own bodyweight in extremely rich but lovely food and smiled a lot. I'm sure if I could have spoken fluent French Monique and I would have got on like a house on fire, but it was more a thumbs up, inane grin and appreciative noises kind of weekend. The house was incredible; full of original features like stone floors, beautiful mosaic tiles and great, high ceilings. Sash windows and shutters with billowing sheer white curtains completed the look. It was beautiful.

Between June and July, Gautier spent half his time in France and half of it in Brighton. We were both a bit worried about what he'd do for a living, particularly given that I had barely any work coming in. Two of the travel magazines I wrote features for had closed down. I couldn't afford to pay for both of us to get by, and increasingly, the worry gave way to stress. I was planning the wedding and half the time he wasn't even the same country as me. I didn't know what dress I wanted, where we should be married, how to even go about getting married and by July, whether we should even *be* getting married. I was panicking about everything. I didn't even really know him, yet I was willing to commit to spending the rest of my life with him? He'd insisted on getting married that year, whereas I thought it more sensible to wait until the next year.

We began pulling apart, and I told him I wasn't sure we should do it. 'I want to,' he said, giving me a hug, 'I love you. But it's not going to be easy. I don't have a job, you don't speak my language, I have to leave all my friends and family in Limoges... it's hard. It's going to be really hard.'

That's what I mean,' I said, 'and if it turns out that it's a big mistake, and you miss France, and your family, and your friends, I'll feel like I've failed you. I wouldn't leave a country with all those cheeses and really good bread for England. I think it's too much for me to live up to. I don't know if I can make you happy. You might regret this forever.'

I was in tears, but it needed to be said. He insisted that we'd be OK, and gave me a kiss. I felt as though I'd spent my entire life making enormous impulse decisions - sometimes really stupid ones - and didn't want this to be something I'd end up regretting. On the other hand, I couldn't imagine my life without him.

He made me a cup of tea.

'We'll be fine,' he said, lighting a cigarette and leaning out of the kitchen window, 'we will. I love you, monkey. Please don't worry.'

Don't worry? Was he kidding?

I continued to worry, but I continued to plan. Gautier went back to France for the month of August. He had designed our invitations - black card with a tattoo style heart and banner with our names in and I was busy trying to find the right venue. I plumped for the Royal Pavilion, as I'd never wanted a church wedding. I didn't like being in church. It was cold, for a start, and I wasn't really big on religion. In retrospect, it would have saved a lot of money, but I couldn't be a hypocrite. I only prayed when I was watching important football matches and I didn't want to pretend otherwise. I didn't *not* believe in God per se, but I thought he'd see it as a bit of a piss take if I turned up at his house asking for his blessing.

The Pavilion would be perfect. It was an amazing building steeped in history and would make for some great photos. I booked it for Sunday 23rd September as spring, summer and autumn Saturdays were booked for the next two years. I was going for midnight blue silk taffeta for my dress, a just below the knee, full skirted 1950s style creation made by a local dressmaker (I had wanted to buy vintage from eBay but Mum had insisted on paying for me to have one made. To this day I still wish I'd bought an original '50s dress as it'd have been around a third of the price) and inspired by a picture I'd seen of Dita Von Teese at some fancy awards do, impossibly high heeled red suede shoes with pom-pom flowers on the toe and red roses for my bouquet. I'd bought the shoes in the January sales for £15 and hadn't yet worn them. It was all built around the red shoes (I have a fixation with Dorothy's ruby slippers from *The Wizard of Oz*). Gautier would wear an off-white suit with blue silk shirt. The red, white and blue theme, I thought, was pretty apt for the joining together of a Frenchman and his English bride.

On the morning of the wedding I woke in quite a bit of pain. Actually, a lot. That wasn't good. I think it was down to all the running around I'd been doing and all the stress of worrying about what everyone else was doing. I had some breakfast and a couple of painkillers, then a hot bath. Charlie had stayed that night, and was gathering her things so that she could get ready at the hotel. Gautier was his usual laid-back self. I threw some things into an overnight bag, and drove the three of us down to the seafront. I dropped him off at the hotel - both his mum and Christophe and my family were already booked in - and I drove to the hairdressers with Charlie. Only I would drive on my own wedding day. I mean, come on. I could have got a cab but no, that would have been too easy!

I'd been so afraid that getting married was the wrong thing to do that I'd not enjoyed the process of getting ready for it at all. I hadn't spoilt myself one little bit, so conscious was I that this was Dad's money and I didn't want to waste it. He'd insisted I spend some on some nice treats, but I never got around to it. I just didn't feel like I deserved it. I don't know why, but I've always felt like that. I punish myself constantly. I think it was because I wasn't working. If I don't work, I don't deserve anything. I have to earn something. It's just how it is. Despite it not being my fault that I wasn't earning, despite my body already punishing me enough, I still managed to punish myself further, make myself feel worse, rather than better. Where this sense of worthlessness comes from I have no idea. Mum went bananas when I told her I'd not booked myself in for anything. No manicure, not even a massage. It's actually really depressing me to write this, to admit how weird I was about all that. As if I didn't deserve to have my nails done. Honestly.

I picked the first hairdresser who said they'd open on a Sunday, and spent half an hour deciding how to have my hair. My friends could have done a better job between them. He was hopeless. By the time Charlie and I had reached the hotel, the back of my hair was coming loose. I'd asked him to pin it to one side so it draped over one shoulder, Cinderella style. He'd just sprayed it with hairspray instead. It was so windy, despite the temperature that it was a mess by the time we'd got to the room. Bo met us at the hotel - she'd come down from London that morning - and did a great job of phoning around to see if everyone was OK.

The table arrangements were wrong, so instead of painting my nails and getting dressed in my room, I was downstairs in the restaurant moving name cards around. It was so stressful it was untrue. I hadn't even done my make-up, or got changed. I had an hour to do everything. Bo offered to paint my nails but my hands were shaking so much I declined. There were so many people in the room that I felt suffocated.

At one point, I was in there with Bo, Charlie (who was in and out of the bathroom getting herself ready), Toby, my photographer friend, Phil and Cherry who'd come to drop off 'something borrowed' (Cherry's garter from her wedding), my parents who were bringing the box of things to decorate the restaurant with for the evening reception, and my friend Kate, who was also changing her outfit and dragging a huge suitcase around with her as she was off to Kenya on a press trip right after the wedding! I couldn't find my bra, even though I knew I'd packed it and, can you believe, hadn't tried my dress on since I'd brought it home two weeks before. It was utter chaos.

I really felt as though my life was spiraling out of control as I was tipping everything out of my bag trying to find my bloody bra. The idea of marrying a man I barely knew didn't just worry me, it utterly terrified me. Now, it makes me really sad that I didn't have any excitement before the big day, just worry. If I could go back in time, I'd go back to that summer, knowing what I know now, that Gautier was right and we would be OK, and enjoy it. It breaks my heart that I had such a hard time of it.

The ceremony was hilarious - the registrar marrying us was named Trevor Love, and as he said, 'We are gathered here today to witness the marriage of Juliette and Gautier,' I let out an almighty squeak, like this, 'Eeeeeeeeeeek!' because I was so nervous. It broke the ice, and I'd always said I hated the idea of a stony silence during my wedding anyway, but Mum looked like she was going to smack me! I finally feel at peace, if a little nervous, and when I looked at Gautier, I knew it was the right decision and all my worries went out the window.

We had a lively ceremony. There were claps and cheers - I could easily have typed that wrong, as 'jeers' - I giggled incessantly, grinned inanely, waved my hands about a lot and pulled silly faces unintentionally. I got the giggles when I put the ring on Gautier's finger, and he looked so terrified at that point that I just wanted to stop everything and take him outside and give him a cigarette. I don't think he understood half of it and he was so nervous about repeating his vows that his hands were shaking.

We drank Pimm's at the reception, but I'd forgotten to give my MP3 player to the hotel staff and hadn't noticed that we were missing the 1930s Parisian jazz which Gautier had spent an entire afternoon downloading until half way through dinner. It was at that point that I regretted not asking Cherry or Bo – or both - to be my maids of honour. Again, without delegating anything, it's no wonder I forgot bras and music. The food was great, and all in all it was a wonderful day. Dad's speech was fantastic, as was Jonathan's. Dad's had a bit of sadness to it when he touched briefly on how ill I had been and how he and Mum at one point never thought they'd see me again, never mind see me get married. Jonathan's speech was worthy of an Oscar; he finished by saying how proud he was of his brave, inspirational sister. I had no idea he thought that. He's never said that. He never really says anything unless it's about football. It meant the world to me. I suddenly saw him as a man, not a boy, too. He'd got a good job, was saving up for a flat, and here I was, becoming a Mrs. I shed a little tear, and held Mum's hand on one side, my husband's on the other. My husband! I couldn't believe I was saying it.

We had the best rockabilly DJs in the entire country doing the music for the evening reception that was held at a glass-fronted restaurant on the beach. Of course, it poured with rain the minute we arrived so nobody even saw the beach. I ended the night with a dance with Dad to his favourite Gene Vincent track. On the buffet table were two chocolate caterpillar cakes. Mum thought I was an idiot; I said, 'I'm having chocolate caterpillar cakes if it's the last thing I do!'

After the wedding, Gautier went back to France for a few days to collect some more of his things. We didn't have a honeymoon, didn't even go out for dinner. We couldn't afford to and I refused Dad's offer of a little money so that we could do the latter. I'm an idiot; it would have been nice to have celebrated at The Grand Hotel with a seafood platter and some cocktails. Instead, we got a cat.

She was the last one left in a litter of seven, and sometimes I can see why nobody had chosen her. She's mental. She eats the dishcloth, eats plastic, eats rubber bands, hides in the bath, scratches every bit of carpet apart from the bit on her scratching post and is partial to broccoli, spinach and homemade banana muffins. We called her Squeaky, because she squeaked. As we lived two floors up, I bought her a little lead and took her for walks outside. We took her to Mum and Dad's house at

Christmas when she was just a few months old and she had a lovely time, her little tummy full of turkey and salmon. She had great fun exploring their huge garden and I made sure she had a few days up there each month so she could have adventures and some exercise. In the flat, I played with her two or three times a day, both of us chasing bits of paper up and down the hallway. Gautier and I were planning on moving soon anyway; the block we lived in was getting noisier and noisier. We were surrounded by teenage mums with screaming kids, insanely noisy Chinese students packed 10 to a flat, and below us, a woman who had a baby and a toddler and penchant for drum and bass music as well as a never ending stream of tracksuit-clad male visitors who all seemed to provoke her into screaming obscenities at them for hours on end. I was heading for a nervous breakdown.

Spring 2008

I'm standing half way up the Eiffel Tower with Gautier, the song 'Bye Bye Paris' by The Ray Collins Hot Club running through my head. I don't want to leave. Monique and Christophe have brought us here for a couple of days. They are brilliant. The wind is blowing ferociously, and Gautier is telling me to hold on tight to Pantouf. I block out the whining American voices of the other tourists, some of whom are so large I worry that the Eiffel Tower will soon resemble the leaning one of Pisa. The view is breathtaking, and I'm so excited I start yapping away like a small dog.

'It's well brilliant, I didn't think it'd be this brilliant, it's brilliant.' Another moment of contentment - I seemed to have them in France more than I did in England. No surprise there - I am absolved of responsibility. I barely have to think, never mind do.

Once home, the pain kicks in again. I am taking dihydrocodeine and anti-nausea tablets some days, codeine and Diazepam on others. I don't have the strength to do this anymore. I can barely move. Gautier helps me into bed and out of it. He helps me get dressed. He had found part-time work at a French-speaking company testing games for phones, so he was working three days a week. The money was terrible but at least it was something. Two weeks later my rheumatologist tells me that if I get a relapse as bad as the one I'd just had, I'd need to come in for a steroid injection. I shake my head. He looks exasperated.

'I'm not having that stuff in my body again,' I explain.

'But it will reduce the inflammation and get you through it,' he says, clicking his pen in and out as the nurse makes notes behind me.

'It might, but I'd rather take painkillers and just not do anything than have steroids again. Honestly. I just wanted to know whether any other patients on Etanercept have had this problem. Has anyone else said that it seems to have worn off?'

He looks blankly at me, and shrugged.

'Is that a yes, or a no?' I ask, leaning forward in my chair, trying to get comfortable.

'We'll try you on something else if this doesn't get better,' he says. 'Come back in...'

I cut him off.

'Six months, I know.'

I was still awake at 3am. Again. Had the drug stopped working, or had I stopped working? Was I becoming immune to it, or was the disease getting worse, and finding a way through the drug? At 7am, I gave up trying to sleep and hauled myself out of bed, trying not to scream out in pain and wake Gautier. I ran a bath. Once the heat had found its way through to my bones, I got out, got dressed and had loosened up enough to bend down and grab Squeaky's bowl, lean into the cupboard to get her food, and feed her. Despite it being possible, it was still an effort, and every movement hurt. She's so rubbish she doesn't even cuddle me or sit on my lap in return for me waiting on her hand and foot. I woke Gautier with a coffee and he told me I looked tired.

'I am tired,' I said, rubbing my eyes, wondering how my wrinkle-decrease eye cream had a hope in hell of working. Being in constant pain is exhausting. Not sleeping, on top of that, is unbearable.

Something needed to change, but what?

'I can't cope with this,' I'd say to Mum, 'sometimes I wish I could just come home and go to bed forever, but I'm married now. There isn't just me to think about. I've got a husband, and a stupid cat.'

My emotions were all over the place. I was sad, I was angry, I was frustrated at being held back, because I'd never known what it was like not to take risks, take on challenges and succeed. My dad never fulfilled his potential, and I saw how the frustration of being forced out of the army hung on his shoulders. I wanted to seize every opportunity which came my way, and create those which didn't. Yet there we were, both with our careers on track when we were young - him in the Royal Electrical & Mechanical Engineers in the army, me as a sports journalist. Within a few years of us doing what we'd always wanted to do, our dreams were cut short. It was uncanny.

When I was 18 and working at the advertising agency in London, I remember filling in a performance-related form sent down by our head of department. I got called into her office because she found it amusing that I had awarded myself more 10 out of 10's than any other secretary. I pointed out that I also gave myself 0 out of 10 for remembering to pass on messages, 1 out of 10 for my appearance (I was always, without fail, in jeans or leggings and Doc Marten boots) and only 1 out of 10 for getting in on time, and she conceded that it balanced itself out.

I've always seen everything in black and white; I was up or I was down, things were brilliant or terrible; I loved something or someone or I hated it, or them. There was no in between. Right now, I was definitely down. I think I had been for a long time, but it had finally come to a head after the wedding. The question was: would I ever get back up?

CHAPTER TWENTY
'THE GIRL CAN'T DANCE'
BUNKER HILL

Spring 2009

For the last six months, Gautier has been working in a new job, with Disney. No, he's not dressing up as Mickey Mouse; he's working in their computer games division in Brighton. He goes to Canada for a month's training; of course, it coincides with our first anniversary - just our luck. I miss him like hell, but at last he has a decent job with a decent wage and we feel we've actually got a chance at some kind of future.

I make a decision that we must move. The noise from the flats surrounding ours was becoming unbearable; I couldn't stand it any longer. We sold the flat and bought house in the Brighton suburbs, moving in on my birthday in July. Gautier's dad, Victor, comes over to work on the house (we communicate in thumbs-up gestures and cups of coffee - me to him). We fill it with Mid-Century furniture from eBay (cheaper than buying new furniture, which is crazy), elaborate vintage-style wallpaper and dark wooden floors - it reflects our mutual love of the 1950s and 1960s.

That summer, Charlie has a baby girl. I'd been trying to get her on the phone for months, but she never returned my calls. I was going to visit her a couple of weeks after the birth, but I didn't feel as though she wanted to see me. I called, but never heard back. After a few months of trying, I gave up, wondering what I'd done wrong. Eventually she emailed to say that she felt our friendship had been one-sided because I'd never visited her in Southend. That was true, but she didn't have a spare bedroom and Southend by train or car was a long trip from Brighton. I was in such bad pain so often I didn't do any long journeys. Having bowel disease also meant I was wary of getting caught out on the motorway needing the loo and being miles from a service station. Even just sitting in the car for more than an hour made my back go into a pain flare-up. If I'd woken up at her flat suddenly unable to walk I'd have no way of getting back home as she didn't drive. All in all, I much preferred to have my friends visit me than me visit them. I would have thought that was obvious to my best friend of all people.

Charlie also said she felt she couldn't talk to me about her pregnancy or her baby because of my 'hatred of children.' Wow. I emailed her back, told her what I thought of that, had a massive cry and thought, 'well, that's me told.' I didn't try to get in touch again.

Still reeling from the shock of losing my best friend, Squeaky went missing. Gautier and I had been in town and she wasn't in when we arrived home at 11.00pm. It was freezing out - the first spell of ice and bitter cold. I was worried sick. Gautier and I looked for her, but it was pitch dark. She could have been anywhere. We went to bed at 2am, and to this day I'll always regret not sleeping downstairs. We both went to sleep and at 7am Gautier went downstairs to find her curled up under the sofa on the wooden floor, shivering. He went to stroke her and she howled.

She had either fallen off a roof (she was always up high, in trees or up on neighbours' roofs) or been hit by a car, or a bus. She had obviously tried to get up the stairs; there were traces of blood on the bottom step. She must have been trying to get home all night. It was utterly heartbreaking. The vet told us she'd broken her pelvis, and she had deep cuts to the backs of her legs. I was in floods of tears. She was bandaged and sent off for an X-Ray. Luckily the vet is two doors down from us, so I was able to pop in and see her a few times over the five days she was in. When we collected her she had to go in a huge crate; she couldn't walk or stand so Gautier and Victor made her a special platform with a sunken litter tray, so she didn't have to balance on it. We slept downstairs with her for three nights, administering painkillers and keeping her warm with a hot water bottle and blankets on the cage.

Mum and Dad came down for Christmas Day, after which we took Squeaky to their house a few days later so that we could go to France to see Gautier's mum and Christophe! It wasn't easy transporting a fragile cat in a two-seater car. I had a pink Nissan Figaro by this time that was great for summer but awful in winter. Ice melted through the roof, the heater didn't work, there was no rear wiper and I could barely see a thing out of the frozen, tiny windows. We were going to cancel our trip but we'd already paid for the Eurostar tickets and I knew Squeaky would be in safe hands at her grandparents, so we decided to go.

Mum sent regular text updates on Squeaky's progress ('she's had some prawns and stood up today!) we had a lovely break in France. Monique and Christophe serve a five-course, Michelin-star worthy dinner. Chomping on scallops and caviar (I like scallops, I don't like fish eggs) then wood pigeon, I'm thinking how much I wish I had faith that things would be better this year; that I'd just get a break from pain, a break with some work, anything. For me, so little has changed over the past year. Everyone else's lives get richer and more fulfilling while mine goes in the opposite direction. Their world opens up as mine closes. Their careers take off, they have children, and essentially they have purpose. My life is a black and white, silent movie; theirs is a glorious 3D Technicolor blockbuster. It's like being a mannequin trapped in a window display; I see life pass me by while I'm stuck in the same position, day after day, week after week, year after year. I feel almost as left behind as I did when I was in hospital, except then I had things to look forward to when I got better. The problem is I didn't *get* better.

When we returned from France in a blizzard, we should have stayed at Mum and Dad's. Instead we made the decision to go home during a brief snow gap, and set off with Squeaky and her cage folded in the back for home. The journey was so perilous I don't know how we did it. We were sliding all over the motorway, Gautier holding firm onto Squeaky's box and me screaming that I 'couldn't see shit'.

We pulled up outside the house in a foot of snow; the car was pretty much sideways in the road but there was nothing I could do about it. When we opened the front door we were met with the coldest rush of air imaginable. I think you know what's coming next: the pipes had frozen. Seriously. I hadn't set the heating high enough and despite giving the neighbour a key 'in case of anything, just go in' he hadn't thought to check up on that (which I would have done had we had their key). The house had just frozen whilst we were in France. The boiler was broken. Nobody could come out because the snow was too heavy and the roads, where we were, just beside the South Downs, were too icy.

We spent 48 hours wrapped in blankets, wearing everything we could. We had a lousy fan heater that pumped out dusty hot air. With no hot water we couldn't shower or do much of anything. Squeaky was still recovering from her accident; we made sure she was warm with two hot water bottles, all the towels we could find and blankets draped over the cage. It was awful. We didn't know our neighbours well enough to seek refuge and couldn't drive to anyone else's place because the roads were black with ice. I was on the verge of asking the police to come out in a land rover and take us to a hotel. You can imagine how bad my pain was at this point. We had no food, either, because we'd been away for a week. We found a few things in the corner shop but my God, that was rough. Eventually an engineer came out and fixed the boiler. I think I said 'I wish we'd stayed at Mum's where it was warm and full of food!' around 4857 times.

Spring 2010

Gautier and I plod on, as ever. I finally get some proper work with a PR agency, working on two fashion accounts. I'm working two days a week, from home, and really enjoying it. I'm so excited as it's something completely new to me; I feel challenged for the first time in years. Unfortunately one of the clients appears to be mentally ill and keeps falling out with me and the director of the agency. In the end she refuses to pay for the work I've done. Turns out she'd not paid them for the past three months; you've got to wonder why they were still working on her account, but there you go. It all ended rather nastily and I was out of a job a few months later through no fault of my own. The other client was lovely and I managed to get them featured in glossy fashion magazine

Grazia several times - and that's no mean feat for an independent fashion label - but as their sales grew, they sacked the agency I was working for and hired a much more expensive agency who'd come in on the back of the press I'd got them and snatched them from under my nose! No matter what I did and how hard I worked, nothing *ever* seemed to go my way, and we were back to square one.

In September Monique and Christophe treated us to a week at a rented house in Provence. I was blown away by how pretty and peaceful it was. We ate great food, drank great wine and sat by the pool all day long. It was just what we needed. If it weren't for their generosity, we'd never have had a break. Gautier spent all his time working, I spent all mine cleaning, cooking, doing really mundane stuff. We went out for the occasional dinner but we could never have afforded a holiday. It was also the only chance his mum got to spend time with him, so I just took advantage of that and enjoyed myself, reading books and indulging in a cheeky beer in the afternoon before getting ready for dinner. I was content, for the first time in years. I thank them by going crazy nuts at Christmas when they come over and cooking three-course dinners three days in a row. On Christmas Eve I spend the entire day baking and peeling vegetables. It's a wonder I had the energy to eat.

Mum and Dad visit more often now that we're settled in the house. They're thrilled that I have the peace and quiet I was longing for and we sit in the garden listening to the birds singing, eating Mum's apple cake and trying to entice Squeaky over for a cuddle (never happens). Dad is so much happier since he retired a couple of years ago and now has all day to watch RAF videos and old westerns he's already seen 448 times and get on with doing the garden. They go to the theatre in London with their friends, they go to nice restaurants, they have a way better social life than I do and it's lovely to see them both so relaxed and enjoying life. I know they spend a lot of time worrying about how I'm doing, but we speak on the phone every day and I know that if I need a break, I can go to their place and be fussed over by Mum.

I love Brighton, but sometimes I think that moving here was the most idiotic thing I have ever done. I know that Mum and Dad wish I were near them, too. And my friends were in London. Who in their right mind would move away from everyone and everything they know when they've just had their heart broken and found out that they have an incurable disease? I mean, really? I often think how hard I make things for myself, and I honestly have no idea why I do the things I do. If any psychologists are reading this, do let me know.

Summer 2011
I spend my days writing, cleaning, cooking, food shopping, putting

things on eBay and going to the Post Office. I meet friends for a coffee if they're not at work, but more often than not, I'm on my own all day. I don't get bored, but I do feel lonely and really miss the camaraderie of being in an office.

In June, Bo announces the birth of twin girls. Soon after, she announces me as one of their godparents. Imagine that! Me! A godmother! I am both stunned and excited at the prospect. She leaves me alone with them for 20 minutes when they're a few months old to go and buy milk. None of us are injured or missing when she gets back. She pronounces my role a resounding success. I'm truly so honoured to play a part in their lives; I wait eagerly for them to start talking nonsense so I can join in with them.

Gautier and I plod along, him working hard at Disney and pushing for promotion while I work on my book and chase my tail looking for freelance work that never materialises. We do manage a trip to Spain for the High Rockabilly weekender in September, as Gautier is playing there with Ana so his flights and our accommodation is paid for, but I really struggle. I also get my bag stolen at Barcelona train station - I'm amazingly lucky, really I am. Off went my bank card, phone, anti-allergy mosquito medication, make-up, new sunglasses... the lot. Thankfully my passport wasn't in there, but it wasn't a great start.

I love watching Gautier play, and seeing him up on stage still sends shivers down my spine. The problem is that with rockabilly weekenders comes non-stop noise due to non-stop drinking. The hotel walls are so thin I can hear people zipping up their suitcases, so imagine how loud a rowdy after-party of Swedish rockabillies is at 7am. It's boiling hot and the air-conditioning doesn't work, so there's no respite from the relentless heat. Weekenders are full-on party zones where everyone is out until the early hours drinking and dancing, and I can't dance anymore. I don't want to stand on the sidelines watching other people dance; it breaks my heart. I've walked away in tears plenty of times. When I drink too much it properly upsets my stomach so I kind of stand there like a spare part, not really knowing what to do with myself. Oh, and I'm constantly chewed at by mosquitoes, too, which I'm allergic to. In other words, as much as I love it, it's bloody hard work when you're not well. Bit by bit I can feel my life just slipping away from me; everything I love becoming further out of my reach until I have nothing left. Cherry and Phil have a baby girl in November, Alice and Ryan have another little girl. Even though that's not what I want, I can't help but feel left behind, somehow.

Monique and Christophe visit again at Christmas; this year I really push the boat out and do a fancy dinner on Christmas Eve as well as Christmas Dinner and Boxing Day lunch. I'm exhausted, but I enjoy cooking and it's my way of saying thank you to them for holidays, and I like to show Monique that her son is being well fed, as I'm sure every mother worries about that!

March 2012

I finally ask for a referral to a different rheumatologist. I'm tired of being told there's nothing that can be done to manage my pain. I feel as though my upper body is packed with bricks. It's a solid, heavy feeling. It's horrendous; as uncomfortable as it is painful, as though I'm wearing a bullet-proof vest, have a suitcase on my back and a pile of books on my head. It's awful. I have an MRI scan, and to compound the confusion about my symptoms, the new rheumatologist tells me that he thinks most of my pain might actually be down to a scoliosis (curvature of the spine). Well, two of them, to be precise: one in my lumbar spine, one in my thoracic spine, both of them leaning to my left with a straight bit somewhere in the middle. Apparently I've had this for the past 12 years, and although I suffered with lower back pain in my early teens, no doctor or consultant thought to mention it to me despite it showing up on scans way back in 2001.

In April Gautier and I go to Bath's Hospital of Rheumatic Diseases, where the specialist consultant (who is lovely) confirms, whilst running his hand down my spine, that along with the AS, I have a 'palpable' scoliosis. If you're not familiar with scoliosis, here's a brief description:

'Scoliosis is an abnormal curvature of the spine to the sides. Patients with scoliosis that is left untreated are more at risk of developing arthritis in their spine (uh, hello). In severe cases of scoliosis, the ribcage can be pushed against the heart and lungs, causing breathing problems and making it difficult for the heart to pump blood around the body. Strain or damage to the heart and lungs increases the chances of lung infections such as pneumonia and heart failure.'

Nice, huh? I have had pain around my ribcage for more than a decade. I can barely lean to my right as I have severely limited mobility on my left side. I have burning pain in my spine and shoulder blades. My spine is pushing against my ribcage. I stand wonky, my left shoulder dipping, my hips out of kilter. My clothes don't sit straight; they never have. Waistbands twist, the legs of my jeans are uneven. It is so obvious that my spine isn't straight it's bordering ridiculous.

The consultant recommends I consider spinal surgery; I recommend that I don't. He reads my notes, nods sagely and agrees that, yes, after all the surgery I've already had, not just on my bowel but my heart and everything else, it's not an option. Nobody in their right mind would perform such complex, lengthy and risky surgery on me after all I've been through. There are so many lesions throughout my body from all the surgery I've had; they'd never be able to see what they're doing and I would never make it out the other side. I talk to Mum and Dad about it; Mum says, quietly, 'no.' I couldn't put them through it, couldn't put Gautier through it, and last but not least, I couldn't put myself through it. It would be absolutely futile. So. I no longer have any hope that I will be free of this pain, and that's quite a statement, because hope - however dwindling - was all I had.

I wouldn't have buried my head in the sand for so long had I actually known how intensely these conditions would take hold, and how much it would change my life. If I'd known I had scoliosis on top I'd have made it my mission to have physiotherapy to attempt to halt its progression. I'd imagine that leaving it completely untreated all these years hasn't really done me much good. In fact, I know it hasn't. I may well have moved back to Mum and Dad's in 2003 rather than buy another place by the seaside. Maybe I'd have bought a place near them, so at least I'd have my independence when I wanted it, but be close by when things were particularly tough. I wouldn't have tried to fight so much. I'd never have given up, nor given in, but a realistic outlook would have saved me a lot of trouble. The National Ankylosing Spondylitis Society have done great work in getting GPs more training so that they are able to differentiate - hopefully - between a 'bad back' and Ankylosing Spondylitis. Faster diagnosis means faster treatment, and that's essential when faced with long-term illness.

When people I've known for years don't understand how frustrating, boring and difficult it is to live with constant pain, it's no wonder that complete strangers have trouble grasping the concept of invisible illness. I've had run-ins with people on the street who've openly accused me of 'faking' my disease to claim a blue badge. A few years ago I was struggling back to my car with a single bag of shopping from the supermarket. A man was locking his bicycle to the lamppost next to my car. I politely asked him to take his bike off the lamppost because it was inches away from the driver's door and I couldn't open the car door enough to get inside. Instead of saying, 'oh, sorry, I'll move it,' he sneered and said, 'you've got plenty of room.' I told him I needed more than other people and pointed to my blue badge on the dashboard.

He told me that I 'didn't look like I had mobility issues' and made a face as if to say, 'pfft, liar'. I pointed out that since he's not a rheumatologist, he probably shouldn't try to diagnose me. He eventually made a big show of holding the bike away from my car while I got in. When I pulled away, sometime later (it takes a while to get in) he looked slightly embarrassed, and waved goodbye. I gave him the finger out of the window.

When I wrote a piece for a Sunday newspaper about living with AS, I had comments on their website ranging from 'thank you for bringing this awful condition into the open' to some real nice ones along the lines of 'I have AS and it's not *that* bad' and 'this is a negative portrayal of having AS, I ski and go mountain biking, clearly this lady is not trying to beat her disease.' Seriously. Dude, I'm happy for you if you can do that, but a lot of us can't walk up the stairs. Actually, I'm not happy for you, because you're so incredibly obnoxious and have no idea how lucky you are. Come back to me in a decade and let me know how you feel then. Maybe your vertebrae will have fused by then, like mine has, and your sodding mountain bike will be on Gumtree.

AS affects everyone in different ways, as any illness does. It's like someone who has recovered from breast cancer telling someone who is dying from breast cancer, 'well, I don't know what you're doing wrong, but it didn't kill me.' Nobody would dare say that, so why is it acceptable to tell me or anyone else who is in constant, debilitating pain what we should or shouldn't be achieving? Life is hard enough as it is without perfect strangers telling me that I too could run a marathon or get on a mountain bike. Here's the thing: I can't even run for a bus! If I suddenly regained full use of my battered, frail body, I'd be in London every weekend dancing myself silly, not running. That's what I used to do before I fell ill; that's what I miss, and that's why I can't bear what has happened to me, because I miss it more than you can imagine.

CHAPTER TWENTY-ONE
'BANANAS IN PYJAMAS'
CAREY BLYTON
(Because it turns out that my spine is bent like a banana and the theme tune to this cartoon show was brilliant in the 1970s)

August 2012

The London Olympics: I manage to get tickets for me, Mum, Jonathan and his girlfriend, Kelsey, through a friend who'd applied for everything and disastrously, got everything. She was about six grand down on her credit card and panicking, so I jumped at the chance. Mum and Dad pay for my ticket as a 40th birthday present. Yes, I am 40. I can't quite believe it. On my *actual* birthday in July Gautier and I went to Ashdown Forest Llama Park to see Llama Tom, their best llama. I had a massive cuddle with him and he even had the grace not to spit at my hideous cold sore, which was lovely of him. I don't think I've ever been happier in my life, other than when I rode a camel at London Zoo when I was three.

Anyway, I digress. We watch Jessica Ennis in the heptathlon and then back home on TV a few days later, squeal with joy when she wins gold. What a mad day out. It nearly killed me to sit on the plastic seat but we were prepared for that; we brought along a cushion and I rolled up Jonathan's jacket to lean against. Every time there was a break in something or other I stood up, stretched and said, 'sorry!' to the people behind me. The journey, however, wiped me out. We were advised to get off at the tube stop that wasn't actually that near the stadium; the walk was horrendous for me. By the time we got there I was almost in tears. By the time we got home... well, Dad had to pick us up from the station and help me down the steps and into the car. And out of the car. And into the house. You get the idea. I spend the next three weeks barely able to do a thing. You'd think I'd actually taken part in the heptathlon, not just watched it. Once again, that's the pay off for having a good time, but I wasn't going to miss an opportunity like that for anything. Thanks again, parents - you're the best!

I never really feel better after that. I know that's quite a sweeping statement, but it's true. I'm perplexed. I ache all over. I feel faint, I feel more exhausted than ever before, and yet I lie awake night after night, unable to sleep. Something else is creeping up on me. I have numbness in my left hand and my fingertips burn. My neck feels as though someone is pushing down on it; a heavy, unbearable weight that makes me nauseous. I'm really, really scared. I go and see an Alexander Technique teacher; he offers great guidance and I feel much better after just a couple of sessions. The trouble is, within a couple of days the pain is back. I lie on the floor, knees bent, remembering what he taught me about how to relax (I have trouble with that) and make myself more aware of my movements and what I'm doing with my body. It helps, and I can sit at the computer a little longer than normal just by thinking about my posture, but the pain in my neck is still there. Nothing seems to shift that other than being on the floor for half an hour, and that's a bit inconvenient. I make friends with next door's dog, Cookie, a lovely little Norfolk Terrier, and at least have him for company. I take him for a walk on the green opposite the house when I'm up to it (slowly, mind) and he sits on the bench with me halfway round so I can rest. Just climbs up on my lap and comforts me. His mum, Clare, gives me a key after a couple of weeks so that when they're at work I can go in and see him, let him out into the garden for a bit, then make myself a coffee and sit on the sofa with him for an hour. I chat to him; he's my best friend, my one true companion and I love him as if he were my own.

In September 2013 I pay a visit to the rheumatology nurse. She examines me, pressing on certain points of my body with her fingers. Each one feels tender, like I've got sunburn or a bruise.

'I think you have fibromyalgia, Juliette,' she said, sitting down at her desk. 'You have all the symptoms: the chronic fatigue, the long-term insomnia, the tender points and the unexplained pain.'

I was almost speechless, but not quite.

'So I've had ulcerative colitis. I have Ankylosing Spondylitis. I have two scoliosis. I've had heart surgery, surgery on my cervix, surgery on my womb and three bouts of bowel surgery, and now I have fibromyalgia?'

I was beginning to wonder what the flip I had done in a former life. Had I been Hitler's mistress? Did I wipe out dinosaurs? Perhaps I pushed a baby out of a lifeboat as the Titanic sank? Oh wait, I know, I must have invented polio.

She tells me that it stems from the body going through emotional or physical trauma; that it kind of breaks down, that the pain receptors 'imagine' pain where there is no reason for pain; that the signals between the nerve endings and the brain get confused, and create these pains.

I've been pushing myself so hard all these years that my body has simply had enough. While I've not quite been in denial, I've never rested for one minute. I don't stop unless my hips actually prevent me from walking. I have never just spent the day on the sofa reading a book or watching a film. Not once. I've done this to myself. I didn't listen to my body. I think the Olympics day out was the last straw. I'm just stuck in the middle, trying to figure out what to do when there really aren't any answers. I want to live my life. I want to do things. I want to have adventures, to have things to look forward to, but my body keeps telling me I can't. I feel like I'm playing Scrabble with hieroglyphics; nothing makes any sense. I've never had a cold sore or weird skin infection (I got impetigo last summer, the week after the cold sore debacle) so it just shows what a terrible state my immune system was in, and how much damage I'd done to myself over the years by never resting.

I left with some information on the condition and with a lump in my throat. I got to the car, I shut the door and I just threw my head back and howled, like a wild animal. I took a deep breath, through the tears, and drove home. I put my foot down on the dual carriageway and considered, for a full five seconds, just ploughing into the bridge that was coming up in front of me.

Right after that diagnosis my symptoms escalate. I spend three nights unable to sleep at all. I go 32 days with no more than two hours' sleep per night. Sometimes I have less than that. I feel as though my brain is detached from my body. I go into town one morning and my legs just give way suddenly. I had to sit on the floor in Marks and Spencer, catch my breath and wait five minutes before I was able to stand up and walk, very slowly, back to the car. I find myself barely able to lift a cup of tea some days; my left arm becomes redundant. I struggle to clean the bath with one hand, my spine contorted and my left arm hanging limply by my side. When I can't clean the bath I figure that's time to admit defeat.

In October Gautier goes to France for 10 days. I like him to have a break from his life here. He works hard, he comes home to someone who tries her best but isn't really the same woman he married five years ago. I feel guilty, I feel sad, and above all else, I feel angry. One night I find myself sitting on the living room floor at 4am, scrunched into a ball in the dark, trying desperately to free myself from this hideous pain. I've been lying in bed for four hours, trying desperately to sleep, but it's all around my body, even in my face. It feels as though my skin is too tight, as if someone is pulling a rope right through the middle of my muscles from the soles of my feet and out through the palms of my hands. It's a strong, squirming sensation so disturbing I really can't do it justice with words. Imagine a rat running all around your insides. It's absolute hell. I stretch, I kind of hop up and down on the spot, I rub my limbs; in the end I just bawl my eyes out, wishing someone would shoot me. After a couple of hours, it subsides. I have a drink - yep, that kind of drink - to calm myself down. I go back to bed. It's 6.45am. I don't sleep.

I spend the rest of the weekend in a daze. I call Mum, and the same day, head to their house for a rest. I still don't sleep.

I am going insane. I mean, more insane than I already am, and remember, I can have several conversations at once - out loud - with stuffed toys. I read everything there is to read about fibromyalgia. Everything I do read says there is no cure. Every group or forum reiterates that. People are suicidal. People 'can't take it'. People are in so much pain.

I posted a comment on a fibro support group on Facebook one afternoon with a photo of Cookie saying how I had felt well enough to go for a little walk that day, and how pretty the autumn leaves were, basically appreciating the little things when the bigger picture was so terrifying. I suggested that even five minutes' walk around the block getting some fresh air beats sitting on the sofa watching TV. Apparently it doesn't. All I received in response were comments like: 'Yeah well lucky you cos you obviously don't have fibro cos you wouldn't of been able to get out of bed wait until you are as bad as me then see how you feel' and another, 'stop posting on here you make me sick telling us what to do if I want to sit on the sofa all day watching telly I will I can't move I'm in pain you don't know how that feels anyway its none of your business what we do f*ck off'. They appeared to sit around all day on Facebook having 'I'm more ill than you are' competitions. I left after someone posted: 'fed up today really bad pain cant see how I'm gonna make dinner fink its pizza n chips for me n hubby lol'.

I have been through too much to end up like this. I am determined not to have this and refuse to read anything else on the subject unless it's from a strictly medical point of view. There are some good support groups out there, but there is also plenty of negativity surrounding chronic illness and I don't think it helps anyone to wallow in self-pity and spend all day discussing your pain on the internet. You become your disease that way, and nothing else. It wins, you lose, end of.

Gautier is still away. I finally see my doctor. I turn up without lipstick on, without eyeliner, without a smile. This is the first time I have allowed myself to be like this, to look as bad as I feel, to not put on a show, to not make jokes, to actually say: HELP ME.

I explain that I haven't slept in over a month. I tell him that when I lie down at night it's like a jukebox starting up - I have four or five songs going around in my head along with random thoughts such as 'should I have my toes broken and shortened?' to 'I need to paint the garage' or 'Are we out of dishwasher tablets?' I can't switch my brain off and if you could see what was going on, I'd probably be advised to have a lobotomy. He prescribes anti-depressants 'for the anxiety, to calm you down, to induce sleep'. I've had insomnia since I was a teenager. That's roughly 25 years of not being able to sleep. I later find out that they're the same tranquilisers that Lindsay Lohan and crazy Carrie in *Homeland* takes. Blimey.

For the first three days, I'm completely manic. Totally 'up', driving myself nuts with ideas, getting over-excited about buying milk, even. 'I'm going to the shop!' I exclaim to nobody in particular. 'Let's watch the news!' I holler to Pantouf. Everything is rushed, in technicolour, at full volume. Cherry calls to see how I'm doing and I'm pretty much at full throttle, shrieking with excitement at all the new ideas I have for world domination in one breath and what I'm going to have for dinner in another. She says, 'Look after yourself, monkey.'

Two days later I crash. I sob until I can't breathe one night, on the floor, in the pitch dark, for three hours. A few weeks later I would find out that you're not supposed to be alone when starting this medication because, essentially, it can make you feel much worse (and when you're talking about someone who felt suicidal in the first place, that's a special kind of worse) before it makes you feel better. My doctor neglected to mention that. I was very much alone. Had I known how they would make me feel I would have gone to Mum and Dad's while they kicked in.

A couple of weeks after starting the medication I feel better. I start to sleep again. Not for long, but I drop off, which hasn't happened for years. I wake up at 5am, still tired, unable to go back to sleep but it's better than nothing. After a week, it settles down even more. I feel less teary, more able to hold it together. My physical symptoms are no better, but I'm sleeping. Well, I'm sleeping a bit. Better than not at all. I make up my mind that this Christmas will be spent at Mum and Dad's. I need a break. I get one. I help Mum but she keeps ordering me to sit down. Jonathan's girlfriend, Kelsey joins us and it's nice, there are six of us at the table and Squeaky in the corner. I finally relax. Well, almost.

We go to France for New Year and have another spectacular feast. This time, when we return, there are no blizzards. Hoorah!

Although I'm sleeping much better than I ever was, I'm still getting periods where the fibromyalgia floors me. I say that, though, and by flooring me I mean I keep going despite my legs wobbling or the burning sensation in my arm reducing me to tears. I decide that the Enbrel might be to blame. There are so many side effects of anti-TNF treatment, all of them pretty sinister, and I've been on it for nine years. Lymphoma is a big one. Multiple sclerosis is another. Then there's tuberculosis and 'other cancers'. I was terrified. There's no research on long-term use in patients because it was only just invented when I started taking it.

I talk to my parents and to Gautier about stopping it. I talk to the rheumatology specialist in Bath and even he agreed that it might be worth coming off it. I have absolutely no idea what will happen if I stop taking it. I have no way of knowing if it will work again if I stop and then decide I need it. The body has a way of rejecting treatment once it becomes too used to it, but it can also reject it full stop if after cessation, it sees it as an intruder. I'm in so much pain that I decide to see what happens. Even my GP looked concerned when I told him how long I'd been on Enbrel. 'Oh, that's a long time,' he said, rubbing his brow, 'it's probably a good idea to see how you get on without it.'

I reason that as I was in pain most days anyway, it can't be doing me much good.

It turns out that it was one of the worst decisions I've ever made. On day thirteen the pain hit me with such force that I almost threw up. It was 4.30am, exactly the same time as I used to be woken by the pain. I couldn't move. I couldn't draw breath. I couldn't quite believe what was happening. Gautier woke up and I was in tears. I still wanted to push through it and see if it eased off, but when I couldn't get in the bath without screaming in pain, I decided I clearly did need it. Funnily enough, the numbness had gone. Oh well. Numbness and a useless arm had to be better than screaming in pain, right?

On day 16 I started injecting again. Within two days my pain was almost bearable (with a cocktail of painkillers, mind). A week later, it was sort of bearable. A couple of months after that and I'm back to how I was before. Well, I guess I won't be trying that again.

December 2013

I up the dosage of the anti-depressants. I wasn't sleeping at all now and I could feel the black cloud descending once more. Just before Christmas I end up in A&E because my arm hurts so much. That's right, my arm. It feels as though it's on fire. The burning pain goes from my shoulder to my fingertips. When I lightly touch the skin, I flinch. I can't drive, I can't make dinner, I can't do much at all. Frankly, I'm too scared to even think about dinner. I have an MRI scan the following day; the results, which I get a couple of months later, are clear. There is no tumour pressing on my cervical spine, causing the pain in my neck. There's nothing sinister going on anywhere, just the usual stuff (crumbling discs, fused vertebrae, adhesions and what not) I see a neurologist who tells me 'to relax' and I will feel better. I laugh. I have to.

I visit a consultant at The Pain Clinic, hoping for an answer. He suggests I take Gabapentin, an anti-epilepsy drug. I say I'm already on enough medication and that I'd sooner have the pain. How could I possibly benefit from putting another strong drug with potentially dangerous side into my system? If you don't believe how awful these drugs are, here's a few of the side effects listed. These are under the header 'common side effects' and they affect around 1 in 100 patients:

'Abnormal gait, acne, back pain (really?!), blood and bone marrow problems, breathing difficulties, confusion, convulsions, coordination problems, depression, diarrhea, double vision (!), anxiety, feelings of hostility, flu, headaches, itching, join pain, memory problems, muscle twitching (amazing, seeing as that's what the drug is prescribed for), muscle pain, nausea, speech problems (really, this is incredible), swelling of the face, tooth problems and last but not least, vertigo, vomiting and weight gain'

How confused would my brain be by all these different medications? Even the consultant in Bath is keen for me to try it. I know it's used for fibromyalgia 'with some success' - not even great success - but I said there was no way in hell I was taking anything else. I was convinced I could make myself better. I just had to find out how.

Ridiculously I agree to Monique and Christophe coming for Christmas. I can hardly say no, but I'm beginning to think that neither Gautier nor his mum actually understand how ill I am. They know how much work I put in - I have to clean the entire house from top to bottom, buy all the food for five days straight (for four of us, with three-courses for dinner along with lunch and breakfast, that's a lot of food), bake, chop, peel, roast... It's never-ending. I wish we'd booked Christmas lunch at The Grand Hotel. That's what I wanted to do. Mum is upset because she worries about me doing so much, Dad worries too, and I worry about them worrying. I still don't say no, though. Instead I get my MasterChef recipe book out and take a deep breath.

In the end I cook mental amazing food - for Christmas Eve I make pan-fried monkfish with shrimp, a butternut squash fondant, green beans wrapped in pancetta and a sauce vierge (no, I didn't know what one of those was either) followed by vanilla panna cotta with a stupid chocolate crumb (that bit was a disaster) and tuile biscuits. What an idiot. I spend all day cooking. Oh yeah, and I have Christmas Dinner to prepare for, too, so the in-laws help with peeling and chopping while I do the dinner. Gautier helps me, thank God. On Christmas Day I really push the boat out - I'm such an idiot that along with the turkey I do roast saffron potatoes, pan-fried Brussels sprouts with pancetta and chestnuts, roasted baby parsnips and carrots with thyme and honey, bread sauce and proper gravy. For dessert I made a dark chocolate and espresso trifle which was dreadful. Not my fault, just the recipe used so much cream we all felt sick after one spoonful! Because we don't see my parents for Christmas (they had a great time at Kelsey's parents' enormous house in the Kent countryside), I invite them for dinner on New Year's Eve.

'Are you sure you're up to it?' asked Mum.

'No, but let's give it a go,' I replied. That night we had a fancy (but not homemade) black truffle spaghetti starter followed by wood pigeon with pommes mousseline, pancetta peas and onion gravy. For dessert I made a dark chocolate and ginger torte (Dad loves dark chocolate and ginger) with a ginger cream. Sometimes I really wonder what I'm doing, but then I think, 'don't think, just keep going, keep going!' and that's exactly what I do. It's nice to be appreciated, and it's nice to treat my family to something special. It's my way of saying thank you for all they do for me, at least until we win Euro Millions and I can just buy them a bloody house instead.

In spring I decide it's time to cure myself of fibromyalgia, or at least have a go. I can't believe I needed to take more medication and flatly refused when my GP suggested it for the third time.

'It works well for fibromyalgia,' he told me.

'If it does, then how come all the people who are taking it still feel awful?' I asked. I didn't go on. Instead, I went home, made a cup of tea, took it upstairs to my office and googled 'muscle cramps' and 'twitchy muscles' along with 'extreme fatigue', 'dizzy spells' and 'neck pain'. The same thing kept popping up - that all of those symptoms can be attributed to magnesium deficiency. Obviously no doctor had suggested that, so I thought I'd have a go myself. I reasoned that it was unlikely to do me any harm, anyway. Within two days of taking it, the hideous skin-crawling sensation and the wobbly legs business stops. Within a week I'm sleeping a bit better. I can shower and dry my hair without having to lie down afterwards. I can walk Cookie on the green without needing to sit on the bench and draw breath. Not only that but the pain in my arms seems to dissipate, too. In other words, it worked.

Here's what I read about magnesium: after oxygen, water, and basic food, magnesium may be the most important element needed by our bodies; vitally important, yet hardly known. It is more important than calcium, potassium or sodium and regulates all three of them Magnesium deficiency can affect virtually every organ system of the body. With regard to skeletal muscle, one may experience twitches, cramps, muscle tension, muscle soreness, including back aches, neck pain, tension headaches and jaw joint (or TMJ) dysfunction. Also, one may experience chest tightness or a peculiar sensation that one can't take a deep breath.' I urge anyone suffering from fibromyalgia to give it a go before you even consider picking up a prescription for something which might make you feel worse after taking it, not better.

What's more, the neck pain went too, after a couple of weeks. I haven't had any of the fibro symptoms since taking magnesium other than occasional numbness and pain in my left hand, and that's after hours of typing. I haven't felt wobbly whilst out and about. I have had no need to consider a lie down. That's it. Of course, no drug company is going to make any money out of me taking magnesium, which is probably why doctors don't bother to check if their patients are deficient in it. And as most patients don't question what their doctor tells them, they go away with their little slip of green paper for a prescription for something or other, and just start popping more pills. On all the fibro support groups, people seemed to be on handfuls of different medication yet nobody reported feeling any better. I didn't understand why nobody questioned what they were taking and why.

As relieved as I am to have found something natural which works, I'm so angry at having been instructed to pop more pills with potentially dangerous side effects that I just want to scream. The rheumatology nurse who also suggested Gabapentin no longer works at the hospital, so I can't tell her how I've managed to pretty much cure myself of an incurable condition, but it's a pretty astonishing turn of events, don't you think? One supplement, twice a day, with no side effects and I'm better. OK, so the anti-depressants mean I sleep better than I did, but still. I'd always advocate going down the 'what nutrients/vitamins might I be missing?' route first than just throw a load of pills down your throat because your GP makes money from each prescription they give you. They don't make money telling you to pop to Boots and buy some capsules. Maybe it won't work for everyone, but it also worked for my dad who'd had night cramps in his legs for years.

I read a very interesting book called *Bad Pharma* by Ben Goldacre that everyone should read, regardless or not of whether they are unwell. It explains so much about the pharmaceutical industry and is a real eye-opener. I'm not bad-mouthing all medication, by any means. I know that I need to take Enbrel to survive - that was made abundantly clear. I also know that the anti-depressants have played an enormous part in regulating my sleep, which in turn means I feel better in general. However, I believe a combination of the addition of magnesium to my diet, along with a slight change in what I eat, has also been a factor. I swap my usual breakfast of cereal (we're talking cereals such as organic cornflakes or Weetabix, not rainbow-coloured lumps of sugar like Cheerios, by the way) for porridge with blueberries, walnuts (massive dose of Vitamin C and magnesium and calcium right there) and honey. Within a few days I feel less bloated, even if the walnuts do give me a bit of grief in the pouch (so itchy!)

We have chicken once a week, and it's organic. I'd rather starve than eat cheap chicken or battery eggs. Everything we eat for dinner I cook from scratch aside from fish-fingers (my favourite comfort food). I don't buy jars of anything except (organic) peanut butter and 'emergency' pesto. Even our jam is homemade (by my mum). I have never drunk Diet Coke or anything containing aspartame. I don't drink fruit juice (high in sugar and too acidic for me) and I never buy ready meals or shop cakes or anything like that. Never have. I don't like the taste of anything that has preservatives in it, including sliced bread. I hate processed food. I hate junk food. I couldn't eat a KFC if you put a gun to my head. I won't deny that I like a drink - it'd be a miracle if I didn't, right? - but we're talking a couple of glasses of red wine four or so nights a week, a rhubarb gin and ginger ale when I'm out and the occasional gluten-free lager, not bottles of Smirnoff hidden in the airing cupboard or the in the toilet cistern. Not yet, anyway.

So while I don't believe that a healthy diet will *cure* all my ills, I do believe that things could be a whole lot worse for me if I the rubbish that most people eat, day in, day out. It's like putting custard into your petrol tank and wondering why your car won't start.

Back in 2010 I sent the first draft manuscript of this book to literary agents before I self-published it as an eBook. They all say that the book needed 'a happy ending'. That I need to show that I have 'overcome my illness'. One of them says, 'can't you run a marathon at the end, something like that?' I kid you not. I had explained in the outline letter that chronic, debilitating illness is not curable, that you do not 'get better'. They clearly didn't understand the concept of it, and were expecting a dramatic 'triumph over tragedy' ending.

Here's how I see it: people understand cancer. It will either kill you, or it won't. There's a terrible ending or a happy one. But even in the darkest moments there *is* often hope. The horrendous things people go through during treatment - the chemo-induced sickness, the hair loss, the sheer pain and exhaustion, the financial implications, the ripple effect it has on family and the fear, well, I wouldn't wish that upon anyone, nor the years of medication and check-ups that follow. What someone diagnosed with cancer *will* have, however, is a fantastic support network of doctors and nurses, Macmillan Cancer Support on hand and everyone understands that you're very sick so they generally want to help you. And nowadays you even get your breast rebuilt after a mastectomy; you're not left with a flat space where your breast once was. When you have your colon removed, and have your insides on your outsides, nobody says, 'Hey, here's some counselling, this is a big deal and you're bound to feel frightened and somewhat traumatised. Oh, and someone will come and visit you at home for a few weeks to see how you're doing, physically and emotionally. Finally, we'll do a bit of plastic surgery on those huge long scars of yours and find a way to stick that revolting red blob protruding from your stomach back in.'

Uh, no. None of that. You're just sent home with a couple of pamphlets and the realisation that there's no cure, and unless some miracle comes along, you've got it for life, and that's it. If I'd had the money and could have put my body through another operation I think I'd have liked breast augmentation; I have the tiniest boobs in the world and hated how my body looked – all I could see where scars and reminders of the worst time of my life. At least having slightly bigger boobs might have given me a little confidence back, but I wasn't about to put my body through any more surgery (plus I couldn't afford it anyway).

The 12-inch scars have faded, but you can still see them, along with all the other ones which came about from tubes being inserted this way and that, and from the stoma itself (which has left an ugly, bumpy scar on my right side) and from my heart surgery in 1976. I look like a road map of the North East.

A good friend of mine who had AS and colitis, was on the same drug treatment as me and was practically housebound ended up with cancer. It was only at this point that friends rallied round and took care of him. Up until then, his conditions and were simply not taken seriously.

'I didn't realise you were that ill, mate' said one friend.

'Only for 15 years,' he said to me from his hospital bed, 'but now that I have cancer I'm suddenly taken seriously. Where were all these people when I couldn't walk because my pain was so bad, or leave the house because my colitis meant I had to be by the bathroom all day?' He put up a brave fight and died a year later. We talked up until the day before he passed. He'd lived with such discomfort and pain for so long that he admitted he couldn't take anymore and was ready to go. He was 48 years years old. I miss him terribly.

Cancer terrifies people. People with cancer *look* like they've got cancer. There is no hiding from it. You wouldn't say, 'hey, get well soon!' to someone wearing a headscarf with no eyebrows and a complexion the colour of concrete. But you'll say it to someone with ulcerative colitis, Crohn's disease or ankylosing spondylitis; conditions for which there are no cures and no respite. The thing is, we won't get well soon. We might have good days. Maybe we might not have a flare-up for a while, but essentially, we're not going to get better, or 'get over it'. All we can learn to do is accept it, and that's one of the hardest things to do.

Publishers require a happy ending, but there isn't one.

When I read about someone with AS or arthritis who *has* just run a marathon or climbed a mountain I can tell you in no uncertain terms that it does *nothing* to make me feel better. In fact, it makes me feel worse, more inadequate, more of a failure. Saying, 'Gemma refuses to let arthritis beat her and has just completed her fifth London marathon' for example makes me think that Gemma's arthritis isn't actually that bad. If it was, she wouldn't be able to walk to the bus stop, let alone run 26 miles. It's basically saying that if we can't run a marathon or cycle from Land's End to John O'Groats, we're allowing the disease to beat us, we're weak, we're not trying hard enough. I think that's a very dangerous message to send out to the thousands of people who battle like mad but simply *can't* win the fight.

Maybe my achievement today was making a cake or cleaning the kitchen floor; maybe I managed to go to the Post Office or upload 20 pairs of shoes I can no longer wear to eBay. When you're in pain all the time, everything is an effort. Everything takes longer, and what little energy you have is sapped when you're dragged down by constant pain, discomfort, frustration and fatigue. If I do two loads of washing, make dinner, wash my hair, smile at the postman, load and empty the dishwasher and no matter how bad I feel, always greet Gautier with a kiss and a smile and dinner on the table when he comes home from work, well, guess what? That's *my* marathon.

The exhausted mother with AS or scoliosis or colitis or fibromyalgia or ME or MS and who drags herself out of bed and takes her children to school, that's *her* marathon. The fathers who go to work despite crippling pain because they have a family to support - just as my dad did - same thing. Ditto the kids trying to get through a school day with juvenile arthritis or any other illness for which there is no end in sight, and their parents who hold the family together no matter what; they're the ones whose achievements go unnoticed and uncelebrated, whose stories go untold, but are they any less brave because their battles are ordinary, every day ones which the rest of us take for granted? I don't think so.

I find a few things that help with the pain, albeit only fleetingly: a deep, hot bath with Epsom salts and lavender oil. I get Gautier to rub Tiger Balm or Deep Heat on my shoulder blades and up my spine before he heads to work. I bought a Shiatsu massage cushion from Amazon which is actually really, really good. I use that every evening as I sit on the sofa. I lie on the floor on my yoga mat with my knees up and my neck supported on a half-inflated ball; my spine almost feels straight.

My parents visit quite often; they bring so many nice things with them it often takes two trips to unload the car. Mum will bring a chicken pie or homemade jam and roses from their garden. Dad has given me all his Elvis and Gene Vincent LPs and hands out £10 notes for me to 'buy some wine or something with donkeys on it' and in return I make stupendous lunches and desserts and even clean the kitchen floor. When my back is turned, I'll find Mum drying up crockery or sweeping the floor. I don't know what I'd do without them; they are pretty incredible. With my parents, if nothing else, I have lucked out.

When the sun's shining, things are so much easier. That's when I get in the car and head to Hove beach. I buy a coffee from the Hove Lawns Café, put my own soya milk in it and stare at the sea for as long as my back can stand it. Plastic café chairs and wrought iron benches aren't the most comfortable of seats, so I don't last long. Dad loves their ham, egg and chips and we go there for a treat when they visit. I wave at all the dogs that walk past, crying inside (and sometimes outwardly) because I haven't got one.

I grab every opportunity I can to enjoy the scraps of pleasure life throws at me because I never know how long it'll be before the next one comes along. If I can catch a break two days in a row I feel like the luckiest person alive.

It has come to this: I finally give in to the fact that I can't wear heels anymore. I sell 23 pairs online. I keep my wedding shoes, though. I will try them on from time to time. I buy a pair of parrot boots. P-A-R-R-O-T-B-O-O-T-S. Black ankle boots (with a mid-height heel) with red, yellow and green parrots kind of embroidered on the sides. In leather, I hasten to add, not in feathers. They're the nuts. I love them. Gautier despairs of my taste in shoes; he's lucky I didn't buy the white pair as well (there's still time).

If I've slept the night before, Gautier brings me a cup of tea before he goes to work. He helps me sit up, helps me out of bed and runs me a bath if I need him to. He passes me my tablets, gives me a kiss and off he goes. I get up, just about, get in the bath, then go downstairs and have my breakfast. I usually have it standing up because if I sit down again, I have to start all over with the pain to get to standing.

I'll load the dishwasher if I can, put on some laundry, check my emails and decide what I can manage to do. I might make it to the supermarket, I might decide the pain is too much and order everything online. I rarely do that, though, because I begrudge spending the money on having it delivered (I know, I know) and if there's no food in the house, it's no good waiting for it to turn up two days later.

I sort out things to do with the house and the car, like paying the bills online, sorting out insurance, buying the wrong sized plant pots online, phoning plumbers or paving contractors or garage roof repairers, whatever needs to be done. I write, of course. A lot. I'm constantly looking for freelance work, and that takes up most of my time. I dust stuff. I clean the floors when I can. I sort out more things to sell on eBay or to give to the cat shelter for their jumble sales. I cook dinner. Basically, I am not good at resting. I literally drag myself out of bed, into the shower, into the car, to wherever I have to go. I grimace whilst I'm doing it, but I do it because the less I accomplish, the worse I feel. I don't think I'll ever change, no matter what my body tells me. I'm afraid that once I sit down and stop, I'll never have the motivation to do anything else.

The only time I gave into it was during a particularly bad fibro flare-up when I had that 'someone is pressing down on my head' neck pain which made me nauseous and dizzy. Saying that, even when I had it all day I'd be up and showered, doing some chores, I'd have cooked dinner and probably done some writing, too. Every 30 minutes or so I'd lie down on the floor and close my eyes; that brought me a little respite. I've always reasoned that I'd sooner be in pain doing something useful than in pain doing nothing. For me, that means the pain has won, and I'm not having that.

I am definitely mental, but you knew that already.

Sometimes, though, the pain is too much, no matter what I do, and I start wondering at which point I will not be able to tolerate it any longer. If the anti-TNF therapy did cause something nasty I would have to come off it. Without it, I would be dead inside a week. Don't think I'm being dramatic, either - nobody on earth could take that kind of pain 24/7, even Thor. I think a lot about suicide, yet can't think of a single way in which I could do it to guarantee being absolutely dead, and I couldn't do it even if I did find a way, because I don't want my family to suffer any more than they do already. I can't leave Pantouf and all his brothers. I can't leave Squeaky. I can't leave Gautier, Mum and Dad, my brother, so instead I walk around with a forced smile while suppressing a gigantic, ear-piercing scream, an ever-threatening tidal wave of emotion and despair that lurks just beneath the surface.

The pain never goes away; neither does the overwhelming sense of loss. If I can't drive to the beach because of the pain, I sit in the garden for a little while with a cup of tea, listening to the chatter of the birds in the trees, watching snails eat my hydrangeas. I think to myself, 'My spine is killing me, but at least the sun's out and I've got hydrangeas and teabags. And snails.' I see the positives in everything, no matter how small. I have to, because the little things are all I have, and I'm not even as ill as some people are. I know someone who spends her entire time taking care of her family despite being on crutches, snacking on liquid morphine with a brain tumour lurking in the back of her head. I'm still the unluckiest person among my friends, my peers, the people whose lives intertwine with mine (or used to), but there is always, always somebody worse off than me, and I never forget that. I read about a soldier who's returned from Afghanistan and lost a limb, or plural, and believe me, I feel like the most despicable person on earth for complaining about my life.

So, this is the deal: my spine is not going to straighten itself out. My colon is not going to grow back. My vertebrae won't suddenly un-fuse. I'm fairly likely to end up with lymphoma, or 'other cancers'. I may well end up with an ileostomy again in the near future; there is no guarantee that my bowel surgery will hold out forever. And please, don't tell me that all I need to do is eat only daffodils and leeches or drink owl's saliva twice a day or stop wearing cotton or pray or whatever. It is what it is, and if there *was* a way to be free of pain, I'd have worked it out by now.

As far as diet goes, that's a tricky one. Advocates of a starch-free diet advise patients with inflammatory illness to cut starch out of their diet as it they believe it is a contributing factor in inflammation. Firstly, a lot of my pain is mechanical (the scoliosis) and no amount of starch-free food is going to make my spine straight. Secondly, a high-fibre diet is the worst diet I can follow. My favourite foods are the things which I can't digest properly, or which get stuck between the adhesions in my small intestine and cause blockages. These are foods which are either too 'woody', such as pineapple, so the stomach acid isn't enough to break it down and it stays just as it did when it went in, or foods which get stuck because they're too, um, 'leafy'.

Here's a list of things I love which I can no longer eat under any circumstances for fear of getting another blockage: carrots, leeks, mushrooms, pumpkin seeds, nuts (apart from walnuts), sweetcorn, bean sprouts, popcorn, celery, mange tout, baby corn, lentils, pineapple, runner beans, apples, peppers, chick peas, black beans (even as brownies) sprouts like alfalfa and beansprouts. Then there are foods I love but avoid because they cause terrible bloating and painful gas issues, and they are: onions, wheat-based pasta, couscous, hummus, pizza, bread, granola, garlic, pears, plums, artichokes, avocados, dairy and on a smaller scale, biscuits and my mum's lovely cakes.

I struggle, too, with skin on fruit or vegetables, so now peel cucumber scrape the seeds out of tomatoes and don't eat blackberries because the seeds get stuck (it's true, you can see it when the camera goes up my insides). I even have bother with salad leaves and blueberry skins, with olives and spinach, all of which just get a bit stuck on their journey from tummy to toilet. When you look at that exhaustive list, it's incredible. It's so hard to find anything to eat, much less anything I want to eat. I crave popcorn and mushrooms the most, weirdly. Basically, at every meal I'm either crossing my fingers that the food goes through me without issue, or sighing because I just want a pile of hot, buttery corn on the cob NOW.

I can, without issue, digest eggs in all forms, potatoes, rice, chicken, fish, prawns, steak, gluten-free pasta, sheep's and goat's cheese, courgettes, squash, peeled cucumber, dark chocolate, oat crackers and porridge oats. Great.

I had my most recent blockage this week, and am currently on 'bowel rest'. I'm at home drinking hideous build-up drinks from the chemist and not actually eating anything. It's been five days of that and I'm climbing the walls with frustration and am craving macaroni cheese like you wouldn't believe. This blockage caused 10 straight hours of the worst imaginable pain ever, and I was convinced that this one would lead to a perforation and kill me. I passed out with the pain, but still didn't ring an ambulance. Even when I was sweating buckets and shaking with cold while it felt like a bull was trampling over my stomach I didn't ring an ambulance. I just writhed and clutched the sheets and cried out in agony. That was after stupidly eating a really nice salad with nuts, alfalfa sprouts, miniscule diced carrots, green beans and buckwheat. I ate a beef bourguignon for dinner that I'd made and threw the whole lot up four hours later because it had nowhere to go; my intestines had twisted and blocked the salad already, so that was sitting halfway down my small bowel, trying to get out. As far as passing the time goes, I wouldn't recommend it.

When Gautier goes away on tour, as he does for a couple of weeks each year, I feel such an overwhelming sense of loneliness I wonder if I might actually die from it. I keep myself as busy as possible – I visit my parents, go to the beach with a book, invite myself to someone's house for dinner if they'll have me and if nobody else is around, I spend most of my time with Cookie, the light of my life who was always there for me. That's right, my best friend is a dog.

This is What Needs to Happen

Gautier and I need to win Euro Millions. I'd build a spa for people with scoliosis and AS and fibromyalgia and IBD bad enough that they can't run a marathon or go mountain biking. They could come and sit in a nice Jacuzzi and have thermal wraps (whatever they are) and a sandwich.

Next I'd set up an alpaca farm and make really soft jumpers for stray dogs, install a carousel in the garden so I could eat my toast whilst going round and round on a pretend horse and have a chef (Francesco Mazzei, please) cook our dinner and also to prepare meals for Squeaky. We'd have a cleaner (no, wait, a team of chimps would be better) and a chauffeur (I want the one from *Crocodile Dundee* - no interview necessary).

I'd open a massive animal sanctuary for cats, dogs, chinchillas, guinea pigs, all woodland creatures (except for worms and slugs), elephants rescued from the circus and horses and donkeys and alpacas. And anteaters. I'd have a moat around the house with a sandpit circling that, and komodo dragons would roam around, their long tongues picking off unwanted visitors, such as Jehovah's Witnesses or people with flyers for nasty fried chicken shops. I would go from room to room by gondola or miniature railway. I'd have a hollowed-out Lancaster bomber or a full-sized replica of Barbie's house, haven't decided yet, where I could eat Reese's Peanut Butter Cups and drink pink lemonade whilst reading pop-up books for four-year-olds and watching re-runs of The Sooty Show from the late '70s. I actually bought a vintage '80s Sweep puppet the other day; I love that show so much it hurts. I'm just not sure how Pantouf will react to having a new brother with such a strong personality enter the house.

We'd have a Lamborghini with a stereo I could actually work (I've never mastered it on any car I've ever owned) and a yellow and black Camaro, just like Bumblebee in *Transformers*, as well as a midnight blue and white-striped one because that'd be my Spurs-coloured car. I'd have indoor trees, parrots, a couple of koalas and an incubator for premature pandas. Out the front I'd have a proper dinosaur park with moving, roaring dinosaurs (models, I don't think I can get real ones no matter how many pound coins I had) and the postman would put our letters into the mouth of a T-Rex. I'd have a cinema room that played *Top Gun* on a loop. I have been in love with Tom Cruise for 26 years. He has no idea. I'm sure he'd like me if he met me. It proper does my head in. If you're reading this, Tom, I love old planes and fast cars. I'm shorter than you by five inches, younger than you by a decade and I really like the way you run, with your elbows tight to your sides. It's very professional. I would even embrace Scientology for you. Well, maybe. We should talk, anyway. Call me!

That Elusive Happy Ending
(I still haven't run a marathon)

Will this do? Six years ago today an English idiot (me) married a French idiot (Gautier). We had met only six months earlier and weren't even living in the same country. Neither of us had a proper job; subsequently neither of us had any money. We couldn't afford a honeymoon and could hardly pay the bills. Gautier had left his friends and family for a nutcase who was riddled with scars and painful diseases, who conversed with stuffed toys and whose only saving grace was being able to make a decent roast dinner. Where a lesser man might have given up on me, especially during those first few months, Gautier would take my hands in his and say: 'I love you, monkey, we'll be OK.' And do you know what? He was right.

As they say in *Transformers*:

'Hope for the best, prepare for the worst', because at the end of every rubbish day, there is always tomorrow.

Please hop by Amazon and leave a nice review of this book if you enjoyed it. If you didn't, take on board what my lovely nanny Marge always told me:

'If you can't say anything nice, don't say anything at all'. Thanks

ABOUT THE AUTHOR

Juliette Wills is a journalist and broadcaster. She is fond of donkeys, cats and dogs of all shapes and sizes and Tottenham Hostpur FC. She loathes green sweets of any kind. This is her third book.

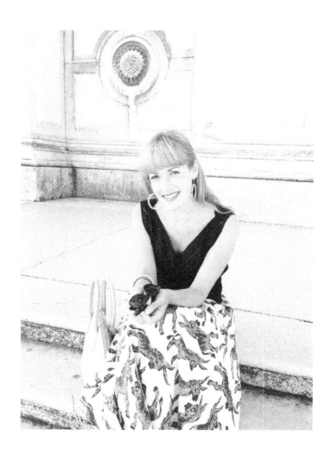

Mostly Cloudy With Some Bright Spells

Made in the USA
Coppell, TX
29 November 2020